Psychiatry
and
Mysticism

Stanley R. Dean, M.D.
Editor

Psychiatry and Mysticism

Nelson-Hall nh Chicago

Library of Congress Cataloging in Publication Data
Main entry under title:

Psychiatry and mysticism.

Includes bibliographies and index.
1. Psychiatry—Congresses. 2. Psychical research—Congresses. I. Dean Stanley R.
RC454.4P785   133.8'01'9   75-8771
ISBN 0-88229-189-0

Manufactured in the United States of America

DEDICATION

To my beautiful wife, Marion—
for her blessed noninterference

Also by Stanley R. Dean, M.D.
Schizophrenia: The First Ten Dean Award Lectures

Contents

Section II

Section III

Section IV

Contributing Authors

PAUL L. ADAMS, M.D., a leading child psychiatrist at the University of Louisville, Kentucky, was earlier associated with Florida and Miami universities. He has authored and coauthored articles and books dealing with social and child psychiatry, including *Primer of Child Psychotherapy* (1974), *Obsessive Children* (1973), *Humane Social Psychiatry* (1972), and *Academic Child Psychiatry* (1970). A Quaker for most of his adult life, he is a "nontheistic meditator who finds the inner and outer lives of great importance, equally, in his daily happenings."

JAMES B. BEAL, B.S., M.E., was an aerospace engineer for the National Aeronautics and Space Administration (NASA) at the Marshall Space Flight Center near Huntsville, Alabama. He is a specialist in biosystems research, bioelectric field effects, and paraphysics, and has lectured and written extensively on these subjects.

JOHN F. BEARY, M.D., was a fourth-year medical student at the Harvard Medical School during the preparation of the paper on the relaxation response. He is currently a medical officer in the United States Air Force.

HERBERT BENSON, M.D., associate professor of medicine at Harvard Medical School, is a cardiologist specializing in hypertension. He was among the first to do extensive research on meditation in this country, and his numerous reports on the subject have been an important factor in its current popularity.

MALCOLM B. BOWERS, JR., M.D., a diplomate of the American Board of Psychiatry, is associate professor of psychiatry at Yale University

School of Medicine and chief of psychiatry at Yale-New Haven Hospital.

FRANCIS J. BRACELAND, M.D., is editor of the *American Journal of Psychiatry,* chairman of the Planning and Development Board of the Institute of Living, past president of the American Psychiatric Association, and holder of honors and awards too numerous to mention.

MARK P. CAROL was a premedical student at Amherst College, Amherst, Mass., during the preparation of the paper on the relaxation response. He is now a medical student at the University of Rochester.

STANLEY R. DEAN, M.D., editor of this book, is a clinical professor of psychiatry at both the University of Florida in Gainesville and the University of Miami. He is a diplomate of the American Board of Psychiatry and a fellow of the American Psychiatric Association, the American College of Psychiatrists, the Royal Society of Medicine, and the National Association of Science Writers. Dr. Dean has published numerous articles and book chapters, including several on psychic subjects, and has edited a book entitled *Schizophrenia: The First Ten Dean Award Lectures.* He founded Research in Schizophrenia Endowment, Inc., and is currently organizing the American Metapsychiatric Association.

JAN EHRENWALD, M.D., had his psychiatric training at the University Clinics at Prague and Vienna. During World War II, he practiced psychiatry and held various professional appointments in England, where he was elected a fellow of the Royal Society of Medicine. He is a diplomate of the American Board of Neurology and Psychiatry, fellow of the American Psychiatric Association, fellow of the New York Academy of Medicine, and consulting psychiatrist at Roosevelt Hospital, New York. His published work includes more than 150 articles and several books on psychiatry and parapsychology.

JULE EISENBUD, M.D., a diplomate of the American Board of Psychiatry and a fellow of the American Psychiatric Association, is an associate clinical professor of psychiatry at the University of Colorado Medical School, Boulder. He has written several articles on parapsychology and two books entitled *The World of Ted Serios* and *Psi and Psychoanalysis.*

J. NORMAN EMERSON, PH.D., professor of anthropology at the University of Toronto and president-elect of the Canadian Archaeological Association, is a well-known authority on Canadian Indian antiquities. He is currently working on a book about his experiences with archaeological psychometry.

NORMA ESTRADA has had extensive training in psychiatric administration and has played an active role in the conception and development of the Everett A. Gladman Memorial Hospital. She is an associate of Dr. Gladman in biofeedback research and therapy.

DANIEL X. FREEDMAN, M.D., is a psychiatrist, research scientist, educator, and author, who has received many awards and honors. He is professor of biological sciences and chairman of the department of psychiatry at the University of Chicago. He is a coauthor of a leading psychiatric textbook, *The Theory and Practice of Psychiatry,* and is chief editor of an American Medical Association journal, *Archives of General Psychiatry.*

ARTHUR E. GLADMAN, M.D., AND NORMA ESTRADA collaborated in the development of the Everett A. Gladman Memorial Hospital, Oakland, California, and have done intensive research on biofeedback techniques for the treatment of psychosomatic illness. Doctor Gladman is a diplomate of the American Board of Psychiatry and a fellow of the American Psychiatric Association.

ALYCE GREEN received her B.A. in psychology from the University of Chicago in 1962. Her present work, which focuses on creativity, is supported by the National Institute of Mental Health for the study of alpha-theta brain wave feedback, reverie, and imagery. She is president of the Association of Transpersonal Psychology and training director of the Voluntary Controls Program of the Research Department of the Menninger Foundation.

ELMER GREEN, PH.D., is head of the Psychophysiology Laboratory at the Menninger Foundation. He received his Ph.D. in biopsychology at the University of Chicago and was research associate in the Department of Medicine at the University of Chicago before going to the Menninger Foundation. In 1964 he established the Voluntary Controls Project, combining disciplines of autogenic and biofeedback training and yoga. He is a director of the Psychosynthesis Institute, the Transpersonal Institute and the Academy of Parapsychology and Medicine.

STANISLAV GROF, M.D., is chief of psychiatric research at the Maryland Psychiatric Research Center in Baltimore and assistant professor of psychiatry at Johns Hopkins University. At present, he is on leave of absence to conduct research in parapsychology at the Esalen Institute, Big Sur, California.

JOHN HUBACHER graduated from the University of California, Los Angeles, with a degree in psychology. Currently he is a graduate student at Sonoma State College. He has co-authored several articles on Kirlian photography, and has done experimental work with the "phantom leaf effect" and healing. Recently he has been involved in the development of Kirlian cinematography.

SHAFICA KARAGULLA, M.D., is a member of the Royal College of Physicians (Edinburgh), and a former assistant professor of psychiatry at the State University of New York. She is president of the Higher Sense Perception Research Foundation and author of *Breakthrough to Creativity* (1967).

LAWRENCE L. LESHAN, PH.D., is a noted career parapsychologist, educator, and author of four books and over fifty articles on parapsychology. His latest book is *The Medium, the Mystic and the Physicist: Toward a General Theory of the Paranormal* (1974).

JULES H. MASSERMAN, M.D., is a renowned psychiatrist, research scientist, author, editor, teacher, and recipient of numerous offices, honors, and awards. He is president of the International Association for Social Psychiatry and secretary of the American Psychiatric Association.

EDGAR D. MITCHELL, SC.D., Apollo 14 astronaut, became the sixth man to walk on the surface of the moon in February, 1971. He is the executive director of the Institute of Noetic Sciences and senior author of *Psychic Explorations* (1974).

THELMA MOSS, PH.D., is a research psychologist at the Neuropsychiatric Institute, University of California at Los Angeles, Center for the Health Sciences. The members of her laboratory staff made possible the first investigations of electrical photography in the United States. Dr. Moss visited the Soviet Union in 1970, where she obtained much literature, schematic diagrams, and invaluable information from Soviet scientists working in the fields of bioenergy, biocommunication, and Kirlian photography.

JOHN C. PIERRAKOS, M.D., is the director of the Institute of Bioenergetic Analysis in New York City and vice-president of the Center of the Living Force. He is a practicing psychiatrist in New York City and has made an extensive study of the phenomena of the energy field in nature and man.

J. B. RHINE, PH.D., is executive director of the Foundation for Research on the Nature of Man, Durham, North Carolina. He was director of the Parapsychology Laboratory at Duke until he retired in 1965. J. B. Rhine founded the *Journal of Parapsychology* in 1937 and the Parapsychological Association in 1957.

WILLIAM G. ROLL is project director of the Psychical Research Foundation, Durham, North Carolina, and editor of *Theta*, a publication of the foundation. In 1964 he was president of the Parapsychological Association, which he helped found in 1957, and editor of its publication, the *Journal of Parapsychology*.

FRANCES SABA is a graduate of the University of California, Los Angeles, and holds an associate degree in fine arts and a bachelor's degree in psychology. For the past three years, she has done experimental work at the Neuropsychiatric Institute at UCLA using the Kirlian method of photographing bioenergetic interactions between people and working with dermoptical perception.

GARY E. SCHWARTZ, PH.D., is an assistant professor of personality psychology in the Department of Psychology and Social Relations at Harvard University. He is chief of psychophysiology, Clinical Psychophysiology Unit, at the Erich Lindemann Mental Health Center, Massachusetts General Hospital, Boston. He is a past president of the Biofeedback Research Society.

BERTHOLD E. SCHWARZ, M.D. is a diplomate of the American Board of Psychiatry, a fellow of the American Psychiatric Association, and a consultant of the Brain Wave Laboratory, Essex County Hospital Center, New Jersey. He is the author of several articles and books on parapsychology.

JULIAN SILVERMAN, PH.D., is the director of Esalen Institute at Big Sur, California, a consultant to the Surgeon General's office of the U.S. Army at Fort Ord and to the California Department of Mental Hygiene, and a staff member of the University of Chicago Medical School. Dr. Silverman has been an editorial consultant for a number of psychiatry and psychology publications, including the *Journal of Nervous and Mental Disease, Journal of Schizophrenia,* and *Journal of Abnormal Psychology.*

CARL SIMONTON, M.D., was chief of radiation therapy at David Grant USAF Medical Center, Travis Air Force Base, from 1971 until recently. He interned at Santa Barbara County Hospital and spent his residency in radiology at the University of Oregon. He is presently engaged in cancer research to evaluate such areas as the will to live versus the will to die, mechanisms governing biofeedback, physiological aspects of meditation, and the fear of death.

DENNY THONG, M.D., is the director of the Bangli Mental Hospital in Bali, Indonesia. He recently visited the United States through the courtesy of the State Department and the Indonesian government.

E. FULLER TORREY, M.D., a psychiatrist and anthropologist, is currently serving as special assistant to the director of the National Institute of Mental Health. He is the author of over sixty professional publications, including two recent books, *The Mind Game: Witchdoctors and Psychiatrists* and *The Death of Psychiatry.*

Acknowledgments

The editor wishes to thank the following for their permission to reprint material:

The American Psychiatric Association for "Metapsychiatry: The Confluence of Psychiatry and Mysticism," by Stanley R. Dean. A shorter version of this article was published with the title "Metapsychiatry: The Interface Between Psychiatry and Mysticism" in the *American Journal of Psychiatry*, Sept. 1973. Copyright American Psychiatric Association.

The American Psychiatric Association and Dr. Francis J. Braceland for "Psychiatry and the Science of Man," by Francis J. Braceland. *American Journal of Psychiatry, July 1957.*

Psychoanalytic Review for "Telepathic Humoresque," by Berthold E. Schwarz. *Psychoanalytic Review,* Vol. 61, No. 4, 1974.

Journal of Parapsychology for "Security Versus Deception in Parapsychology," by J. B. Rhine. *Journal of Parapsychology,* March 1974.

New Horizons Research Foundation for "Intuitive Archaeology: The Argillite Carving," by J. N. Emerson. Published with the title "Intuitive Archaeology, A Psychic Approach" in *New Horizons,* Jan. 1974. Copyright New Horizons Research Foundation.

Psychology Today for "Positive and Negative Aspects of Meditation," by Gary E. Schwartz. Published with the title "TM Relaxes Some People and

Makes Them Feel Better." Reprinted from *Psychology Today Magazine,* April 1974. Copyright © 1974 Ziff-Davis Publishing Company.

Psychiatry for "The Relaxation Response," by Herbert Benson, John F. Beary, and Mark P. Carol. *Psychiatry,* 37:37–46, 1974.

The Viking Press, Inc., for "Toward a General Theory of Psychic Healing," by Lawrence LeShan. Chapter 7 of *The Medium, the Mystic, and the Physicist,* by Lawrence LeShan. Copyright © 1966, 1973, 1974 by Lawrence LeShan. All rights reserved. Reprinted by permission of The Viking Press, Inc., and the author.

The Academy of Parapsychology and Medicine for "Mind Training, ESP, Hypnosis, and Voluntary Control of Internal States," by Elmer E. and Alyce Green, *APM Report,* Spring 1973; and for "The Role of the Mind in Cancer Therapy," by Carl Simonton, *Proceedings of the Academy of Parapsychology and Medicine,* 1972.

Journal of Transpersonal Psychology for "Varieties of Transpersonal Experience: Observations from LSD Psychotherapy," by Stanislav Grof. Copyright *Journal of Transpersonal Psychology,* Vol. 4, No. 1, 1972. Reprinted by permission of the Transpersonal Institute, 2637 Marshall Drive, Palo Alto, Ca. 94303.

The American Medical Association for " 'Psychedelic' Experiences in Acute Psychoses," by Malcom B. Bowers, Jr., and Daniel X. Freedman. *Archives of General Psychiatry,* 15:240, 1966. Copyright 1966 American Medical Association.

Special thanks for the painstaking task of preparing the indexes are due to R. Alan and Marilyn McConnell. R. A. McConnell is Director of the Psychotronic Workshop and Program Advisor of Life Laboratory at Miami Dade Community College.

Introduction

THIS BOOK is intended for the general reader as well as the professional, and is part of a major multidisciplinary project aimed at bridging the gap and establishing rapport between medical science and psychic research. Without such rapport many believe that psychic research, a perennial stepchild of science, may never achieve the first-class status that it so richly deserves but that has so far eluded it.

The apostle Paul once asked, "What is man that thou art mindful of him? Thou crownedst him with glory and honor, and didst set him over the works of thy hands. Thou hast put all things in subjection under his feet. But we see not yet all things put under him" (*Hebrews,* 2:6–8). That phrase, *"not yet,"* commands attention, for it implies an eventuality—and we may even now be on the very threshold of its realization. So, if we adopt integration as our watchword, and if modern technology discourages factionalism and welcomes fresh involvement, recognition and status will be the result. Projects such as ours shall then be viewed as a competitive stimulus rather than a competitive hazard. The old guard will realize that lighting one candle from another does not diminish the glow of the first, but increases the total available light.[1]

Fortunately, *timing,* which is so often the essence of endeavor, has never

---

[1]Dr. Alan Gregory, one of psychiatry's most constructive critics, advocated the extension of psychiatry into many fields beyond the office and the hospital, and urged that psychiatry should be concerned with "optimal performance of human beings as civilized creatures." (Quoted by Robert L. Robinson, Director of Public Affairs, American Psychiatric Association, in a lecture, CRITICISMS OF PSYCHIATRY, presented at a meeting of the American College of Psychiatrists, January 26, 1973)

been more propitious. Aggregate knowledge is more accessible than ever, and worldwide interest is at an all-time high. Colleges and universities are beginning to list psi subjects in their curricula, and scientific bodies are including them in their programs. It is only a matter of time before portions of the new technology will be incorporated into the practice of medicine. In fact, that has already been done by some prominent physicians.

PSYCHIATRY AND MYSTICISM is an outgrowth of three historic panel-symposia on psychic phenomena that were presented at consecutive annual meetings of the American Psychiatric Association in Dallas (Schul, 1972; Smith, 1972), Honolulu (Dean, 1973), and Detroit (Dean, 1974). Participants in the first were physicians Howard Rome (moderator), Berthold Schwarz, Jan Ehrenwald, and Jule Eisenbud, together with astronaut Edgar Mitchell and behavioral scientist William Roll. In the second were physicians Ramon Parres (moderator), William McGary, George Ritchie, Aristide Esser, and parapsychologist Brendon O'Regan; and the third included physicians Bernard Glueck, Fuller Torrey, and Shafica Karagulla, together with psychologists Thelma Moss, Lawrence LeShan, and research engineer James Beal. It was my distinct privilege to arrange and participate in all of them. These three symposia plus a few invitational papers by other experts make up the substance of this volume.

It has been said that many people glimpse visions of the truth, but few jump out of their armchairs to pursue them. Our distinguished authors have made that leap, and it is inevitable that many more will follow their example. At this writing, more than 200 psychiatrists and other physicians are included among our 2000 correspondents, and similar ratios exist among doctors who have applied for membership in a new multidisciplinary organization—the American Metapsychiatric Association (AMPA)—that we are in the process of organizing (see Chapter I).

A few firsts in connection with our project may be worthy of mention from a historical viewpoint. Our 1972 and 1973 panels were sponsored by an official branch of the American Psychiatric Association—its Task Force on Transcultural Psychiatry, of which I was a member. Our 1974 program in Detroit attracted an audience of 650 lay and professional people—the largest panel attendance in APA history (*Psychiatric News,* 1974).[2] And this book is the

---

[2]"Metapsychiatry panel draws overflow audience in Detroit," *Psychiatric News,* 1974 9:17, June 19.

first comprehensive record of psi lectures on any APA agenda. None of this, however, implies that the project was initiated or sanctioned by the American Psychiatric Association. It is a wholly independent endeavor which, though greatly enhanced by such a prestigious and impartial forum, is my sole responsibility. Some of my psychic friends, of course, will say that the inscrutable role of synchronicity and predestination played its part—but that is a conjecture that they, rather than I, are left to ponder. I can only express my gratitude for being a member of such a progressive organization, with so many farsighted friends within it.

Compiling and editing a volume of this kind, consisting of highly individual manuscripts, is an arduous and time-consuming task, but it is also a labor of love and a lesson in humility, for it puts into sharp perspective the indispensable roles played by so many others, and gives me an opportunity to acknowledge publicly my gratitude to them.

My heartfelt thanks go to the participants in our panels, to all the authors who have contributed to this book and to the editorial staff of Nelson-Hall Inc., especially Janet Elliott, for an overwhelming task well done. At the same time I must ask forgiveness from others whose excellent papers were omitted only because of space limitations.

I also thank the following for their moral support: Editors Francis Braceland and Evelyn Myers *(American Journal of Psychiatry)*, Robert Robinson *(Psychiatric News)*, Julius Stulman *(Fields Within Fields)*, and James Bolen *(Psychic* Magazine) for first publishing some of my articles; Drs. Melvin Sabshin, Henry Work, Keith Brodie, and their perceptive APA program committees for their cooperation in assigning our panels; convention manager Dominic Deriso and his capable deputy, Kathleen Bryan, for their expert staging of our programs; and many other colleagues in the American Psychiatric Association and in the American College of Psychiatrists, whose temperate advice and encouragement enabled me to steer a conservative and ethical course through a potentially controversial subject.

Many people helped to spread the news about our programs, thus insuring a large attendance, and I owe thanks to all of them, but especially to Floyce Korsak of Dallas; Patricia Diegel of Honolulu; Dr. Elaine Rogan, Sadhu Grewal, Mrs. Bertha Colon, reporter William Clark of Detroit, and Dr. Raymond Killinger, Fort Lauderdale, Florida.

And first, last, and foremost, thanks to my unflappable secretary, Valerie Joy Anders, whose goodnatured firmness, patience, and expertise were indispensable factors in putting it all together.

References

Dean, S. R. Metapsychiatry. *Psychic* July-Aug. 1973, 5.
_____. Metapsychiatry: the confluence of psychiatry and mysticism. *Fields Within Fields,* Spring 1974, 11:3–11.
Schul, B. D. Science and psi: transcultural trends, a symposium at the American Psychiatric Association convention. *Psychic,* Sept. 1972, 40–42.
Smith, S. Science and psi—a symposium. *Parapsychology Review,* Sept.-Oct. 1972, 5–8.

Section I

Metapsychiatry was selected for a number of reasons as a name for the developing branch of psychiatry that deals with psychic phenomena:

1. Metapsychiatry is congruent with psychiatric terminology.
2. Metapsychiatry encompasses a much wider area than parapsychology.
3. Metapsychiatry calls to mind and strikes a harmonious chord with metaphysics, which by definition deals with first principles, and seeks to explain the nature of being or reality and of the origin and structure of the universe.
4. Metapsychiatry is more palatable to psychiatrists than parapsychiatry, which was also considered. The prefix "para," especially since World War II, has come to have a subordinate connotation, as in paramedics, parapsychiatric aides, and so forth. Hence, parapsychiatry seemed inappropriate to designate a major specialty.

Metapsychiatry is strongly interdisciplinary, having synergistic relationships with parapsychology, philosophy, religion, and empirical logic. These mutually supportive components can produce results that neither could produce alone. It is therefore important that one discipline should not disparage another, a tendency that I found to be strangely prevalent in psychic circles, especially in extolling the virtues of psychic healing over medicine. Such disparagement is unnecessary, and is bound to be self-defeating in the long run. A mature person ought to be able to feel right without the need to proclaim that others are wrong.

It is fitting to begin this section of the book with a definition of mysticism. It simply means that very exceptional kinds of knowledge and awareness may reach consciousness through channels other than those known to us at present.

1

These channels have been postulated as being intuitive, divine, chemical, and/or electronic. A prevailing tendency has been to regard them as forms of energy with field properties, which, like magnetic or gravitational fields, are amenable to scientific research. Others believe that they are latent—inborn higher sense perceptions—spontaneously accessible to some, requiring special training in others, or awaiting the course of evolution in most. But whatever their nature, one thing seems certain—that it is only a matter of time before those channels are identified—a matter of time before the mysticism of yesterday, as so often happens, becomes the science of today.

We are not at all deterred by the fact that we are dealing with a controversial subject. For is not religion controversial? And psychiatry? There will always be doubters, and we welcome them, for they keep us on our mettle. But we distinguish between doubting and prejudice—as in Voltaire's definition of apparitions: "Supernatural visions permitted to him or her gifted by God with the special grace of possessing a cracked brain, a hysterical temperament, a disordered digestion, but, above all, the art of lying with effrontery." Yet wasn't it the same Voltaire who said, "I disagree with what you say, but will defend to the death your right to say it."

We are not even deterred by ignorance, for as Norman Hackerman pointed out: "in the sense of the unaware and as yet unlearned, our ignorance and our recognition of that ignorance may be the best motivation both for problem-solving and for creative activity. . . . For to some to whom truth is an unvariant, that is, something engraved in stone, it must be unsettling to be told that even long-standing natural 'laws' are subject to alteration in light of fuller understanding."[1]

---

[1]Editorial, Ignorance as the driving force. *Science,* 1974, 183, March 8.

Stanley R. Dean

Metapsychiatry: The Confluence of Psychiatry and Mysticism

IT SEEMS STRANGE that I should have become involved in psychic matters, for my orientation is decidedly pragmatic, and I have never experienced any psychic manifestations stronger than an occasional flash of intuition common to all of us. My psychic friends, of course, think differently; they believe that powerful "forces" are at work. Be that as it may, my approach has been that of a professional observer—impartial but not indifferent, an advocate but hardly a fanatic.

My initiation was quite unpremeditated. It occurred during a visit to Tokyo in 1963 when two Japanese colleagues invited me to accompany them to the institute of Zen Master Ishiguro. That renowned sage, after a lifetime in Zen, had in 1957 simplified the arduous rituals of Zen meditation to a point where its basic techniques could be learned in a matter of days (Ishiguro, 1964). I had the opportunity of observing and filming his classes on that occasion and on several subsequent visits to Japan. The psychological and physiological effects of his system of meditation were being studied by several Japanese investigators, among them my two mentors, Koji Sato, then professor of psychology at Kyoto University (Sato, 1958) and Akira Kasamatsu, professor of psychiatry at Tokyo University (Kasamatsu, 1963). Their findings, also reported here (Dean, 1965), were remarkably similar to those published more recently on transcendental meditation. The latter is currently enjoying a burst of popularity, excellently summarized by Ornstein (1972).

At first my interest was purely that of a privileged sightseer witnessing something a bit more extraordinary than the usual tourist attractions. But somewhere along the way I was pricked by the thorn of awareness, and as a result, have become more and more dedicated to the proposition that psychiatry should at long last embark upon a systematic investigation of this related area of the mind, hitherto preempted by psychology, religion, and philosophy. That determination was strengthened by subsequent observations of psychic healing in Bali (Dean, 1972) and by intensive interviews with psychics and sensitives at home and abroad.

I was impressed to find that great numbers of sensible, rational people in all walks of life, lay and professional, believed in mystical states of consciousness, had themselves experienced various manifestations of it, and had derived constructive benefit from it. We psychiatrists are conditioned to equate hallucinations with schizophrenia and other psychoses, but throughout history there have been instances of nonpsychotic individuals—ordinary people as well as sages and seers—who have heard voices, seen visions, and experienced other supernatural phenomena.

I am currently conducting intensive psychiatric evaluations on a series of such individuals in order to obtain a factual determination of their mental and emotional status.[1] As a physician I am particularly interested in any healing factors that clinical development of the ultraconscious may contribute to psychotherapy.

Ten short years ago psychic research was still so controversial that I felt some trepidation in emphasizing its psychiatric importance. Fortunately, the groundwork had been laid by a handful of contemporary psychiatrists: Kelman (1960), Ehrenwald (1966), Eisenbud (1970), Ullman (1973), Stevenson (1965), Schwarz (1965), and Karagulla (1971) are among the better known. Many other psychiatrists, including some in high places, were privately interested, and willing to back an ethical spokesman. As a result, I encountered scarcely any obstacles. My papers were readily published, and some were reprinted in the *Congressional Record* (Dean, 1971). I was invited to show my films and to lecture at medical meetings in Japan, Argentina, Yugoslavia, and Canada, as well as in the United States. And recently the American Psychiatric Association activated a Task Force on Meditation in response to the widespread interest in that area.

There is no question in my mind that psychic research needs greater recognition from medicine and psychiatry in order to achieve the first-class status that it deserves, but that has so far eluded it. In pursuing that premise, I was at first appalled by the vastness of the subject and my relative ignorance of it. But I was reassured by the wisdom of such physicians as Sir George

---

[1]This study is partially supported by a grant from the Academy of Parapsychology, Healing, and Psychic Sciences.

Pickering (1965), former president of the British Medical Association, who candidly stated:

> The older I have become, the more sure I am that an awareness of ignorance is the *sine qua non* for a good scientist. One begins scientific work by asking a question, and one proceeds to gather material to try to answer it. . . . Becoming familiar with a set of phenomena is a necessary preliminary to understanding them: the next step is the realization of how ignorant we all are as to how and why the events happen . . . and then the collection of information and the formulation and testing of hypotheses. You will see then that I am contrasting ignorance and indifference.

Man has always been fascinated with the world of the spirit. There is a natural tendency for the uncluttered mind to drift toward the abstract, and we need not fear that science will be compromised by it, for many scientific facts began as abstract theories. The more man's mind is liberated, the more it will pursue its age-old contemplation of the enigma of the spirit. Alan Watts (1960) developed the thesis that psychotherapy should not be restricted to the relationship merely between man and society, but should also try to uncover the interactions between man and cosmos, for beyond society are universal phenomena transcending all cultures.

Mysticism, according to Aldous Huxley, is the only effective method that has yet been known for the radical and permanent transformation of personality. And a modern philosopher, George Plochmann, (1964), cautions that mysticism is neither an asylum of ignorance nor a place where logic leaves off and forces us to keep quiet.

Discussion

"Metapsychiatry" is a term born of necessity to designate the important but hitherto unclassified interface between psychiatry and mysticism. Metapsychiatry encompasses not only parapsychology, but also all other supernatural manifestations of consciousness that are in any way relevant to the theory and practice of psychiatry. Thus, metapsychiatry may be conceptualized as the base of a pyramid whose other sides are psychiatry, parapsychology, philosophy, and mysticism. First proposed by me (Dean, 1971), the term "metapsychiatry" has found its way into the newest edition of the official psychiatric glossary of the American Psychiatric Association.

It stands to reason that psychic research is a legitimate concern of psychiatry, the specialty best qualified to investigate phenomena, assess validity, and expose fallacy in matters of the mind. As yet there is no general agreement, even among parapsychologists, as to what is psychic and what is not. The term encompasses a heterogeneous assortment of superstitions, beliefs, and procedures ranging, for example, from witchcraft at one extreme to biofeedback-monitoring at the other. In between are a large number of diverse elements related to each other only by an underlying current of mysticism. Some are little more than fanciful superstitions; others hover tantalizingly on the very brink of natural law, seemingly within arms' reach of scientific validation. Clearly, an updated system of psi classification is urgently needed. It would help define categories, determine directions, and establish priorities. Here, too, psychiatry, with its taxonomic expertise, could play an important ancillary role.

Psychiatry can even take special pride in becoming involved, for Richard Maurice Bucke, in 1890 the president of APA's parent organization, the American Medico-Psychological Association, was a distinguished leader in the field. In May 1894, he read a paper entitled "Cosmic Consciousness" at the annual meeting of that society in Philadelphia. Four years later, and reprinted often, a book was published under the same title (Bucke, 1964). In it he developed the theory that a seemingly miraculous higher consciousness, appearing sporadically throughout the ages, was a natural rather than an occult phenomenon, that it was latent in all of us, and was, in fact, an evolutionary process that would eventually raise all mankind to a higher level of existence. He predicted that psychic research would eventually become a major concern of psychiatry. Dr. Bucke was ahead of his time, but more and more his book is being rediscovered and acclaimed. Our APA panels were, in a very real sense, a tribute to this brilliant pioneer.

There have also been other leaders in psychiatry, among them Freud and Jung, who were known for their preoccupation with the occult. And Francis J. Braceland (1957), in his presidential address to the American Psychiatric Association convention, said:

> In the light of history this new [Freudian] psychology heralded the end of a purely mechanistic concept of Man. . . . No one approach to psychiatric disorder can claim a monopoly upon wisdom, understanding, and therapeutic efficiency. We espouse a comprehensive form of psychiatry, and integration is the watchword in our emphasis. . . . The net result of the evidence underscores the need to approach psychological problems from the humanistic point of view which affirms Man's spiritual nature [pp. 3, 7, 9].

Cosmic consciousness refers to a suprasensory, suprarational level of mentation that transcends all other human experience, and creates a sense of oneness with the universe. Its existence has been known since antiquity under a variety of regional and ritual terms—*nirvana, satori, samedhi, unio mystica, kairos*— to name but a few. For purposes of standardization, the term "ultraconsciousness" is proposed because it has closer semantic ties to current psychiatric nomenclature (Dean, 1965).

Miraculous powers have been attributed to the ultraconscious, and from it have sprung the highest creativity and loftiest ideals of man. Yet it still remains the greatest enigma of the mind. All but neglected by science in the past, it has in recent years attracted ever-increasing interest for a number of reasons:

1. Accelerated communication and travel have forged closer transcultural links between Western empiricism and Eastern mysticism, thereby creating a cross-fertilizing continuum wherein ancient truths could be reexamined in the light of modern technology.

2. Transcultural psychiatry has become increasingly interested in shamanism and psychic healing (Dean, 1972; Kiev, 1964; Torrey, 1972).

3. Psychedelic drugs, their uses and abuses, have dramatically focused attention upon extraordinary levels of consciousness (Cohen, 1966; Freedman, 1968).

4. Computer technology has made available vast reservoirs of integrated data that have broken down many of the barriers which previously isolated the behavioral from the physical sciences. As a result, it will become feasible for many sciences to coordinate the findings of various centers.[2]

5. Space exploration has ushered in an enormous and imminent awareness of the universe, and with it a corresponding desire to expand the horizons of consciousness. Man has always been fascinated by the unknown. Today he has a greater general knowledge than ever before. It is axiomatic that with enhanced knowledge comes a thirst for ever greater understanding.

6. Today's technology makes possible more sophisticated, scientifically respectable research on consciousness—e.g., REM dream monitoring, modern meditation techniques, and physiological self-regulation through biofeedback training. These developments have added an important and exciting new dimension to psychiatry and psychosomatic medicine (Ornstein, 1972; Shapiro & Schwartz, 1972).

7. The world is in a state of crisis, perhaps even in danger of annihilation. People who have become increasingly disillusioned by the inability of

---

[2]Central Premonitions Registry, Box 482, Times Square Station, New York, New York 10036.

modern technology to stem the tides of war, crime, intolerance, poverty, and pollution are impelled to seek new avenues of universal harmony.

A current bestseller reports large-scale, government-sponsored research in Soviet countries that has allegedly resulted in some startling psychic discoveries (Ostrander & Schroeder, 1971). One with far-reaching political and paramilitary implications is concerned with the possibility of influencing human behavior (brainwashing) and even matter (psychokinesis) by telepathic remote control. Another, of special interest to space exploration, alludes to instant telepathic communication over immense distances via theoretical units of thought approaching the speed of light. There have even been attempts to explain supernatural religious beliefs and psychic healing on a scientific basis. A special high-frequency photographic technique, known as the Kirlian effect, after its Russian proponents (Kirlian & Kirlian, 1961), has allegedly revealed halo-like, pulsating, bioenergetic emanations that are emitted into the atmosphere by all forms of life and presumably intermingle and interact with other emanations, past, present, and future, and can theoretically be detected by properly developed human and mechanical sensors. Thelma Moss and her co-workers at University of California at Los Angeles have succeeded in making similar photographs (Moss & Johnson, 1973). A whole new field of research, *psychotronics,*[3] has sprung up about these and other modern technological developments.

The question naturally arises whether such emanations correspond to the religious conceptions of soul and, in turn, lend credence to the claims of gifted psychics that they are able to tune into the emanations of other souls, cure sickness by the laying on of hands, and so forth. If so, the human mind could be regarded as a supersensitive receiver capable, in its highest development, of tuning into the innermost channels of the universe. Needless to say, if it can be scientifically proved that individuals can communicate with each other by extrasensory means, it could be a discovery of the very highest magnitude.

Edgar D. Mitchell, former Apollo 14 astronaut, now director of the Institute of Neotic Sciences (IONS) in Palo Alto, California, believes, as do most of us, that the attainment of an ennobling level of consciousness, far from being a mere philosophical speculation, is needed for the realization of man's potential as a total human being; it may even be necessary for human survival

---

[3]Psychotronics was first used as a term in Prague, Czechoslovakia, at the First World Congress of the International Association for Psychotronic Research in 1973. Psychotronics is the scientific interdisciplinary study of the biology of consciousness and the bioenergy systems of a living organism, considered as a whole functioning unit within a total pattern of unity.

(Vaughan, 1971). Those reasons alone make it deserving of top priority in scientific research.

There is certainly an urgent need for our own government to initiate such research. It probably has considerable awareness of the problem already. The United States Army Intelligence Agency has for some time recognized the power of mental telepathy. One of the manuals (Norman, 1972) published by the Technical Bulletin Department is entitled "Techniques of Surveillance and Undercover Investigation." The book states, "During fixed surveillance, the surveillant should avoid any action (e.g., staring at the hands or at the individual's head) which would, *through the recognized phenomenon of sixth sense* (mental telepathy perception), compromise the investigator's mission [p. 151]" (Author's italics). In other words, a spy must be careful lest his subject picks up his thoughts and vice versa through ESP!

Description

The full ultraconscious summit, though rare, produces a superhuman transmutation of consciousness that defies description. The mind, divinely intoxicated, literally reels and trips over itself, groping and struggling for words of sufficient exaltation and grandeur to portray the transcendental vision. As yet we have no adequate words. A fragment of a poem *in Four Quartets* by T. S. Eliot, though used by him in a somewhat different context, seems particularly appropriate here:

> . . . Words strain,
> Crack and sometimes break under the burden,
> Under the tension, slip, slide, perish,
> Decay with imprecision, will not stay in place,
> Will not stay still . . . [pp. 7–8].

One cannot help but wonder if the phenomenon is analogous, even remotely, to erotic love, the one other emotion that has inspired comparable paeans of rapture.[4] Gopi Krishna (1971) believes that the ultraconscious which he calls Kundalini is, in fact, a highly developed transmutation of sex vitality. But,

---

[4]"Coital coupling in marriage can be a launching pad for a transcendental experience in which understanding of the divine is unveiled." (W. E. Phipps: Sacramental sexuality, p. 210. *J. of Religion and Health,* 13:207–216, 1974).

if there is a similarity, it is like that between the light of the sun and the glow of a candle. The narrator must therefore be content with a mere approximation, trusting the intuition of the listener or reader to sense the ultimate meaning.

To begin with, there are many *formes frustes* of the ultraconscious spectrum, and they vary greatly in frequency, intensity, and duration in different persons and even in the same person at different times. They may occur at any time, awake or asleep, spontaneously or only after long years of arduous discipline.

From the welter of literature and liturgy, ancient and modern, I have summarized these distinguishing characteristics of the ultraconscious summit:

1. The onset is ushered in by an awareness of dazzling light that floods the brain and fills the mind. In the East, the ultraconscious summit is called the Brahmic Splendor. Walt Whitman speaks of it in "Prayer of Columbus" from his *Leaves of Grass* as ineffable light—"light rare, untellable, lighting the very light—beyond all signs, descriptions, languages [p. 323]." Dante writes that it is capable of "transhumanizing a man into a god" and gives a moving description in the following lines of mystical incandescence from "Il Paradiso" of the *Divine Comedy:*

> The light I saw was like a blazing river
> A streaming radiance between two banks
> Enameled with wonders of the Spring
> And from that streaming issued living sparks
> That fell on every side as little flowers
> And glowed like rubies in a field of gold.

> Fixing my gaze upon the Eternal Light
> I saw enclosed within its depths,
> Bound up with love together in one volume,
> The scattered leaves of all the universe:
> Substance and accidents, and their relations
> Together fused in such a way
> That what I speak of is one single flame.
> Within the luminous profound subsistence
> Of that Exalted Light saw I three circles
> Of three colors yet of one dimension

> And by the second seemed the first reflected
> As rainbow is by rainbow, and the third
> Seemed fire that equally from both is breathed [p. 591].

2. The individual is bathed in emotions of supercharged joy, rapture, triumph, grandeur, reverential awe, and wonder—an ecstasy so overwhelming that it seems little less than a sort of superpsychic orgasm.

3. An intellectual illumination occurs that is quite impossible to describe. In an intuitive flash, one has an awareness of the meaning and drift of the universe, an identification and merging with creation, infinity and immortality, a depth beyond depth of revealed meaning—in short, a conception of an over-self, so omnipotent that religion has interpreted it as God. The individual attains a conception of the whole that dwarfs all learning, speculation, and imagination, and makes the old attempts to understand the universe elementary and petty.

4. There is a feeling of transcendental love and compassion for all living things.

5. Fear of death falls off like an old cloak; physical and mental suffering vanish. There is an enhancement of mental and physical vigor and activity, a rejuvenation and prolongation of life. This property, especially, should command the interest of the physician and psychiatrist.

6. There is a reappraisal of the material things in life, an enchanced appreciation of beauty, a realization of the relative unimportance of riches and abundance compared to the treasures of the ultraconscious.

7. There is an extraordinary quickening of the intellect, an uncovering of latent genius. Far from being a passive, dream-like state, however, the ultraconscious summit can endow an individual with powers so far-reaching as to influence the course of history.

8. There is a sense of mission. The ultraconscious revelation is so moving and profound that the individual cannot contain it within himself, but is moved to share it with all fellow men.

9. A charismatic change occurs in personality—an inner and outer radiance, as though charged with some divinely inspired power, a magnetic force that attracts and inspires others with unshakable loyalty and faith.

10. There is a sudden or gradual development of extraordinary psychic gifts such as clairvoyance, extrasensory perception, telepathy, precognition, psychic healing, and so forth. Though generally regarded as occult, such phenomena may have a more rational explanation. They may be due to an awakening of latent transhuman powers of perception plus the interplay of bioenergetic emanations and forces previously mentioned.

Summation

The ultraconscious summit is a genuine metamorphosis of consciousness which has been experienced by certain sages, prophets, leaders, and men of genius through the ages. The factors producing it are as yet unknown, but the remarkable uniformity of distinguishing characteristics, regardless of origin, should leave no doubt that a common denominator underlies all of them. It is only a matter of time before science will dissociate the ultraconscious from religious dogma and explain it to the satisfaction of the intellect in terms of natural law.

Summarized below are some of the questions that have been raised:

1. Is the ultraconscious a gift of God, beyond human understanding? If so, it should be accepted as a matter of pure faith, and without futher question.
2. Is the ultraconscious state a pathological mental disorder? If so, how could it elicit genius in religion, literature, and the arts?
3. Is it brought on by hypnosis or suggestion? How, then, can one explain its permanence, charisma, and intellectual powers even in the unschooled and irreligious?
4. Does self-mortification and sensory deprivation, as practiced by ascetics, produce metabolic by-products with hallucinogenic properties similar to those of psychedelic drugs? Why then is this phenomenon not encountered more often in connection with disease, surgery, and battle wounds?
5. Is ultraconsciousness all a matter of charlatanism?

Obviously none of these produces a satisfactory answer. Where else can we turn? Lawrence LeShan (1969) reminds us that "it is part of the faith of science that if serious people work diligently on a problem for a long period of time and cannot arrive at a satisfactory answer, they are asking the wrong question, and a new one is needed [p. 36]." In this case, it should be one that appeals both to science and to common sense. It may be framed as follows:

6. *Is the ultraconscious experience a natural biological phenomenon latent in all of us?* Are there areas of perception and cognition in the brain, as yet undiscovered, that can be energized by chemical or other physiological mediators as yet unknown?

In my opinion, it is that question which has the greatest appeal to reason and offers the best possibility of producing a definitive answer.

The developing human mind undoubtedly harbors a rudimentary awareness of cosmic evolution, manifest more in some than in others, that may ultimately evolve into an aggregate understanding of the origin and nature of the universe. Emanuel Walloff,[5] a chemical engineer, suggests the phrase, "Psychogeny recapitulates cosmogeny," to summarize that concept, comparing it with the well-known embryological aphorism, "Ontogeny recapitulates philogeny." A similar idea was stated by Paracelsus, a mystic and scientist, more than 400 years ago: The microcosm corresponds to the macrocosm. The ultraconscious, even though latent, gives off signals of illumination a good part of the time, faint and subtle in some, strong in others. Kelman (1970) believes that major and minor periods of illumination, which he calls "kairos", could be helped to occur with patients, could be recognized when illumination did happen, and could be used by psychiatrists to augment psychotherapy.

Fortunately, there is no dearth of material. Though total ultraconsciousness is rare, a great variety of lesser manifestations is extremely common. The scientist is already studying them in his laboratory through research on biofeedback, Kirlian photography, physiological effects of meditation, electroencephalographic dream monitoring, extrasensory perception, and so forth. It is only a matter of time before the enlightened clinician will be able to use some of those procedures in his practice. Meanwhile, a simple first step would be to encourage people to disclose any paranormal (supernatural) experiences, and to treat such disclosures with an open-minded, noncynical attitude. The clinician will be amazed at the abundant material thus elicited. And, if the resulting data from laboratory and clinic were collected, pooled and analyzed, it could not help but result in a rational breakthrough of this hitherto inscrutable subject.

Needless to say, we are not dealing with an unmixed blessing. All sorts of cults and commerical enterprises have sprung up exploiting meditation, biofeedback, mind control, and higher states of consciousness. Some may offer free lectures and demonstrations to entice the beginner, then go on to progressively escalating assessments, which, at a fanatical level of involvement, may reach confiscatory extremes. It is important to differentiate true ultraconsciousness from what Freedman (1968) summarizes as the pseudoprofundity, gullibility, and romanticism of the dilettante, the cultist, and the charlatan. A recent article (Peterson, 1973) stresses the dangers inherent in unskilled, unscrupulous, often unlicensed practitioners of various methods of mind control. The article quotes Allen Cohen, director of a drug abuse institute at the John F. Kennedy University at Martinez, California, as saying: "I've seen

---

[5]Personal communication, January 20, 1972.

more than 100 psychic eruptions in people who have gotten in over their heads. By the late 70's we'll have the same need for discrimination in these exotic alternatives for drugs as we now have for drugs themselves." The same article quotes Elmer and Alyce Green, biofeedback researchers at the Menninger Foundation, as saying that unless practitioners are subject to legal and professional regulations, the government may summarily ban many research and training programs that otherwise might become valuable adjuncts to our educational and health systems.

Most experts agree that many movements that end up with secret rituals and cultish overdependence on the leader are potentially harmful. Ethical professionals are doing something about it. For example, at the 1971 meeting of the Society for Psychophysiological Research, David Shapiro (1973) of the Massachusetts Mental Health Center chaired a symposium entitled. "Ethical, Legal, and Medical Issues in Biofeedback Technology." The group was concerned about the explosion of advertisements and headlines about electronic yoga, new states of awareness, alpha waves and creativity, and control of the mind. They have gone on record as expressing that concern to the press and to responsible governmental agencies.

In general, however, the advantages of psychic research in ethical hands far outweigh the disadvantages, and open up unparalleled new worlds to the scientist and physician of tomorrow. In order to give special emphasis to the relationship between psychiatry and psychic phenomena, an American Metapsychiatric Association is in the process of being organized which, though psychiatrically oriented, will be open to all behavioral scientists and responsible laymen. All who are interested should communicate with the author at the earliest opportunity. The American Metapsychiatric Association has no desire to supplant, but rather to supplement, existing organizations. As conceived by its founders, AMPA will create a competitive stimulus rather than a competitive hazard in the field of psychic research. AMPA's goal throughout will be to replace strangeness, sensationalism, and fraud with logic, common sense, and professional responsibility.

Despite my lack of occult powers, I can envision a tremendous upsurge in psychic education and research, with and without government assistance, and in the very near future. Is that clairvoyance or common sense? Perhaps the two are not so different after all.

Psychic Aphorisms
(A personal compendium of psi beliefs and theories)

Faith is not fantasy; it is a form of precognition that has divined for countless years what science is just beginning to understand.

Science and mysticism are fraternal twins, long separated, but now on the verge of reunion.

Psychogeny recapitulates cosmogeny, i.e., the developing mind includes an innate awareness of the origin and meaning of the universe.

Evolution is not homogeneous, but proceeds in two divergent streams; mental and physical. Mental evolution is far ahead of the physical.

The ultraconscious state bridges the evolutionary gap and produces cosmic awareness.

Psi power is latent in all, and an experiential reality to many.

Thought is a form of energy; it has universal field properties which, like gravitational and magnetic fields, are amenable to scientific research.

Thought fields, like the theoretical tachyon, can interact, traverse space, and penetrate matter more or less instantaneously.

Thought fields survive death and are analogous to soul and spirit.

Thought fields are eternal; hence, past existence (reincarnation) is as valid a concept as future immortality.

Psychic research is on a par with other important courses of study; it should be included in academic curricula and lead to degrees and doctorates.

A new age is dawning—the Psychic Age—on the heels of the Atomic Age and Space Age.

References

Braceland, F. J. Psychiatry and the science of man. *American Journal of Psychiatry,* 1957, 114, 1–9.

Bucke, R. M. *Cosmic consciousness.* New York: Dutton, 1964.

Cohen, S. *The beyond within: the LSD story.* New York: Atheneum, 1966.

Dante, A. *The divine comedy.* Translated by H. W. Longfellow. Boston: Houghton-Mifflin, 1913.

Dean, S. R. Beyond the unconscious: the ultraconscious. *Psychologia.* 1965, 8, 145–150. *American Journal of Psychiatry,* Letters, 1965, 122, 471.

———. Metapsychiatry and the unconscious. *American Journal of Psychiatry,* 1971, 128, 154–155.

_____. Shamanism vs. psychiatry in Bali, 'island of the gods.' *American Journal of Psychiatry,* 1972, **129,** 91–94.

_____. Metapsychiatry. *Psychic,* 1973, **July-August,** 5.

_____. Metapsychiatry: the interface between psychiatry and mysticism. *American Journal of Psychiatry,* 1973, **130,** 1036–1038.

Ehrenwald, J. *Psychotherapy: myth and method.* New York: Grune & Stratton, 1966.

Eisenbud, J. *Psi and psychoanalysis.* New York: Grune & Stratton, 1970.

Eliot, T. S. *Four quartets.* New York: Harcourt, 1943.

Freedman, D. X. On the use and abuse of LSD. *Archives of General Psychiatry,* 1968, 18, 330–347.

Ishiguro, H. *The scientific truth of Zen.* Tokyo: Zenrigaku Society, 1964.

Karagulla, S. *Breakthrough to creativity.* Santa Monica, Ca.: DeVorss, 1971.

Kasamatsu, A. *Science of zazen.* Tokyo: Koishigawa Branch of Tokyo University, 1963.

Kelman, H. Kairos and the therapeutic process. *Journal of Existential Psychiatry,* 1970, 1, 233–269.

Kiev, A. (Ed.) *Studies in primitive psychiatry today: magic, faith, and healing.* New York: Free Press, 1964.

Kirlian, S. D. & Kirlian, V. C. Photography and visual observations by means of high-frequency currents. *Journal of Scientific and Descriptive Photography,* 1961, 6, 397–403.

Krishna, G. *Kundalini, the evolutionary energy in man.* Berkeley: Shambala Publications, 1971.

LeShan, L. Human survival of biological death. In *Main Currents in Modern Thought.* Foundation for Integrative Education, 1969, **26,** 35–45.

Moss, T. & Johnson, K. Bioplasma or corona discharge? In S. Krippner and D. Rubin (Eds.), *Galaxies of life.* New York: Gordon and Breach, 1973.

Norman, E. H. *Beyond the strange.* New York: Popular Library, 1972.

Ornstein, R. E. *The psychology of consciousness.* San Francisco: W. H. Freeman, 1972.

Ostrander, S. & Schroeder, L. *Psychic discoveries behind the iron curtain.* New York: Bantam, 1971.

Peterson, J. Science and psychic power. *The National Observer,* 1973, 11/20.

Pickering, G. The great value of ignorance. *Medical World News,* 1965, 6, 74.

Plochmann, G. K. A note on Harrison's notes on "das mystiche." *Southern Journal of Philosophy,* 1964, 2, 9–10.

Sato, K. The concept of 'on' in Ruth Benedict and D. T. Suzuki. *Psychologia,* 1958, **2,** 243–245.

Schul, B. D. Science and psi: transcultural trends. *Psychic,* 1972, **4,** 40–42.

Schwarz, B. E. *Psychic-dynamics.* New York: Pageant Press, 1965.

Shapiro, D. Recommendations of ethics committee regarding biofeedback techniques and instrumentation: issues of public and professional concern. *Psychophysiology,* 1973, **10,** 533–535.

Shapiro, D. & Schwartz, G. E. Biofeedback and visceral learning: clinical applications. *Seminars in Psychiatry,* 1972, **4,** 171–183.

Smith, S. Science and psi—a symposium. *Parapsychology Review,* 1972, Sept.-Oct., 5–8.

Stevenson, I. Some psychological principles relevant to research in survival. *Journal of American Society for Psychical Research,* 1965, **59,** 318–337.

Torrey, E. F. *The mind game.* New York: Emerson Hall, 1972.

Ullman, M. *Dream telepathy.* New York: Macmillan, 1973.

Vaughan, A. Interview: Captain Edgar D. Mitchell. *Psychic,* 1971, **3,** 5–ff.

Watts, A. *Psychotherapy east and west.* New York: Mentor, New American Library, 1960.

Whitman, W. *Leaves of grass.* Philadelphia: McKay, 1891.

Francis J. Braceland

Psychiatry and the
Science of Man

> We are that bold and adventurous piece of nature, which he
> that studies may wisely learn, in a compendium, what others
> labour at in a divided piece and endless volume.
>
> Sir Thomas Browne

I

WHEN THE THEORETICAL physicists, Doctors Lee and Yang, . . . challenged
the principle of parity, their work shattered completely one of the basic laws
which had been built into all physical theories. . . . This had been a philosophically pleasing theory—this idea of mirror symmetry of submicroscopic particles—which they demolished and, worse and more of it, it had consistently
borne fruit in the making of successful predictions about atomic and nuclear
processes. This is worthy of our attention—the theory was erroneous; yet
successful predictions were made from it. Now, suddenly, this attractive theory
was destroyed and we are told that there is no one who can say when or how
the pieces will be put together again. In the early stages of their work, the
young scientists could hardly have suspected the widespread implications their
findings would have, but before long it became apparent that an obstacle was
removed and a way was now clear and, out of the intellectual ferment and
ceaseless reexamination of principles the new discovery had initiated, there

This chapter encompasses the major part of Dr. Braceland's Presidential Address delivered at
the 113th Annual Convention of the American Psychiatric Association, May 13–18. 1957,
Chicago, Illinois. It was published in the American Journal of Psychiatry, July 1957. Though
presented almost twenty years ago, it is so relevant to the spirit and subject of this book that it
is being reproduced here with the author's permission.

might eventuate something which thus far had eluded all scientists. This eventuality hopefully might be a unified field theory encompassing all of the laws of matter, energy and the universe.

This little drama of physical science had its counterpart in the last decade of the last century when Freud challenged the then current ideas regarding the etiology of emotional disorder. These ideas, too, had been philosophically comfortable and they had been held in various guises for many years. Freud's brilliant observations, unrecognized and unappreciated at first, are now seen to have signalled a turning point, not only in psychology, but also in science, and from them another eventuality might also stem—in this case a step toward a unitary or integrated approach to the science of man. Some aspects of the new theory, as propounded first, would have to be changed, but even from these would come some successful predictions about the emotional reaction of man.

While the potentialities of the physicists' ideas were recognized quickly, Freud's revolutionary ideas were missed entirely. They were even overlooked by Freud and his colleagues, for they did not realize that here were the precursors of an entirely new system of thought, one which would require an approach entirely different from that being applied to the formulations of general medicine. Unhappily, this new system was forced into the then extant and waiting molds of scientific thought, though it took procrustean techniques to do it. Had the newness and the significance of these ideas been recognized and had they been followed to their logical conclusion, instead of being pushed into convenient molds, much of the bitterness and opposition which their promulgation engendered would have been avoided. It is only now that the far reaching importance of these ideas and insights are being fully appreciated. Their influence penetrates into many disciplines; they are more by far than a treatment and research method; buried in them are precious creative currents and, in the words of Karl Stern[1], as a result of what we have learned from them, "our image of the interior world of man can never be the same as it was prior to 1894."

The beginnings of a new era are usually not recognized by the pioneers who are working in it. Ordinarily they proceed, thinking and operating in the approved categories of the time, unaware of the revolutionary aspects of their work. It was ever thus. It is the historian who retrospectively sees indications of approaching revolution at a time when few are aware that their traditional world is in rapid change. Though it may seem paradoxical in the light of some present day teaching, viewed in the light of history this new psychology heralded the end of a purely mechanistic concept of man.

Once again ... there are omens and portents which indicate that we are on the threshold of other major changes. The tell-tale symptoms and signs are those of restless inquiry, examination and reexamination. Many of the major medical disciplines are in a state of transition, as are the physical sciences. ... Psychoanalysis is examining itself as a discipline and seeking to evaluate its efforts and its results and its directions, and one might prognosticate that the findings will herald an even closer rapprochement with medicine.

Medical educators are in full scale reassessment of their curricula, due to the realization that, despite their high standards, something is still lacking in their finished product. The practice of medicine itself is changing and, as Atchley[2] puts it, the doctor now, "instead of being satisfied to merely identify his patient's condition with a large group of similar diseases, tries to analyze all the various abnormal components in this one person and thus reach an appraisal, rather than apply a label."

Verily, then, these are times of change—these are the best of times; these are the worst of times—we have everything before us; we have nothing before us. There are sounds of trouble in the distance, but the click of Madame Defarge's needles now is supplanted by the sound of the Geiger counter symbolic of a nuclear age. In this transitional phase, as psychiatry reexamines itself, it seeks to find its place in the scheme of things. Until now it has been lusty, sprawling, verbose and growing space. It is wise to examine itself while there is still an earth for the meek to inherit.

If the present state of psychiatry is envisaged as one of transition or transformation, there arise certain problems of gravity which the psychiatrist has to consider in full consciousness of his responsibility and hence, in seriousness and humility. The future development of his discipline depends upon the solution of these problems, as does the value of the services he will render to mankind. Though philosophers may discuss whether the events of history follow their own intrinsic, inexorable laws, or whether they be directed to some extent by man's doings, we must act, as Ignatius Loyola says, as if everything depended upon us, even though we know that nothing depends upon us alone.

Modern psychiatry, by virtue of its intrinsic developments on the one hand, and by the demands made by society on the other, differs from what it was even a quarter century ago. It no longer focuses entirely upon mental disease, nor the individual as a "mental patient," but rather it envisages man in the totality of his being and in the totality of his relationships. Consequently, the place of psychiatry within the system of medicine, as well as within the complex of all disciplines concerned with man, his nature, his work and his destiny, also has changed. If one designates the totality of all disciplines concerned with the manifold aspects of human being and doing as *humanism,* then psychiatry has become a *humanistic* discipline. It has become an essential part of an over-all science of man, of general anthropology. The movement of psychiatry in this direction and the ensuing transformation of psychiatric thinking is not an isolated phenomenon. It is expressive of a new turn in the manner in which man looks at himself. It was Sherrington who said: "Man in his mood may count himself in his day a brief spectator of his own shaping as it still progresses."

Psychiatry by becoming more humanistic need not in any way become less scientific. Scientific inquiry and methodology must always form the solid foundation of our discipline, but upon this foundation must be erected the edifice of a psychiatry which will be an applied science of man. The humanistic tendencies of our discipline have already proved a stumbling block for some of our medical colleagues. Because of some misunderstanding, they equate the humanistic aspects of our approach with a meddlesome form of do-goodism; yet nothing can be further from the truth. Humanism and a scientific approach to the science of man are not mutually exclusive. By science we mean here not mathematical science in the narrow sense of the term, but the meaning which it had of old: "encompassing and well ordered knowledge." One might even say the ideal goal of the psychiatrist is to achieve wisdom. The best one can do, of course, is to aspire to this attainment and the first step toward it is that of recognizing one's limitations, of being conscious, as was Socrates, that one knows nothing in comparison with what he should know. Psychiatry can be justly proud of its achievements in the relatively short time in which it has functioned as a discipline; yet at the same time it is required to be humble because of what it does not know and because of the enormous problems which still face it. Paradoxically, wisdom is a mixture of humility and legitimate pride.

If psychiatry is to take its proper place in the science of man, it must be aware of its limitations and realize that it is only a part of this science, an important but a small part insofar as the general knowledge of man is concerned. To forget this is to run the danger of scientific imperialism. By this term I mean to indicate the tendency, encountered regularly in the history of knowledge, to credit a special discipline with universal significance. The final result of such enthronement is always the catastrophic dethronement of the apparently supreme branch of knowledge. You have seen this little melodrama even within the framework of psychiatry itself. If you cast about you, you will see it on an even larger scale in the form of a cloud of anti-scientific attitude, "no bigger than a man's hand," but there nonetheless. It is an increasing unwillingness to see in science a world-saving panacea or to believe in the possibility of solving all human problems by means of scientific inquiry. If this cloud enlarges, it is because the scientists, or perhaps better the popularizers of science, have indulged in this imperialism and failed to recognize that human existence shows facets where science and her methodology prove insufficient. The same danger faces psychiatry, if its popularizers become too enthusiastic or its enthusiasts become too popular. . . .

Psychiatry is a part of the science of man; it has a place in it and is a dependent upon it and a contributor to it. It is a part of the science of man because it deals with certain basic and historic problems of man and his society: with thought, emotion, behavior and human relatedness gone wrong. Psychiatry is dependent upon that science, inasmuch as appraisal of the abnormal is necessarily based upon knowledge of what is conceded to be normal, on knowledge of man's intrinsic nature and what makes him function and behave as he does. Psychiatry's contribution comes from the demonstration it makes of certain basic features of the human psyche and their universality.

II

Science builds upon knowledge previously accumulated, not only in its own field, but in encompassing and contiguous areas. All inquiry in a circumscribed area is advantaged by the use of general principles and the data of related sciences. Psychiatry is dependent upon many disciplines concerned with human biology and human behavior. Just as the phenomenon, man, and all that pertains to it is extremely complex, so also is abnormality at the human level. The more abnormality refers to the total human being, as it does in psychiatry, the more necessary it becomes for psychiatry to consider all of the diverse aspects of human nature and human conduct and to examine the knowledge recorded by succeeding generations of thoughtful students of man. We learn today what we may have to unlearn tomorrow and we learn recurrently lessons which were taught before and then forgotten in the changing seasons of science. Today the accumulation of knowledge about man and his behavior is proceeding swiftly along many fronts and from the interpenetration and integration of that knowledge will emerge the new science of man of which we speak. It will be well for us to incorporate into that science the older wisdom and not to neglect it because it speaks of man's eternal preoccupations and so of his future purpose.

Speculative as this all may seem, it is of the greatest importance to us here and now. The organic substrate of the psyche is again a matter of major interest and, if we are not careful, all or part of that vast psychological insight, which Janet, Freud, Jung, Adler and Meyer and their followers gave us, will languish or be minimized. We have already hinted at the dangers of reduction-ism from the complex phenomena with which we deal to any simple formula. The history of psychiatry, which reflects the cultural, as well as the medical, climate of society is testimony to this. Exclusively mentalistic and exclusively biological conceptions have reigned in turn and have contributed in turn to the one-sidedness of psychiatry's preoccupation at various recurring inter-vals. . . .

. . . Not that the value of psychotherapy was lessened in any way, but it became clear and definite, and we now may regard it as axiomatic that *no one approach to psychiatric disorder can claim a monopoly upon wisdom, under-standing or therapeutic efficacy.*

III

It is evident by now that we espouse a comprehensive form of psychiatry and that integration is the watch word in our emphasis. Unfortunately, this term has taken on connotations which are not our consideration here. By integration we mean that all possible aspects of man's make-up and his needs be considered and united with each other in a homogeneous picture. Having discussed the predominantly mental, we should note briefly the activities in the somatic and the social aspects of man's life and what, for want of a better term, we will designate the philosophy of present day existence. This is the material with which, and the field in which the psychiatrist works. . . .

. . . The net result of the evidence we have underscores the need to approach psychological problems from the humanistic point of view which affirms man's spiritual nature.

Meaningfulness of existence is not a by-product of modern science. Science produces no antidote for the trials and tribulations of man in a changing social and industrial order and a rapidly diminishing world. Man is easily upset and thrown off balance when the things on which he habitually relies fail him. The quest for security in modern life is difficult of attainment. For every new security established, another insecurity emerges. Not only does technological development bring its own dangers, but maintenance of security depends on ever closer cooperation and a denser network of social relationships. The more complicated a machinery becomes, the more vulnerable it becomes, and this is certainly true of the machinery of social life, and it is within the bounds of this social life that the psychiatrist works.

Today's society is seemingly dominated by what Riesman calls the "other-directed" man, who finds the motivations of his conduct and the ends he pursues not in himself, but in the dictation of the group. An age of mass production and mass communication gives birth to a mass society, where the individual is as much standardized as are syndicated columns, TV shows and the products of industry. Few dare to be different, and for good reason—for to be different brings them under the condemnation of the group on whose opinion they form their own opinion of themselves. The idolatry of conformity, of being exactly like everyone else in a group which tolerates only "marginal diversity"; the frenzy with which so many people addict themselves to all sorts of superficial activities or passivities—these and other enslavements of contemporary life originate, at least to some extent, from the need to replace beliefs and values and faith in which man once found security. But man's dignity cannot be served in ways that tend to depersonalize him and to deprive his existence of its real meaning. It cannot be served in the "over-adjustment" which is being advocated today, and the attempt to fit all men into a common denominator: the cooperative submitting member of the group. . . .

To serve man's dignity means to consider each man's individuality thoroughly and widely. The necessity of viewing man by means of categories of "historical thinking" is as obvious here as it ever was in the development of new approaches to psychiatry in recent years. These new approaches tend to make both the study and practice of psychiatry much more difficult. Psychiatric practice is not just the application of learned technique, no matter how exclusive or inspired it may claim to be. The practice presupposes a sort of human understanding by the psychiatrist. Human understanding is not merely the ability to explain human actions, attitudes, mental states, in terms of some theory which, as such, is necessarily general. All such theories remain somehow on the surface, for they are incapable of grasping precisely what it is that makes a person this one person, distinct from all others. . . .

But what consequences and what directions may be drawn from all this for the future of psychiatry as a science? Though predictions are as uncertain as prescriptions are presumptuous, we must nevertheless attempt to map out some sort of program, or at least to delineate some sort of picture of what is going to happen in our field in the near future. Such an attempt is less risky the more conscious we are of the preliminary nature of all we may say and the more willing we are to modify our plans in the wake of new experience.

Of one point we may be certain: psychiatry will have to be more than ever a medical discipline. The recognition of the causal role of somatic factors, and of the therapeutic effect of physio-chemical methods, underscores the need for a thorough knowledge of medicine as a prerequisite for doing responsible and successful psychiatric treatment. By the same token, the basic disciplines of psychiatry must be accepted by medicine. Anthropology, social and experimental psychology, the "normal" basic psychiatric science disciplines derive from faculties of philosophy and are not taught in medical schools. Even clinical psychology, an important aspect of psychiatric science, is rarely part of the young psychiatrist's training. As a result, the psychiatrist is handicapped at times when he attempts to think out new methods of approach to disease not already catalogued in his textbook, and the doctor who does not specialize in psychiatry is not adequately equipped to deal with the host of psychiatric problems he encounters in daily practice. The answer to this is as thorough teaching of the basic science disciplines of psychiatry as those of the purely medical sciences.

We may also be fairly certain of another point which, though already discernible, is more of a general vision than a clearly outlined program. We have come to realize that psychiatry, while undoubtedly and strictly a medical discipline, must at the same time be more than this. The psychiatrist in research and in practice is not justified in restricting his endeavors to one aspect of the human being. He has to take account of man as a whole and in the totality of his vital, social, cultural situation. Paradoxical though it may sound, the statement is nonetheless cogent, that to be truly a psychiatrist, one has to be more than a psychiatrist, more than a specialist. As we mentioned above, he must be a humanist. While scientific inquiry and methodology must always form the solid foundation of our discipline, upon this foundation may be erected the edifice of a psychiatry which will be the "applied science of man."

The ideal goal of the psychiatrist is to achieve wisdom, over and above the circumscribed knowledge that science, as it is understood today, affords. Psychiatry could do well with a philosophy of its own. Almost a century has passed since philosophy was formally expelled from psychiatry, but she returns inexorably to remind us that the old problem of the relationship obtaining between mind and body still exists. Philosophy can claim no jurisdiction in matters pertaining to psychiatry and medicine proper. And it would be inappropriate to demand that the psychiatrist be a philosopher in the academic sense. But surely it is legitimate to demand from him an awareness of the fact that the problems in his purview transcend in their ultimate significance the field of purely empirical inquiry and that human existence extends beyond the strictly "natural" into the world of ideas, of truths, of values. The knowledge of man provided by dynamic psychiatry has made it clearer than ever that it is the inner life of the individual which is of paramount importance. . . .

I know the futility of asking overworked and fatigued men to look up from their labors in order to see something grand in the over-all scheme of things;

yet look up we must and, when we do, we can better serve not only the progress of psychiatry, but also the progress of man to a fuller and better life.

If the science of man brings enlightenment to psychiatry, psychiatry can repay this debt amply by keeping in mind the great dignity of man and what human nature really is. The psychiatrist, even more than others, is entitled to make his own the words of the poet, Terence:

> "Nil humani a me alienum puto." (Nothing that concerns a man do I deem alien to me.)

References

1. Stern, Karl. *The Third Revolution.* New York: Harcourt, Brace & Co., 1955.
2. Atchley, Dana W. "The Changing Physician." *Atlantic Monthly,* August 1956.

Jules H. Masserman

Myth, Mystique, and Metapsychiatry

IN AN EXCHANGE of letters with Freud, Albert Einstein once questioned whether a putative death instinct really doomed man to self-destruction, and enquired whether psychoanalysis was not, after all, a compendium of myths. Replied Freud, in effect: "True, but are not all sciences?" Freud thus joined Empedocles, Berkeley, Kant, Hegel, Whitehead, Susan Langer, and other philosophers in contending that we live not in an essentially knowable reality, but in a matrix of individually convenient imagery.

Certainly, classical psychoanalysis is replete with the myths of Narcissus, Electra, Oedipus, and others; unfortunately, however, it often strips them of their more poetic and subtle significance. For example, Narcissis did not fall in love with himself to the neglect of his friend Ameinius and his mistress Echo: instead, after due reflection at a quiet pool, he was lost in admiration of his upward-gazing image, and thereby became an early flower-child. Dour Electra, for the purported love of her dead father, had her mother Clytaemnestra and the interloper Aegisthus murdered while making brother Orestes and practically everyone else miserable—hardly a relevant paradigm for a simple Electra complex of living father-daughter erotism. So also, the Oedipus legend far transcends Freud's personal preoccupation with incest between mother and son; much more comprehensively, it explores almost every poignant human motivation, relationship, tragedy, and hope. Let us reexamine the full Sophoclean trilogy:

> Laius, King of Thebes, is warned by the Oracle of Delphi that his newborn son would slay him—a fairly safe prophecy, since all children will inevitably displace their elders. Fearing punishment

29

for fully preventive infanticide (as most of us do), Laius instead
binds the child's ankles (Oedipus means swollen feet), places him
in a basket and, there being no Nilotic bulrushes about, leaves him
on nearby Mount Cithaeron. Oedipus is found by the seer
Teiresias, and adopted by Polybus and Merope, the royal family of
Corinth—as indeed rejected children are perennially rescued by
pediatricians, nurseries, pedagogues, child psychoanalysts, and other
parental surrogates. But Oedipus retains nagging doubts that he is
really the true Prince of Corinth (for that matter, who can be
absolutely certain of his own paternity?), cannot get satisfactory
assurances from King Polybus or Queen Merope, and is further
perplexed when the Delphic Oracle informs him that he will kill
his father and marry his mother. Trying to escape his fate (as who
does not?), Oedipus vows never to see his supposed parents Polybus
or Merope again, and leaves Corinth to wander in search of what
Erik Erikson would call his true identity. At a crossroads outside
Thebes, an old man blocks his right of way and is killed in the
ensuing contest—as all oldsters who dare too long to challenge
imperious youth will be disposed of in their turn. Oedipus then
vanquishes a Sphinx by solving its life or death riddle as to man's
quadri-, bi-, and tripedal locomotion from crawl to cane (*vide* our
current crop of adolescent omniscients), and thereby emancipates
the Thebans from years of sphincteric terror. For reward he is
given the vacant throne of Thebes and marries the widowed
Queen Iocaste.
    And yet, nagging doubts remain (who is free of them?), and
Oedipus, after more years of restless research (a precarious
occupation), finds sightless Teiresias and learns from him the awful
truth: that he, Oedipus, had indeed killed his father Laius and
cohabited incestuously with his mother, Iocaste—awful, of course,
only because he fears that others regard it so. He blinds (not
castrates) himself in expiation (and thereby becomes a pathetic
rather than reprehensible figure), exiles his former friend Creon
and his own potentially competitive sons Eteocles and Polyneices,
and then preempts the services of his daughters, Antigone and
Ismene, in further wanderings throughout Hellas—as all aging
parents have tried to do ever since Agamemnon sacrificed
Iphigeneia on the perennial plea that this was what a good
daughter should do to please her father's gods. Finally, at Colonus,
Oedipus consults the Fates, pleads for justice, and is himself
granted the status of demigod—thus acquiring the archangelic
status we all believe we deserve.

By preempting such legends, Freud approached closely the Jungian concepts of the mysterious *anima* and *animus*—the core patterns—that imbue
not only man's primal conations throughout the ages, but also his persistently

mythical notions of his cosmic relationships. Nevertheless, dialectic man loves to live by contradictions, and his nature abhors any vacuum of even temporary subservience to capricious fate before achieving omnipotence. Ergo, materialistic-minded Aristotelians or Newtonians among us instead contend that picturesque parables may serve to entertain the oneiric-minded, but have no place in practice. After all, say they, there is an external, palpable world of *real* objects (a tree is not a myth, whether or not anyone calls it a poem), and these objects, inanimate or human, interact in ways that can be observed, measured, and controlled by man alone. In the logical positivist view, knowledge will illuminate the world, free man of his mythologies, and, in a current Oedipal paraphrase, slay the Sphinx and let scientific sunshine in.

The opposing doctrines outlined above echo the classical disputes between Ionic and Athenian academes, the medieval polemics among nominalists and phenomenalists, Henry James' distinctions between soft-headed dreamers and hard-headed pragmatists (said James, in effect, "truth is to both merely an expedient way of thinking"), and C. P. Snow's concept of "two cultural types. . . scientists and humanists." I am tempted to comment that *if* men can be even partially divided into two types, one type seems addicted to such oversimplified dichotomies.

Indeed, although materialistic tenets have had a long and cherished tradition, few scientists, however hard-headed, have really accepted them in pure form. Thus Democritus (460–370 BC) insisted that the world is made of . . . "unchangeable atoms and their motions in space," yet admitted that "sweet and bitter, cold and warm, as well as all [such perceptions] exist but in opinion and not in reality." Leibnitz (1646–1716) likewise qualified his concepts of the ultimate monads, from which both the cosmos and God were constructed, by stating, "I am able to prove that not only light, color, heat and the like, but motion, shape and extension, too, are merely *apparent* qualities." There ensued, through Kant, Hegel, and the German idealists, an increasing recognition of the psychopoetic essence of all knowledge, including the so-called laws of physics, until Arthur Eddington could write:

> It is we (and not any eternal verities) who determine sense-data by our interpretations, who impose structure, and *who regain from nature, which is infinitely varied, that which our minds have put into nature.* We have found a strange footprint on the shores of the unknown. We have devised profound theories, one after the other, to account for its origin. At last we have succeeded in reconstructing the creature that made the footprint. And lo! It is our own!

James Jeans equated space itself with human affect: "It is probably as meaningless to discuss how much room an electron takes up as to discuss how much room a fear, an anxiety, or an uncertainty takes up."

Freud, too, admitted: "Our understanding reaches only so far as our anthropomorphism."

In an even more searching reprise of the psychologic parameters of physical thought, the mathematical physicist Barnett wrote:

> It is meaningless to ask [what] is "really true" . . . in the abstract lexicon of quantum physics there is no such word as "really." . . . It is futile, moreover, to hope that the invention of more delicate tools may enable man to penetrate much farther. There is an indeterminacy about all events of the atomic universe which refinements of measure and observation can never dispel. . . . [But] if physical events are indeterminate and the future is unpredictable, then perhaps the unknown quantity called "mind" may yet guide man's destiny among the infinite uncertainties of a capricious universe.

Utilizing such mentalistic dicta to justify his interest in parapsychology and the mystique of what he termed "confluentiality," Arthur Koestler commented: "The unthinkable phenomena of ESP appear somewhat less preposterous in the light of the unthinkable proposition(s) of physics."

Thus vanishes external reality and a world in which objectivity and certainty were at worst nebulous and at best asymptotic. What recourse then in psychiatry, as well as in mathematics and physics, other than the creation of essential myths to serve man's ultimate (Ur) needs?

Partially on this heuristic basis, in a presidential address to the Illinois Psychiatric Society as long ago as 1953, I formulated three of these essential and thereby universal assumptions or ultimate (Ur) fantasies, here briefly restated as follows:

> First, that man can indeed control the material universe with his sciences and technologies.
> Second, that he can achieve social Utopias of peace and brotherhood.
> And third, that his anthropomorphic philosophies and theologies really define and encompass the infinite.

How necessary these myths are is attested to by their persistence throughout the ages despite tragic evidence to the contrary. To wit: As to the first Ur-fantasy, consider man's delusions of technical mastery while he despoils his planet until his very existence is seriously threatened.

As to his cultural hypocrisy, observe the world in economic, racial and political turmoil.

And as to his metaphysical Ur-seekings, witness the proliferation of astrologers, oracles, faith-healers, gurus, and other seers and prophets in kaleidoscopic profusion—all proclaiming mutually exclusive and often militantly antiintellectual wisdoms. Ponder this comment by the president of the Sloan-Kettering Cancer Center:

> In [such a] climate, it is no wonder that general support for scientific research and training in the biomedical sciences has come upon hard times. There is an unmistakable loss of confidence in the value and effectiveness of science in general, not just medicine. Doubts have arisen about the capacity of science to solve our health problems, and there are new fears concerning the harmful effects of science in medicine. We are suspected of devising hideous new technologies to engineer ordinary, friendly, everyday man out of existence, [of having] special basement laboratories where we invent ways to control human behavior, transplant heads, raise identical parthenogenetic babies in plastic test tubes, clone prominent political figures and teach computers to think rings around the rest of us. [Instead] all of the major ills are being coped with by acupuncture, apricot pits, or astrology, or transcendental meditation. [to which I would add: transcendental medication.]

Regrettably, psychiatry and psychoanalysis are not spared; some of us still relinquish our birthright to comprehensive and integrative conceptualizations of human conduct and its social vicissitudes in favor of Id-Ego-Superego simplicisms reminiscent of the Loki-Thor-Wotan, Seth-Osiris-Ra, Ahriman-Zoroaster-Ahura Mazda, and other quasi-theologic trinities of counterposed intracerebral *irrational evil vs. practical reality vs. august imperatives.* Alternatively, we opt at one extreme in viewing man as a programmed Skinnerian automaton and at the other as an existentialistic, evanescent, quasi-Platonic abstraction whose principle Sartrean virtue is to deny death. Or, with chimeric wishfulness, some of us join the Christian Scientists and Tom Szasz in regarding disease as merely error, thus permitting us to heal individual and social ills through doctrinal distance or a thaumaturgic form of ESP. And as more of man's sciences and social systems fail and his hopes for mystic succor become more pressing, the whimsical plea of an erudite ministerial friend becomes increasingly urgent:

> For twenty years I built a magnificent church in this university community by presenting God as the Prime Mover and Transcendent Mathematician; but for the past five years, university community or not, I have had to support His church by putting a beard back on the face of the Lord, getting Him interested again in falling sparrows and playing up His compassion for all sinners—except variably, Catholics, Communists—and occasionally, some Republicans.

In summary, then, we have no more scientific evidence for the reality of Thanatos, orgone energy, UFO sightings, extrasensory perception, umbilical enlightenment, or other such phantasms than we have for the existence of devils, souls or angels; however, we have incontrovertible data that such beliefs have ever greatly influenced human behavior. And myths will continue to do so, since man seeks fulfillment of his yearnings for security (and with covert insistence, immortality) not only through his solipsistic sciences and social compacts, but through an eternal recourse to wishful mysticisms that to him represent the ultimate realities.

I myself, therefore, make no claim to be immune to the need for the same quietly desperate yearnings with regard to the triune Ur-anxieties we all share. Accordingly, I concluded my presidential address to the Fourth Congress of the International Association for Social Psychiatry in 1972 with my own trinity of compensatory Ur-faiths:

> *Technical:* Despite the advanced despoiling of our planet and the fact that we have at hand, with no known defenses against them, enough nuclear devices to kill everyone on earth thirty times over, I believe—I must believe—that with spreading indignation and concerted effective action, we shall rein in our Frankensteinian technology in time to save our species and, hopefully, others also.
>
> *Social:* As to our current racist turmoil, since *homo habilis* is a single, universally fecund species, differences of race or color will eventually become about as distinguishable as Lombard, Hittite, or Etruscan strains are in us, their Mediterranean descendants. Foreswearing the insanity of wars, man will become progressively more cognizant of the necessities of mutual respect, concord, and cooperation—and thereby move closer to a world community.
>
> *Philosophic-theologic:* Finally, when we develop a deeper sense of cosmic identity that will transcend our current ideologic

parochialisms and the animistic myths and rituals of our primitive religions, we shall become humbler, kinder, wiser—and perhaps more deserving of a happier future.

It was at this point in my writing, as the rays from a setting sun glowed through a shade in my library on books ranging from Charles Darwin's *Origins of Species* and George Sarton's *History of Science* through Sigmund Freud's *Collected Works*—not failing *en passant* to illuminate James Frazier's *Golden Bough,* Lewis Carroll's *Alice in Wonderland,* and E. K. Thompson's *Great Religions*—further prose seemed no longer sufficiently expressive, and gave place to a monody accompanied by a haunting refrain of yearning and mystic hope, with cadences peculiarly different from all else I had ever composed. May I end this opus with this coda?

References

Barnett, L. *The universe and Dr. Einstein.* New York: Mentor, 1956.

Douglas, A. V., & Eddington, A. E. *A biography.* London: International University Press, 1957.

Glass, B. The ethical basis of science. *Science,* 1965, 150, 1254–1267.

Masserman, J. H. *Practice of dynamic psychiatry.* Philadelphia: W. B. Saunders, 1955.

―――. Or shall we all commit suicide? *Current Psychiatric Therapies,* 1962, 2, 273.

―――. Man's eternal anxieties. *Illinois Medical Journal,* 1966, 127, 375–561.

―――. *Modern therapy of personality disorders.* Dubuque, Iowa: W. C. Brown, 1966.

―――. *Biodynamic roots of human behavior.* Springfield, Ill.: C. C. Thomas, 1968.

―――. *A psychiatric odyssey.* New York: Science House, 1971.

―――, & Schwab, J. (Eds.). *Man for humanity.* Springfield, Ill.: C. C. Thomas, 1972.

Nunberg, H., & Federn, E. *Minutes of the Vienna Psychoanalytic Society.* New York: International University Press, 1960.

Schilt, P. A. *Albert Einstein, philosopher, scientist.* Evanston, Ill.: Library of Living Philosophers, 1949.

Whitehead, A. N. *Science and the modern world.* New York: Mentor, 1925.

LIFE IS STRANGE
(For and by Jules Masserman)

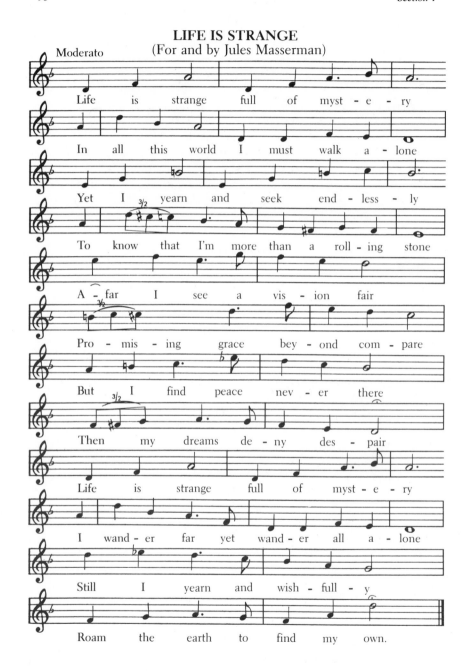

Moderato

Life   is   strange   full   of   myst - e - ry

In   all   this   world   I   must   walk   a - lone

Yet   I   yearn   and   seek   end - less - ly

To   know   that   I'm   more   than   a   roll - ing   stone

A - far   I   see   a   vis - ion   fair

Pro - mis - ing   grace   bey - ond   com - pare

But   I   find   peace   nev - er   there

Then   my   dreams   de - ny   des - pair

Life   is   strange   full   of   myst - e - ry

I   wand - er   far   yet   wand - er   all   a - lone

Still   I   yearn   and   wish - full - y

Roam   the   earth   to   find   my   own.

Edgar D. Mitchell

Awareness and Science

In THE EXCELLENT work of Shklovskii and Sagan (1966), a long-standing expectation of the scientific community is cogently enunciated, that all of nature's functioning can eventually be explained with the complex properties of atomic and subatomic particles. Even before Niels Bohr successfully developed an elementary model for atomic structure in 1913, the atomic character of matter had been predicted as the basis for all natural phenomena. The characteristics of energy and matter, as explained by quantum mechanics, wave mechanics, relativisitic mechanics, and the uncertainty principle, lend credence to this expectation, even though there are dualities and philosophic inconsistencies apparent in current models of energy/matter transformation (Reiser, 1966) when applied on a cosmic scale.

In spite of the philosophical problems, contemporary thinking based on these concepts has provided important pragmatic results which have found their way into every branch of engineering, science, even philosophy itself. The biological and behavioral sciences, as well as the art and science of medicine, base their model for life processes firmly on physical theories surrounding molecular structure and the electromagnetic nature of molecular fields. It is not, therefore, the purpose of this paper to find fault with those tools of science, or the applications that provide a basis for the most spectacular growth of knowledge in recorded history. For without that knowledge there would be no opportunity to explore beyond it. However, for many reasons, only one of which is the success of atomic theory, many aspects of nature which do not fit comfortably into classical concepts of physical science have been discounted or, at best, have been temporarily set aside pending better data. It is to some of these aspects of nature that this paper is addressed.

37

To gain insight into the historical course of scientific inquiry, one should recall that less than four centuries ago, scholars were divided on the cosmological issue of heliocentric versus geocentric theory of planetary motion, a debate temporarily won by the Inquisition when Giordano Bruno was burned at the stake in 1600. Certainly Bruno and the Copernican theory were subsequently vindicated, but continued opposition of theological scholars to concepts that challenged religious dogma has been an important force in shaping the path of scientific history. To a large extent, objective inquiry into the higher order functioning of man and into metaphysical topics has been sufficiently hindered by clerical opposition, by the difficulty of the problem, and by the inadequate experimental tools of earlier days. Many scientists have rejected such inquiries as being unproductive and unworthy of continued interest. In fact, the lack of interest has solidified into a dogma that is almost as dangerous as the religious view it opposes. This unwritten but often enunciated view is that all basic physical laws have been discovered, and we only need apply them correctly to understand all of nature. The unfortunate result is that science speaks only of the physical nature of man, while philosophy and theology address the intrinsic man, producing a duality of concept that has yet to be bridged.

However, in contemporary thought, we are increasingly directing scientific effort and resources toward the understanding of life processes and, beyond that, to the understanding of behavior and then consciousness. In this we find that the genesis model of nature that serves well to explain the structure and functions of inanimate matter and low order life processes becomes less and less satisfactory. The intelligent being should not be too surprised at this turn of events. If the inanimate aspects of the universe could be represented as a tenfold multivariant problem, then it is necessary to deal with at least an order of magnitude of greater complexity when considering the physiology of living systems, and an order of magnitude greater yet when confronted with the behavioral aspects.

Recently, it has been shown that the elements carbon, nitrogen, oxygen, and hydrogen can be synthesized under the proper flux of solar energy to form spontaneously amino acid molecules, a class of primordial materials necessary for the evolution of living matter. However, amino acids do not possess life. They behave strictly in accordance with known laws of organic molecular behavior. The most elemental forms said to live, that is, to reproduce and to mutate, are the DNA and RNA matrices. Even these life forms seem amenable to molecular synthesis, but have not as yet been satisfactorily synthesized solely from primitive materials, although it appears reasonable that they can be. Thus, it is plausible that elementary forms basic to all known terrestial life can form spontaneously from elementary atomic particles, given the proper environment. But let us turn attention now to the macroscopic scale, to the highest form we know—homo sapiens. Is it possible, as contemporary science suggests, that man is only a complex compilation of organic molecules synthesized from elemental compounds, or as has been postulated during less sophisticated times, is there more to it than that? Surely there are few men who, if they do not have a conviction, at least harbor a subconscious hope that in an ordered, evolving universe, man is more than simply a chance synthesis of matter. The subjective awareness of man almost demands it, in spite of scientific skepticism. We should remember, however, that conjecture does not change the reality, and neither point of view has been proven convincingly with empirical techniques. We can agree though that somewhere along the complex evolutionary chain of molecular compounding, culminating in homo sapiens, consciousness took place. It is precisely the acquisition of consciousness (in the sense of self-awareness) by the living organism that becomes a pivotal issue of scientific versus theological dogma.

Consciousness, awareness, reason—attributes long considered solely the characteristics of man, seem particularly unyielding to analysis with the tools of physical theory. One must concede that the complex properties of molecular electromagnetic fields may possibly account for these characteristics and that a physical model to explain them lies only beyond the horizon of current analytical techniques. As will be discussed in subsequent pages, however, there is reason to doubt this supposition. Furthermore, recent research with animals and plants (Braud, unpublished) causes one to consider whether subjective attributes are even uniquely the property of mankind in the manner we have presumed. The Backster results (1968) offer exciting implications in this area.

This line of thought, strengthened by the results of parapsychological (psi) research, leads one to the conclusion that perhaps all life *cannot* be explained by extending current molecular–electromagnetic models. If such is the case, where do we begin the search for a concept that will augment and improve understanding of the life process? In this investigator's opinion, we should start to look at living organisms and the phenomena they produce, beyond the physical laws as now understood. Some of the phenomena that have been discounted or set aside for later examination should be reexamined. There is now sufficient evidence to warrant this reexploration, and scientists, however skeptical, have the obligation to examine the evidence.

Studies of normally functioning individuals (Braud, unpublished), individuals subjected to altered states of consciousness, and the "gifted" persons we call "psychics" suggest that certain conditions of awareness permit the production of phenomena that are unpredicted and unexplained by physical theory.

The evidence is still only suggestive with respect to some of these occurrences, because they fall short of the demands for empirical proof. However, in other areas proof has been offered for the existence of these phenomena, even though there are those who still do not accept it as such. Somehow these occurrences must be explained by formulating a predictive construct of the life mechanism.

What phenomena must be considered in this instance? For years many investigators (Rhine, Pratt, Smith, et al., 1966) have sought to compile sufficient statistical evidence that General-Extra-Sensory-Perception (GESP) faculties exist. There should be no doubt to the informed observer that the case has been convincingly stated, using standards far more severe than demanded for most scientific research.

In the literature, in this author's opinion, the case for telepathy (Rhine et al., 1966) is unassailable; the case for contemporaneous clairvoyance (McMahan, unpublished) is almost as well documented. The cases for psychokinesis and precognition are strong, but present special problems of proof that have not been totally resolved. (Domert, unpublished) The cases for healing and psychic surgery are suggestive, but have not as yet been adequately dealt with in the scientific literature, although certain unpublished works and anecdotal material from impeccable sources are under study.

Although these phenomena do not, by any means, exhaust the list of provocative occurrences, they are sufficient for the purpose of illustrating the problem science encounters in explaining life.

Let us examine for a moment some of the problems posed by psi evidence. In the case of telepathy, the problem is one of information transfer over distances and under conditions difficult to understand by acoustical or electromagnetic means. Osis and Turner (1968) have performed experiments suggesting that telepathic signals do not propagate inversely proportional to the square of distance as would be the case for electromagnetic events. This investigator's work (Mitchell, 1971), if considered a telepathic event, casts doubt on an electromagnetic hypothesis by virtue of the power required of the brain for transmission over Earth-lunar distances (Adamenko, personal correspondence). Various experiments not yet published in scientific literature suggest that materials capable of attenuating or shielding em radiation do not affect telepathy. These are curious results, but the problem becomes even more perplexing when precognition is considered, since time becomes a parameter in addition to distance. For the present, let us accept that telepathy/distance relationships may be indeterminate if results can be foretold. For example, my experiment could be considered precognition at Earth distances rather than telepathy at lunar distances.

Contemporaneous clairvoyance does not pose problems significantly more difficult than telepathy and, certainly, they are less difficult than precognition; therefore, let us move on to discuss precognition.

Precognition is defined as the knowing of an event prior to its occurrence and by a mechanism which precludes the knowledge being obtained by a process of reason. One implication is that information is transmittable at speeds faster than the speed of light. Another is that the nature of time may be entirely different than we perceive it. Both of these possibilities are very disturbing in terms of physical theory. The philosophic implications are equally upsetting. If the future is knowable, is it predetermined and unchangeable? What happens in this case to the free will of man?

These are difficult and disturbing questions that will not vanish simply by ignoring the evidence for precognitive functioning. And that evidence is surprisingly strong.

Psychokinesis is an equally puzzling phenomenon, that is, the ability of mind to influence matter remotely. In particular, the work of Schmidt (1970) is fascinating and well-documented, suggesting that even lower forms of life are capable of producing psychokinetic events.

Physical theory includes no mechanism that would permit such occurrences; moreover, the existence of psychokinesis casts doubt on our ability to design any experiment, the result of which is not subject in some measure to the preconceptions of the experimenter. This is a profound and perplexing idea.

In the medical sciences, cases of inexplicable healing have been known for years and usually discounted. However, recent films and accounts presented by qualified physicians of healing and even surgery under bizarre conditions, cast doubt on the completeness of our medical knowledge. It is my hope that some of this evidence will be presented in the near future to appropriate medical authorities.

The range of phenomena mentioned here seems to be closely related, if not indeed the functioning of a unitary process. They are causing repercussions in nearly every branch of modern science. It appears that if the various manifestations of psi activity are to be explained, our model of living organisms based solely on pyramiding of active and interacting atomic particles and their associated electromagnetic fields, must be modified to a large degree. It is the opinion of this investigator that current models cannot be extended to encompass these proven phenomena.

To the theoretician, the implications of psi verification are manifestly clear, but what is the potential effect in the day-to-day functioning of individuals in society? Certainly a major benefit is the assurance to thousands who are troubled by psi occurrences that they are not simply suffering from an aberration of mental processes. In a social structure where the existence of psi has been denied by material science, and acknowledged but denounced by religious teachings, it should not be surprising that individuals who experience such events are confused and disturbed. An informal sampling of published results would lead one to believe that those who experience psi are a large portion of the population. How many individuals, one wonders, have been suspected of aberrant mental functioning because of an encounter with one of the psi manifestations? We must also ask whether or not those encounters are normal experiences of the human organism. This question cannot be answered until these phenomena are studied on a larger scale than at present. However, this experimenter's bias is that a natural explanation, probably involving an unknown mechanism, is available and that possibly all living creatures, certainly those of a higher order, utilize these same processes.

But what are the applications to our mode of living? The answer must be considered carefully, since it is obvious that we are not just dealing with another sensory mechanism such as the tactile or visual senses. The implications of being able to perceive another's thoughts or to control another mind with thought are certainly infinitely more profound than touching or seeing another person's physical being. For this reason, we must project the future utilization of psi cautiously, with due regard for our current lack of knowledge and for the philosophical ramifications.

It is possible that psi events are not amenable to consistent control, that is, they are not completely replicable. In such a case, a future of applied psi does not exist, and we will continue to deal with spontaneous, sporadic events. It is also possible that psi is another sensory mechanism being spawned by natural evolutionary processes, which can be trained and applied to communication, mind control, control over matter, etc., in ways similar to the application of our five other senses. Such an eventuality would fit comfortably into a cybernetics approach to life functioning, since it is a mechanistic approach. In this case, there are potential applications which can prove immensely beneficial to mankind. There are also other applications which one would prefer not to see developed, but they will be, nevertheless.

It is entirely possible, however, that psi occurrences represent a step in the evolutionary process of life forms toward an ultimate predestined goal—a distinctly different view from that of a chance origin and evolution of life. In this case, the moral, ethical, and theological ramifications of psi development are too numerous to be dealt with here.

Whatever the answer, we cannot delay the search any longer. As a start in understanding the higher order functioning of life processes, it seems imperative that all branches of science must first objectively examine the puzzling and illusive psi phenomena in order that the apparent contradictions and seeming violations of physical law be understood. In addition, this investigator contends that the subjective examination of the consciousness of living beings is likely to provide important clues. It is impossible to deny that individuals in altered states of consciousness produce both physiological (Wallace, Benson & Wilson, 1971) and psychological behavior that is extraordinary in terms of current knowledge. Objective empiricism has always been the strength of science; in fact, some will say it is tantamount to a definition of science. However, homo sapiens, at least, is subjective. To each man, reality is as *he* perceives it, even the scientist. One only need look at various interpretations of the same objective data to recognize that all of us are primarily subjective creatures. Experimentation may be objective, experimenters are not. Sensing, whether it be tactile, visual, or ESP, is a subjective experience.

Consider, for example, a social order such as ours where the sense of touch was just evolving in a few individuals of the species, the remainder having only the four other senses, or at best, a fleeting sensation upon physical contact with an object. The individuals so blessed (or cursed) by nature would have a difficult time convincing the rest that something different was happening to them. They would undoubtedly be castigated for their peculiarities. By blind-folding the "sensitives," science could objectively discover that the phenomenon existed by noting the subjects' response to tactile stimulation—providing the subject had a reliable tactile sense. (Whereupon all who had even the slightest feeling would come forth and admit that they had perceived such sensations for years.) But, none of the objective tests would be possible without the subjective awareness of the "sensitive", and certainly the "sensitive's" impressions would be necessary to establish the concepts of warm, soft, hard, rough, smooth, etc. The point is that subjective empiricism is as important to science as objective empiricism if we are to understand life. With all its seemingly aberrant behavior, the mind is the most remarkable sensor and most complex computer available. It is the only instrument capable of understanding itself. The search for understanding of consciousness should give credence, therefore, to the overwhelming subjective opinion "I am"—"I am aware of the realities of my existence."

Theologians and philosophers have examined these ideas for eons, but the pragmatic theoretician, desiring to perceive the physical world objectively, does not incorporate such concepts into his constructs of the universe. Perhaps, however, it is time to do so. Perhaps the current models of matter cannot be extended to explain the higher order functions of life any better than Newtonian physics could be extended to relativity—the former being a subset of the latter.

The "I am," the being, the personality, life itself, may indeed be distinct from the physical organism it controls. If this is so, no amount of reworking current atomic and electromagnetic theories without a new postulate will produce an acceptable understanding of nature.

Let us therefore take a large step and propose models for living creatures that incorporate a distinct, energetic mechanism that interacts with matter to produce that higher order functioning of life—consciousness. Let us deduce from these models the types of experimental evidence needed to verify or deny the hypothesis. Then let us set out to obtain that evidence using the best objective and subjective techniques modern thought can provide. Such a construct must allow for the currently verifiable psi functioning, as well as those for which evidence is less strong, if the construct is to be viable and of any lasting utility.

The world's intellectual resources, whether from the objective disciplines of the physical, biological, and behavioral sciences, or from the subjective endeavors of a searching consciousness, must find common ground if the riddles of universal existence are ever to be explained.

References

Adamenko, V., Soviet physicist, personal correspondence.

Backster, C. Evidence of a primary perception in plant life. *International Journal of Parapsychology,* 1968, 10.

Braud, L. Psychological correlates of psi. Mind Science Foundation (unpublished research report).

Braud, W. G. Physiological interactions and infrahuman research. Mind Science Foundation (unpublished research report).

Domert, W. Precognition, prophesy, and retrocognition. Mind Science Foundation (unpublished research report).

McMahan, J. B. Clairvoyance—a review of the literature. Mind Science Foundation (unpublished research report).

Mitchell, E. An ESP test from Apollo XIV. *Journal of Parapsychology,* 1971, **35** (2).

Osis, K. & Turner, Jr., M. E. Distance and ESP; a transcontinental experiment. *Proceedings ASPR,* 1968, 27 (9).

Reiser, O. L. *Cosmic humanism.* Cambridge, Mass.: Schenkman, 1966.

Rhine, J. B., Pratt, J. G., Smith, B. M., Stuart, C. E., & Greenwood, J. A. *Extra-sensory perception after 60 years.* Boston: Humphries, Brandon Press, 1966.

Schmidt, H. PK experiments with animals as subjects. *Journal of Parapsychology,* 1970, **34.**

Shklovskii, I. S. & Sagen, C. *Intelligent life in the universe.* San Francisco: Holden-Day, 1966.

Wallace, R. K., Benson, H., & Wilson, A. F. A wakeful hypometabolic physiologic state. *American Journal of Physiology,* 1971, **221** (3).

W. G. Roll

ESP and America's Occult Upsurge

In 1967 the Ouija board surpassed Monopoly as America's favorite board game. This event in the games industry reflected a wider conflict that is continuing to fragment our society. On the one side we have the "Counter Culture" (Roszak, 1969), "Consciousness III" (Reich, 1970), and "a new wave of American mysticism" (Godwin, 1972); on the other side we have the mechanistic approach to man of industrialized Western society.

The conflict can be traced back to the "two cultures" division seen by C. P. Snow in 1963 between science and the humanities. The confrontation discussed here, however, is more an outgrowth of the two cultures' dispute than it is synonymous with it. To some extent the present division cuts across Snow's because some scientists have joined the counter culture, and certain writers and artists are vehemently opposed to it.

A central issue is the nature of man. Many followers of the counter culture are believers in the occult; that is, they believe, without the benefit of scientific evidence, that there are imperceptible forces or relationships in the world which connect man to his environment (occult comes from a Latin word meaning to cover up or to hide). They think that man can control these forces and thereby cause changes in his environment without direct physical contact or instruments. In contrast, the biological and behavioral sciences restrict the human entity to whatever goes on within the skin. When man observes things in his environment or interacts with it, he does so by means of his organism or the tools he has built to extend its range.

Parapsychology has been straddling the fence between the two camps: its subject matter is imperceptible forces and relationships, but it explores these by means of established scientific methods. It therefore has something in common with both sides, and could help to create a working relationship between them.

The Occult and the Establishment

One thing all agree on. There has been a striking upsurge of interest in the occult. John Godwin, a journalist and author (1972), sees a wave of mysticism "rolling over the entire American horizon."

Samuel McCracken (1971), an editor of *Change* and an assistant professor of literature and humanities at Reed College, says, "Something has been happening to the youthful intellect. . . . The symptoms are familiar enough: the growing and uncritical admiration for and acceptance of the esoteric and the occult, indications of breakdown in critical abilities, explicit rejections of rationality in politics. The *I-Ching* becomes a best-seller; colleges admit witchcraft and astrology to the paracurriculum . . . if interest in Zen wanes, there is the rise of Transcendental Meditation and the lunacies of the Hare Krishna cult" (p. 81).

Harvey Brooks (1971), dean of the engineering and applied physics division of Harvard, says there is "a flight toward antirational cults. . . . Astrology, once the refuge of the ignorant and the illiterate, is now gaining favor among many intellectuals, even young scientists. . . . The national investment in astrology is between ten and twenty times that in astronomy" (p. 24). Brooks fears that the current "antiscientific and antirational ideology" may contribute to the disintegration of science and technology and thereby to the disappearance of part of the world's population with a decline in the material conditions of the rest.

Alvin Toffler (1970), writer and visiting scholar at the Russell Sage Foundation, speaks of a "garish revival of mysticism. Suddenly astrology is the rage. Zen, yoga, seances, and witchcraft become popular pastimes. Cults form around the search for Dionysian experience, for non-verbal and supposedly non-linear communication. We are told it is more important to 'feel' than to 'think,' as though there were a contradiction between the two. Existentialist oracles join Catholic mystics, Jungian psychoanalysts, and Hindu gurus in exalting the mystical and emotional against the scientific and rational" (p. 450).

Others claim that far from a breakdown of culture and society, we are seeing the birth of a safer and saner world. Charles Reich (1970), the Consciousness III advocate, encourages nonrational thought—drug-thought, mysticism, impulses. But he believes these are not really nonrational at all; they merely introduce new elements into the sterile, rigid, outworn rationality that prevails today" (p. 315).

John Godwin (1972) finds a factual claim here and there among the superstitions and promotional efforts which mainly constitute "America's occult upsurge." He also sees a revival of an old American dream: "the idea that somewhere on earth there is room for the kingdom of Heaven. . . . When the land became filled from east to west and lay locked in the armor of its technology, the dream turned inward and became mysticism. But the basic theme is unchanged and unshaken: belief in the perfectibility of the human condition" (p. xvif).

Theodore Roszak (1969) says that Oriental religions, Dadaism and American Indian folklore, romantic *Weltschmerz,* and so forth may be a "garish motley" but are "all we have to hold against the final consolidation of a technocratic totalitarianism in which we shall find ourselves ingeniously adapted to an existence wholly estranged from everything that has ever made the life of man an interesting adventure" (p. xiii).

In this controversy between accustomed Western ways of looking at things and the ways of Consciousness III and the Counter Culture, little is said about the nature of man and his world. Before we can determine what is a rational way of looking at things, we must have some idea of what the real world is like.

Parapsychology has something to say which may be relevant to this issue. First a few general remarks about this field.

Parapsychology in USA and USSR

Parapsychological or psi phenomena fall into two main types: extrasensory perception (ESP) and psychokinesis (PK). We talk about ESP when people obtain information about their social or physical environment without using the known senses or rational inference. PK refers to cases where people seem able to produce physical changes, again without known means. One of the most gifted ESP subjects studied by us is Lalsingh Harribance, a citizen of Trinidad, British West Indies. In one experiment (Roll & Klein, 1972), he made 1000 attempts at identifying cards located in an adjoining room. Half the cards had pictures of men and the other half, women. The chance score was therefore about 500 correct guesses. Instead he got a score of 622, a figure with odds of about ten billion to one against chance. In this experiment, somebody was looking at the cards at the same time Harribance was guessing, so he was possibly using telepathy. To see if Harribance could succeed under clairvoyant conditions, that is, if there was no one looking at the cards, the test was repeated with the cards turned upside down. This time he did even better with a score of 677.

In testing for PK, the most prominent subject today is perhaps Nina Kulagina of Leningrad. In the presence of both Russian (Rejdak, 1971) and American (Ullman, 1971) parapsychologists, she has been able to move small objects such as matchboxes and cigar containers across a table, supposedly by PK. It should be added, however, that there are no detailed reports of Russian PK experiments conducted under fully controlled conditions.

The positive attitude toward parapsychology in Russia is a recent development (Krippner & Davidson, 1972). The 1955 edition of the *Soviet Encyclopedia,* which gives the official viewpoint on science, defines parapsychology as "the non-scientific idealistic consideration of supernatural abilities of perceptual phenomena." In the 1970 edition, however, parapsychology has become "the area of psychical and biophysical research dealing with the informational and energetic possibilities of living organisms. Parapsychology considers the newest forms of sensitivity, the results of those sensitivities, and the possibilities of the human organism."

The current ESP and PK work in Russia and America are only recent examples of a stream of research which in Russia goes back to the ESP experiments conducted with dogs in the 1920s by W. Bechterev (1949) and the ESP tests in the 1930s and 1940s by L. L. Vasiliev (1963), Bechterev's pupil and a professor of physiology at Leningrad University. In America and nations of Western Europe, the beginning of serious work in parapsychology is usually traced to the founding of the Society for Psychical Research in London in 1882.

Another important year was 1927, when J. B. Rhine (1954) began his ESP tests at Duke University under William McDougall, the first chairman of the psychology department. One of the most striking early card-guessing series was conducted by J. G. Pratt with Hubert Pearce, a divinity student, as the subject. While in a building one hundred yards from the one where Pratt handled the cards, Pearce guessed seventy-four packs of ESP cards. This was a clairvoyance test since Pratt kept the cards face down. The total score gave odds of more than a sextillion to one against chance. Pratt has remained active in the field; he is now at the division of parapsychology of the University of Virginia. In England, a lecturer of mathematics at London University, S. G. Soal (1954), heard about the Duke University work and tried unsuccessfully to repeat it—until he came across two subjects whose performance gave odds of billions to one against chance in telepathy tests. The precautions that were taken against sensory cues, cheating, faulty statistics, recording errors, and other ordinary explanations seem to leave no other explanation than ESP in the results of these tests by Pratt and Soal. And there are many more such experiments reported (Pratt, 1969; Rhine & Brier, 1968; Rhine & Pratt, 1962).

Even more convincing than the purely statistical argument of astronomical odds are the many indications that ESP is closely integrated with the rest of human personality. As is true for the familiar sensory processes, ESP is not something odd and discontinuous but operates as part of the total organism. This has been evidenced in many ways. As psychologists are well aware, a person may not "see" or remember a disliked event; similarly in ESP tests, it has been shown that a skeptic about ESP is likely to score negatively, that is, he will tend to avoid the ESP targets, while a believer will tend to score positively. This discovery was first made by Gertrude Schmeidler (1958) in her sheep-goat tests with students at the City College of New York—the sheep were believers in ESP, goats disbelievers. Similarly, M. L. Anderson and Rhea White (1958) found that children tested for ESP in the classroom tended to score negatively when teachers they disliked conducted the tests, while popular teachers elicited positive results. And ESP scores may also be a measure of the success of psychotherapy (Hudesman & Schmeidler, 1971).

ESP responses are influenced by memory functions (Roll, 1966) as are familiar perceptual processes. And ESP has been found to be related to several personality traits (Johnson & Kanthamani, 1967; Kanthamani & Rao, 1972; Mangan, 1958; Schmeidler & McConnell, 1958). Dreams that allow other unconscious material to come to the surface also appear favorable to ESP (Ullman, Krippner & Feldstein, 1966). In addition to man, other species, including cats (Osis, 1952) and mice (Schouten, 1972) have shown evidence of ESP. And some subjects seem able to revive anesthetized mice by PK (Watkins & Watkins, 1971) or to heal their wounds (Grad, 1965). Physical instruments are no barrier to psi and wide use is made of automated equipment for testing ESP (Schmidt, 1969a, 1969b) as well as PK (Cox, Feather & Carpenter, 1966; McConnell, Snowdon & Powell, 1955; Schmidt, 1970).

Nevertheless, parapsychology is a modest enterprise. It often comes as a surprise that all the universities and research institutes around the world can only muster about thirty full-time parapsychologists with perhaps twice that number of unpaid volunteers. The psychic tide sweeping the country can hardly be construed as the outcome of the work of this small group. Indeed, parapsychologists themselves are sometimes alarmed about the popular interest. It seems to them that their hard-earned results are drowning among announcements by present-day prophets, the dramatized ESP on TV, and the promoters of psychic development courses. Parapsychologists seem more comfortable with their critics, whose language, after all, they speak, than with the supersheep of the aquarian age. Nevertheless, parapsychologists and others who use the scientific method may yet have something to learn from the practitioners of the occult.

Occult Technology

It is true that the practitioner of the occult is generally not interested in evaluating his procedures scientifically. In part this can be attributed to a disillusionment with Western science, which sometimes has led away from significant human goals rather than towards them. But this does not mean that the occult is beyond scientific inquiry. If such energies exist, they may turn out to be hidden only in the way that most electromagnetic waves are hidden from sense perception. From the point of view of orthodox physics, perhaps the main distinguishing mark of the occult is that these hypothetical forces are psychological, at least to a degree, and directly controlled by an individual without the use of intermediary physical instruments, such as radio transmitters. Instead of physical mechanisms, the psychic practitioner relies on himself as the principal instrument. He believes that certain psychological and physiological procedures will increase his potency as a transmitter or receiver of these forces. His procedures may include esoteric rituals, consciousness-altering drugs, dancing, chanting, and so on.

The Counter Culture has spawned a counter-technology, the purpose of which is to establish man's relationship with the forces in the universe that Western technology has ignored. Most of the occult practices of today are not new. We can detect elements from the magical practices of tribal societies, medieval Europe, spiritualist seances, and religious rituals.

Whatever the origins of occult techniques may be, scientific observation and experimentation are not among them. This by itself does not make them anti-scientific. The emergence of a technology without the support of a basic science is not new in the history of man. Inventions as basic to modern life as the compass, the smelting of metals, and irrigation systems were made well before the scientific age. In fact this nonscientific technology did the spadework for science. It was the alchemists, during their hit or miss attempts to produce gold and the elixir of life, who discovered many of the important facts about metals and chemical compounds and thereby laid the foundation of chemistry and physics. In a similar way, we may come to look on the occult techniques of today as prescientific rather than antiscientific.

There is an important difference between occult techniques and mechanistic technology. This difference has to do with purpose, rather than with scientific method. In general, Western technology and science are directed toward securing the survival and well-being of man as a physical organism. Occult practices appear to be directed toward another purpose, to secure the survival and well-being of man as a psychical organism.

In much the same way that our mechanistic technology often does not serve our physical well-being and even directly threatens it, there are also dangers in the occult. It is no less important to identify superstitious and pathological elements in psychic beliefs than it is to verify valid ones. False beliefs are not for that reason impotent. History has enough examples, from witchcraft trials to gas ovens, of sacrifices on the altar of the occult.

Testing the Occult

One of the most recent developments in occult technology is mind control methods for developing psychic powers. Sometimes biofeedback equipment is used or other psychophysiological devices. Promoters of these methods claim that striking ESP powers result and that there are all kinds of beneficial effects, including success in business ventures. There is insufficient scientific evidence to support the claims, but multitudes enroll in the courses. Metapsychiatry could serve an important function by testing such claims.

Though the field of parapsychology may utilize some of its skills for extracting such facts as there may be in occult claims, it is not equipped to track down the fictitious aspects. The task is not only to identify the superstitious and pathological elements but to find the psychological, social, or other conditions that fostered these elements and then to redirect them into positive channels. This is one of many areas where metapsychiatry, an interdisciplinary effort between psychologists, anthropologists, and parapsychologists, is needed.

In their approach to the occult, parapsychologists are best equipped to deal with practices that are believed to involve ESP and PK because they have developed procedures to investigate such phenomena scientifically. Sometimes a single practice entails several beliefs which have to be treated separately. For example, people who use the Ouija board may believe that spirits of the dead move the pointer across the alphabet board, thereby spelling out messages, but it can easily be shown that the entities who move the pointer are the living people whose fingers are on it. It can also be fairly easily determined whether or not the information produced by the operators of Ouija boards goes beyond their ordinary knowledge, in other words, whether or not the spellings contain evidence of ESP. However, parapsychologists have not so far been able to design experiments—with or without Ouija boards—to determine whether or not such ESP information sometimes originates from deceased but surviving personalities. But many of the simpler claims made by the practitioners of the occult could easily be tested and, in fact, occasionally have been tested. Exploratory studies have been made where the Ouija board (Gauld, 1971) and the *I-Ching* (Rubin & Honorton, 1971) were used to elicit ESP responses. A brief study has been made of the claim that a Yogi could enhance the ESP score of a group of students after instruction on meditation and breathing (Schmeidler, 1970). A "psychic healer" has been tested using plants and animals (Grad, 1965), and the claims of sensitives and mediums that they could "read" people—that is, make verifiable statements about them—without sensory contact have also been explored (Pratt, 1969; Roll, Morris, Damgaard, et al., 1972).

In their studies of the occult, parapsychologists may come across new ways of exploring and perhaps controlling ESP and PK. If such methods are found, this could obviously be of great scientific and practical importance. Such discoveries, however, may not make much difference to man and his view of himself in the world. New ways to improve ESP and PK may amount to little more than new ways in which man can manipulate the environment and other people. This would be an addition, not an alternative, to present-day technology and is not likely to ameliorate the conflict we are concerned with here. As Godwin (1972) says in his chapter on witchcraft, "in an age where everyone except computer cards gets duly stapled, folded and mutilated, one of the greatest attainable boons is the feeling of being a manipulator instead of the eternally manipulated" (p. 75).

ESP and Expansion of Consciousness

There is one aspect of occult practices that may be more relevant to the issue at hand than methods solely intended to enhance psychical powers. Occult practices, including witchcraft, operating the Ouija board, and the *I-Ching,* involve the belief that a person is not an encapsulated entity but extends into the social and physical and even cosmic environment.

In the course of his interviews Godwin (1972) was surprised at the lengthy and apparently pointless ceremonies and rituals used by cult organizations. He soon realized "that for many members these are the most important and satisfying aspects of the creed, that by performing them they achieve a sense of belonging, of worth, that no other function can fully replace" (p. xv).

It seems that the purpose of these practices is often not so much to obtain hidden information or affect distant events as it is to engender experiences of self-transcendence. This may be one reason why psychic practitioners tend to be uninterested in scientific tests of their procedures. If a Ouija board session or a witchcraft ceremony stimulates feelings of unity with the other participants, it may matter little whether or not it was also effective in achieving its ostensible goal. Sometimes an experience of unity seems to be the only purpose. This is true especially for meditation and other methods which are explicity directed towards the expansion of consciousness.

Persons who have such experiences often have a strong conviction of confronting something real and not simply their private dreams and illusions. If this is true, if there are procedures which can help a person to achieve more integrated and meaningful relations, the increasing acceptance of such procedures should have a positive influence on man's attitudes about his social and physical environment. The question for us is whether or not experiences of expanded consciousness can be studied scientifically. Parapsychology is interested in the aspects of the human self which extend beyond the visible organism, and may have the means to explore the problem.

Some parapsychologists look at ESP and PK as evidence of "psi fields" that surround and connect people and objects in ways similar to physical fields (some believe that psi fields will turn out to be physical fields). If we use this terminology, the question becomes whether or not a person's self-awareness or consciousness may include the psi field. The term "field consciousness" (FC) has been used to describe such a hypothetical extension of consciousness.

The issue is whether experiences of transcendence are illusory or whether there is a real sense in which consciousness can extend beyond the organism. If the experience is associated with ESP or PK, that is, if a person can actually apprehend or influence distant events at the time he has an experience of transcendence, this might suggest that these events in a sense are a part of the self. On the other hand, if the world experienced at such times is entirely subjective, such an experience would seem only to be a private dream.

We can explore the question in two ways. One way is to find out if meditators or others who seem to have FC experiences are also unusually good at ESP and PK. Another way is to study people who are particularly successful ESP and PK subjects to see if they report many FC experiences. Reports of

ESP incidents are more common than of PK, so ESP will be emphasized.

In taking the first approach, we need to keep in mind that it is usually not the purpose of persons who seek FC experiences to develop psychical abilities. If ESP experiences arise, they are generally treated as incidental by-products. This is not surprising since such experiences seem as likely to concern trivial events as weighty ones. If ESP incidents are treated seriously, it is usually because they are seen as objective indications that the meditator has attained or is in the process of attaining an FC state. A story (Yu, 1969) from the life of the late Chinese Zen *(Ch'an)* teacher, Hsu Yun, is a good illustration. After many years of meditation, "the master succeeded in realizing singleness of mind, and in his fifty-sixth year, one evening, in Kao Ming monastery at Yangchow, after a long meditation, he opened his eyes and saw everything inside and outside the monastery. Through the wall, he saw a monk urinating outside, a guest monk in the latrine, and far away, boats plying on the river and trees on both its banks" (p. 74).

An example closer to home is told by Richard Alpert, known as Baba Ram Dass (1971a) since his initiation by an Indian teacher of meditation. When he was at Esalen, Big Sur, "being a Holy Man," somebody asked him if he had any psychic powers. He said no and that he was glad he did not since he had a big ego and might misuse them. "Imagine," he said to a man who had just arrived, "if I could look at you, sir, and I could say, 'You were walking up the hill to get here and you looked down on the ground and you saw what you thought was a jewel and you picked it up and you threw it away.' Could you imagine if I could tell about things like that in your life?" The man replied that as he was walking up the hill, he did see something on the ground which looked like jade but "it turned out to be a piece of ginger ale bottle and I threw it away." (1971a, p. 66). Alpert has similar stories about his teacher (Baba Ram Dass, 1971b). They will be found in most other accounts of persons seeking the FC experience, whether these be Hasidic Jews (Buber, 1947), Sufi Muslims (Nicholson, 1966), or whatever their religious or cultural background may be.

In the same way that we find many ESP stories around persons who seek transcending experiences, there are also many accounts of transcending experiences from persons who seem to be endowed with unusual ESP abilities. W. H. C. Tenhaeff (1966), professor of parapsychology at the University of Utrecht, quotes from Alexis Didier, a famous French clairvoyant of the mid-1800s who used the ESP method known as object association (or psychometry): "With the help of a simple lock of hair or a letter, I come into contact with them [the owner of the hair or letter], irrespective of the distance separating us. . . . I see them, I hear them, they live their lives in me. I feel myself suffer their pains, having part in their joys. My soul . . . comes into touch with them and between them and me arises a community of consciousness" (p. 416).

In his own psychological studies of forty-seven Dutch psychics, Tenhaeff found a "great 'sensitivity' for everything coming from the outside world. . . . Also, they endeavor to identify with persons and objects near them. There is an attempt to attain what. . . . Lucien Levy-Bruhl has called 'participation mystique' " (p. 417).

As a result of accounts such as these, parapsychologists at the Psychical Research Foundation and elsewhere have begun to explore meditation as a means to enhance psi abilities. In an ESP experiment with a group of meditators at the American Society for Psychical Research, Karlis Osis and Edwin Bokert (1971) stated that the people who did best in ESP had a "feeling of merging with the others, and a feeling of oneness as if the boundaries between what is 'me' and what is not 'me' were dissolving" (p. 33). At the Foundation for Research on the Nature of Man, Francine Matas and Lee Pantas (1971) did exploratory PK tests and found that subjects who had practiced meditation or similar forms of self-development were more successful than the control group.

In exploring the relationship between meditation and psi abilities, it is interesting to note that persons who have such abilities to a marked degree often use procedures to activate them which are similar to the procedures advocated by many meditation systems. In most forms of meditation (Wallace & Benson, 1972), the meditator seeks a deep state of relaxation, yet remains fully awake. Usually, the mind is either kept blank or is engaged in some task, such as repeating a word mentally or visualizing an object, with the hope that this will reduce discursive thinking and allow the meditator to experience the unity between himself and the rest of the world. Sometimes rhythmic chanting or movements are used instead of silent meditation. ESP subjects may develop comparable procedures. One of Tenhaeff's (1966) psychics "often started tapping his feet more or less rhythmically. This apparently caused a state of relaxation, which facilitated the rising of telepathic impressions. . . . [He] also used to blindfold himself when the impression did not come easily to him. 'I have to shut myself off from the outside world for a moment,' he would say. Thus, blindfolded he then started tapping his feet."

In a survey of eighteen particularly successful ESP subjects, Rhea White (1964) of the American Society for Psychical Research found that they would first try to enter a state of relaxation as a preparation for the test. At the same time, they remained alert and cleared their minds of extraneous thoughts either by keeping their minds blank or by focusing their attention on a mental image. After a period of waiting, this image would be released and an ESP impression would enter consciousness.

Alpha and ESP

Interest in the question of whether or not meditation and similar procedures enhance ESP was increased when it was discovered by Joseph Kamiya (1969) that meditation states may be objectively verified through the presence (or rather predominance) of the alpha brain wave and possibly other slow waves. If meditation is a favoring condition for ESP, we might therefore find alpha to be associated with ESP. In an experiment with Lalsingh Harribance (Morris, Roll, Klein, et al., 1972) at the Psychical Research Foundation, it was found that his ESP was in fact best when the production (percent-time amount) of alpha was highest.

Harribance usually precedes his tests with a period of quiet and prayer. In a study by Rex Stanford and Ian Stevenson (Stanford & Stevenson, 1972) at the University of Virginia, the subject used a meditation procedure before each ESP trial to clear his mind and then tried to develop a mental image of the ESP target. His ESP scores were highest when the alpha frequency was low during the mind-clearing period, perhaps indicating that the more tranquil his state the better was he prepared for the ESP task. Scoring was also good when there was an increase in frequency between the mind-clearing and image development phases, which may suggest that the development of the ESP response involves an increase in mental activity. Kamiya (1969) also found that alpha rhythm may be augmented using biofeedback techniques. This has raised the possibility that ESP scores may be enhanced at the same time. A beginning has been made by Charles Honorton and others (1971) to explore this possibility at Maimonides Hospital in Brooklyn.

Complementarity and the Two Brains

In the findings mentioned here, it appears that the experience of self-transcendence which many people report is in some sense real. It seems that human personality, through field consciousness (FC), infiltrates its environ-

ment so that distant people and things are not only experienced as part of the
self but in a real sense are part of that self.

If the FC experience is not a subjective illusion, the question arises about
how we can accommodate this state of consciousness with the ordinary awareness of ourselves as encapsulated entities separated from others and from our
physical surroundings. In other words, which one is the real world? For
answers to questions about reality, we often look to physics. In the world of
Newton, which more or less corresponds with our common sense experience,
things and people were like billiard balls which only interacted when they hit
each other or when they reacted to physical forces such as gravity or light. But
the world of modern physics is surprisingly similar to the FC world described
by Yogi, Zen teachers, and others. In quantum physics, which many regard
as the basis of physics (and some of all science), the sharp distinction between
the observer and the system observed has disappeared. Werner Heisenberg
(1930) stated: "The traditional requirement of science . . . a division of the
world into subject and object (observer and observed) . . . is not permissible
in quantum physics."

Jan Ehrenwald (1958), draws an analogy between this and the therapeutic
situation. ". . . the very act by which the therapist observes and registers the
patient's productions interferes with the spontaneity and genuineness of the
latter's productions. Yet this interference is just as inescapable as the physicist's interference with the physical object observed on the microphysical
plane."

The interference by the therapist, which possibly includes telepathic leakage, may result in "doctrinal compliance" by the patient. By picking up
sensory and extrasensory cues about the expectations of the therapist, his
patient unconsciously causes his symptoms, dreams, and general behavior to
conform with them. Similarly, in ESP tests, the investigator (Feather & Brier,
1971; West & Fisk, 1953), can apparently influence the results of the subjects
without being physically present.

We do not have to go to the therapeutic situation or the experiments of
the physicists to see that man is an integral part of his world. In our ecology-
minded times, it has become clear that there is an intimate man-environment
relationship. In a sense, the trees and grass which give us oxygen are as much
a part of the human organism as the bone marrow which produces the blood
that carries the oxygen through the body.

Modern physicists agree with another parapsychological observation: the
world is much vaster than our usual sense experience intimates. Hermann
Weyl (1934) says, "Only to the gaze of my consciousness, crawling upward

along the life of my body, does a section of this world come to life as a fleeting image in space which continuously changes in time" (p. 116).

When physicists philosophize, they often treat the world of everyday experiences as an illusion; it is not the real world. One physicist has another solution. According to J. Robert Oppenheimer (1966), the answer to the question, "which world is real?" is not "either/or"; we do not have to regard one world as real, the other as illusory. Oppenheimer accepts "two ways of thinking, the way of time and history and the way of eternity and timelessness, [which] are both parts of man's efforts to comprehend the world in which he lives. Neither is comprehended in the other nor reducible to it. They are, as we have learned to say in physics, complementary views, each supplementing the other, neither telling the whole story" (p. 695). The excerpts from Weyl and Oppenheimer together with many others illustrating the similarity between the world view of physicists and mystics were first brought to my attention by Lawrence LeShan (1969).

The complementarity concept in physics resulted from the fact that the exact position and velocity of an electron cannot both be measured at the same time. The observation of one excludes the observation of the other. Oppenheimer's extension of this concept to our picture of the world in some ways matches recent findings about the human brain. Perhaps the two ways of experiencing the world result from the fact that we possess two brains and not just one. From the split brain work of R. W. Sperry (1968), it appears that the world may be experienced in two ways according to which hemisphere is dominant. Usually the left one is. This hemisphere is involved in speech and in analytic and temporal thinking, while the right hemisphere emphasizes spatial relationships and global configurations. The right hemisphere tends to show more alpha than the left. This new look at the brain suggests new research projects for parapsychology. If the time-ordered and analytical way of experiencing the world goes with left-hemisphere domination, perhaps the more global awareness involved in FC states and ESP are more likely to occur when the right hemisphere dominates. At the Psychical Research Foundation, we are now making comparative studies of EEG patterns from the two hemispheres during ESP tests to determine if ESP or some parts of the ESP process rely on one hemisphere more than the other (it may be that the right hemisphere is mainly involved in the reception of ESP and that the left is mainly involved in expressing this information in speech or writing).

Ehrenwald draws attention to an interesting similarity, first noticed by Pascual Jordan (1958), between the complementarity principle and the Freudian mechanism of repression. In analytical terms, the position or velocity of an electron represses the other, as it were. If we look at the relation between the two brain hemispheres in this way, it may be said that one hemisphere represses the other. Except in patients whose two hemispheres have been severed, one is generally dominant at a particular time at the expense of the other. (But in people who have had this operation, the two brains and the two sides of the body they control can apparently function simultaneously and independently—for these patients, one hand may literally not know what the other is doing.)

Another way of saying this is that the dominant hemisphere is "conscious" and the other "unconscious." In our society the cards are stacked in favor of the left side of the brain: the right side is generally repressed and unconscious.

Conclusion

Let us return to the issue which started this discussion: the conflict between the so-called practitioners of the occult and the followers of Western science and technology. As we have seen, the distinction is not sharp. The theories of modern physics at least share the occult belief that there are more connections in the world than meet the eye. If we adopt the complementarity picture of the universe, there is no longer a conflict, but two views of the world, each of which is valid. We do not ask which is the real world but recognize that under certain conditions of observation or experience, one world is real, and under different conditions the other one is.

It appears that the practitioners of the occult are not necessarily fleeing reality, but may be searching for that part of reality which contemporary science and society are neglecting. This approach need not be antiscientific. On the contrary, science is needed to separate real from false and superstitious elements.

If there are irrational elements in occult practices, by the same token, there are irrational elements in the blind rejection of these practices. If we assert *a priori* that nothing can come of approaching the occult scientifically, we follow our own unproven beliefs and contribute further to the division between the practitioners of the occult and the rest of society.

Today's occult upsurge may well in part be the result of the denial by the main part of society that there is a psychical aspect of human personality. As we know, if part of the personality is repressed and its needs unfulfilled, they are likely to find irrational outlets. If the sciences that deal with man could join forces in dispelling man's illusions, regardless of what form they take, we would help him realize the full scope of his personality. We may then be able to lay a solid foundation for a new technology which, complemented by our present one, would enable man to live fully in all worlds he is capable of experiencing.

References

Anderson, M. L. & White, R. A survey of work on ESP and teacher-pupil attitudes. *Journal of Parapsychology,* 1958, **22,** 246–268.

Baba Ram Dass. Baba Ram Dass lecture at the Menninger Foundation: Part II. *The Journal of Transpersonal Psychology,* 1971a, **1,** 47–84.

Baba Ram Dass. *Be here now.* San Cristobal, New Mexico: Lama Foundation, 1971b.

Bechterev, W. "Direct influence" of a person upon the behavior of animals. *Journal of Parapsychology,* 1949, **13,** 166–176.

Brooks, H. Can science survive in the modern age? *Science,* 1971, **174,** 21–30.

Buber, M. *Tales of the Hasidim early masters.* New York: Schocken Books, 1947.

Cox, W. E., Feather, S. R., & Carpenter, J. C. The effect of PK on electromechanical systems. *Journal of Parapsychology,* 1966, **30,** 184–194.

Ehrenwald, J. Doctrinal compliance in psychotherapy and problems of scientific methodology. *Progress in Psychotherapy,* 1958, **3,** 44–54.

Feather, S. R. & Brier, R. The effect of the checker on precognition. In J. B. Rhine (Ed.), *Progress in Parapsychology.* Durham, North Carolina: The Parapsychology Press, 1971.

Gauld, A. A series of "drop-in" communicators. *Proceedings of the Society for Psychical Research,* 1971, **55,** 273–340.

Godwin, J. *Occult America.* New York: Doubleday, 1972.

Grad, B. Some biological effects of the "laying on of hands": A review of experiments with plants and animals. *Journal of the American Society for Psychical Research,* 1965, **59,** 95–129.

Heisenberg, W. *Physical principles of quantum theory.* Chicago: University of Chicago Press, 1930.

Honorton, C., Davidson, R., & Bindler, P. Feedback-augmented EEG alpha, shifts in subjective state, and ESP card-guessing performance. *Journal of the American Society for Psychical Research,* 1971, **65,** 308–323.

Hudesman, J. & Schmeidler, G. R. ESP scores following therapeutic sessions. *Journal of the American Society for Psychical Research,* 1971, **65,** 215–222.

Johnson, M., & Kanthamani, B. K. The defense mechanism test as a predictor of ESP scoring direction. *Journal of Parapsychology,* 1967, **31**, 99–110.

Kamiya, J. Operant control of the EEG alpha rhythm and some of its reported effects on consciousness. In C. T. Tart (Ed.), *Altered states of consciousness.* New York: Wiley, 1969.

Kanthamani, B. K. & Rao, K. R. Personality characteristics of ESP subjects: III. Extraversion and ESP. *Journal of Parapsychology,* 1972, **36**, 198–212.

_____. Personality characteristics of ESP subjects: IV. Neuroticism and ESP. *Journal of Parapsychology,* 1973, **37**, 37–50.

Krippner, S. & Davidson, R. Parapsychology in the USSR. *Saturday Review,* 1972, **55**, 56–60.

LeShan, L. Physicists and mystics: Similarities in world view. *Journal of Transpersonal Psychology,* 1969, **1**, 1–20.

McConnell, R. A., Snowdon, R. J., & Powell, K. F. Wishing with dice. *Journal of Experimental Psychology,* 1955, **50**, 269–275.

McCracken, S. The fuzzing of America. In Philip Nobile (Ed.), *The con III controversy.* New York: Pocket Books, 1971.

Mangan, G. L. *A review of published research on the relation of some personality variables to ESP scoring level.* New York: Parapsychology Foundation, 1958. (Parapsychological Monographs, No. 1)

Matas, F., & Pantas, L. A PK experiment comparing meditating versus non-meditating subjects. *Proceedings of the Parapsychological Association,* 1971, **8**, 12–13.

Morris, R. L., Roll, W. G., Klein, J., & Wheeler, G. EEG patterns and ESP results in forced-choice experiments with Lalsingh Harribance. *Journal of the American Society for Psychical Research,* 1972, **66**, 253–268.

Nicholson, R. A. *The mystics of Islam.* London: Routledge and Kegan Paul, 1966.

Oppenheimer, J. R. *Science and the common understanding.* New York: Simon and Schuster, 1966.

Osis, K. A test of the occurrence of a psi effect between man and the cat. *Journal of Parapsychology,* 1952, **16**, 233–256.

Osis, K. & Bokert, E. ESP and changed states of consciousness induced by meditation. *Journal of the American Society for Psychical Research,* 1971, **65**, 17–65.

Pratt, J. G. *On the evaluation of verbal material in parapsychology.* New York: Parapsychology Foundation, 1969. (Parapsychological Monographs, No. 10)

Rao, K. R. *Experimental parapsychology: A review and interpretation.* Springfield, Ill.: Thomas, 1966.

Reich, C. *The greening of America.* New York: Random House, 1970.

Rejdak, Z. Nina Kulagina's mind over matter. *Psychic,* 1971, June, 2, 24–25.

Rhine, J. B., & Brier, R. (Eds.) *Parapsychology today.* New York: Citadel, 1968.

Rhine, J. B., & Pratt, J. G. A review of the Pearce-Pratt distance series of ESP tests. *Journal of Parapsychology,* 1954, 18, 165–177.

————. *Parapsychology: frontier science of the mind.* Rev. ed. Springfield, Ill.: Thomas, 1962.

Roll, W. G. ESP and memory. *International Journal of Neuropsychiatry,* 1966, 2, 505–521.

Roll, W. G. & Klein, J. Further forced-choice ESP experiments with Lalsingh Harribance. *Journal of the American Society for Psychical Research,* 1972, 66, 103–112.

Roll, W. G., Morris, R. L., Damgaard, J. A., Klein, J., & Roll, M. Free verbal response experiments with Lalsingh Harribance. *Journal of the American Society for Psychical Research,* 1973, 67, 197–207.

Roszak, T. *The making of a counter culture.* New York: Anchor Books, Doubleday, 1969.

Rubin, L. & Honorton, C. Separating the yins from the yangs: An experiment with the *I Ching. Proceedings of the Parapsychological Association,* 1971, 8, 6–7.

Schmeidler, G. R. High ESP scores after a Swami's brief instruction in meditation and breathing. *Journal of the American Society for Psychical Research,* 1970, 64, 100–103.

Schmeidler, G. R. & McConnell, R. A. *ESP and personality patterns.* New Haven: Yale University Press, 1958.

Schmidt, H. A PK test with electronic equipment. *Journal of Parapsychology,* 1970, 34, 175–181.

————. Clairvoyance tests with a machine. *Journal of Parapsychology, 1969,* 33, 300-306.

————. Precognition of a quantum process. *Journal of Parapsychology, 1969,* 33, 99–108.

Schouten, Sybo A. Psi in mice: positive reinforcement. *Journal of Parapsychology,* 1972, 36, 261–282.

Snow, C. P. *The two cultures and a second look.* New York: Mentor Books, 1963.

Soal, S. G. & Bateman, F. *Modern experiments in telepathy.* New Haven: Yale University Press, 1954.

Sperry, R. W. Hemisphere deconnection and unity in conscious awareness. *American Psychologist,* 1968, **23**, 723–733.

Stanford, R. G. & Stevenson, I. EEG correlates of free-response GESP in an individual subject. *Journal of the American Society for Psychical Research,* 1972, **66**, 357–368.

Tenhaeff, W. H. C. Some aspects of parapsychological research in the Netherlands. *International Journal of Neuropsychiatry,* 1966, **2**, 408–419.

Toffler, A. *Future shock.* New York: Random House, 1970.

Ullman, M. An informal session with Nina Kulagina. *Proceedings of the Parapsychological Association,* 1971, **8**, 21–22.

Ullman, M., Krippner, S. , & Feldstein, S. Experimentally-induced telepathic dreams; two studies using EEG-REM monitoring technique. *International Journal of Neuropsychiatry,* 1966, **2**, 420–437.

Vasiliev, L. L. *Experiments in mental suggestion.* Church Crookham, England: Institute for the Study of Mental Images, 1963.

Wallace, R. K. & Benson, H. The physiology of meditation. *Scientific American,* 1972, **226**, 84–91.

Watkins, G. R. & Watkins, A. M. Possible PK influence on the resuscitation of anesthetized mice. *Journal of Parapsychology,* 1971, **35**, 257–272.

West, D. J. & Fisk, G. W. A dual ESP experiment with clock cards. *Journal of the Society for Psychical Research,* 1953, **37**, 185–197.

Weyl, H. *Philosophy of mathematics and life.* London: Cambridge University Press, 1934.

White, R. A. A comparison of old and new methods of response to targets in ESP experiments. *Journal of the American Society for Psychical Research,* 1964, **58**, 21–56.

Yu, L. K. *The secrets of chinese meditation.* London: Rider, 1969.

Jan Ehrenwald

The Non-Euclidian Mind:
A Neurophysiological Model of
Psi Phenomena

ON TRYING TO formulate a neurophysiological or neuropsychiatric model of psi phenomena, we must begin with two, more or less dogmatic, statements—one factual, the other theoretical. First, we must be satisfied that such psi phenomena as telepathy, clairvoyance, precognition, or psychokinesis do in reality exist. We must be ready to acknowledge the possibility of thought and action at a distance and their attending causal and spatio-temporal anomalies, even though such an assumption brings us precariously close to belief in witchcraft; to the delusions of our paranoid patients; to magic and animistic concepts of preliterate man or the child. Clearly, if the discovery by parapsychologists of a new continent of the human mind were an empty claim, there would be nothing to discuss. There would be no point in trying to map its surface features, to delve into its geological origin, or to speculate about its future.

A second proviso is that we must be ready for a radical revision of our concepts of space, time, and causality; of some of our familiar ideas about the nature of consciousness; about cerebral localization; and about human personality in general.

Above all, we must realize that there is an irreducible gap in our ultimate understanding of how neurophysiological processes are converted into conscious perceptions, or how they trigger acts of volition. The gap, in what can be described as the autopsychic sphere, is admittedly small and usually ignored or glossed over by both scientists and laymen. It is more conspicuous and much larger on the psi level or in the heteropsychic sphere. But it is essentially of the same order. Nevertheless, despite the continued existence of the gap between physical event and ordinary perception or volition, the behavioral sciences have been able to establish themselves as a pragmatic discipline without feeling obliged to agonize at every step about the metaphysical implications of the gap. It is only fair for parapsychology to claim the same prerogative.

With these provisos, it is possible to submit five interlacing and mutually supporting hypotheses, knit together in a coherent neurophysiological model that should promote a better understanding of psi phenomena and serve as a rationale for further experimentation.

The first hypothesis takes off from thoroughly familiar ground. It amounts to a simple linear extension of the basic cleavage between afferent and efferent neural conduction; between input and output; between sensory and motor activity characteristic of our mental organization. It can be described as the extension hypothesis.

The Extension Hypothesis

The starting point of this hypothesis is the elementary fact that the reliability or acuity of cutaneous perceptions or sensitiveness to touch is at its best, say, at the finger tips; that it is less so at the dorsum of the hand; still less on the surface of internal organs; and zero on the fingernails, on the enamel of teeth, or on a lock of hair clipped off by the barber. Psychologically speaking, teeth and hair or nail parings belong to the nonego. They are no longer part of our body image, or at least an expendable part of it.

In a similar vein, I can move my right index finger any time at my whim; somewhat less reliably, I can raise my left eyebrow. With some practice, I can move my right ear lobe. But only a Yogi or a subject trained by special biofeedback techniques can influence his heart muscle on purpose, while nobody can lift a hemianesthetic and paralyzed leg. It too has become nonego as far as the patient's awareness and volitional control is concerned (See Figure).

On the psi-level of functioning, the situation, both quantitatively and qualitatively, is vastly different. What is usually relegated to the nonego is no longer cut off from the ego by a sharp demarkation line. A symbiotic mother may be directly aware of her baby's distress (Ehrenwald, 1971). If she is neurotic, she may be instrumental in having her child act out her own emotionally charged, repressed, antisocial impulses. An analytic patient may produce a dream reflecting some of his therapist's emotionally-charged mental content. A gifted telepathic sensitive may be able to pick a virtual stranger's

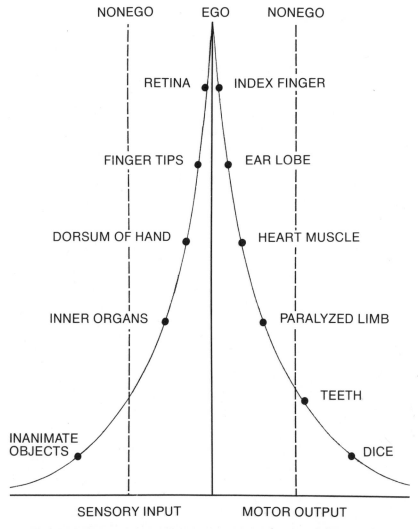

The sloping curves converging at the imaginary point of the ego represent the diminishing return of motor efficacy and acuity of perception as we move from the ego to the nonego. Yet it should be noted that the outer reaches of the graphs do not ever touch the base line. They represent the symbiotic gradient as explained in the text. At the same time, the two curves enclose — but do not seal off from the rest of the world — what is here described as the open, non-Euclidian model of personality structure.

brain. He may do so with special reference to such unique bits of information as names, numerals, or other tracer elements in the agent's mind (Ehrenwald, 1955). Or else he may function under clairvoyant conditions; that is, he may extend his range of sensitiveness to such inanimate objects as ESP cards, numerals, or letters of the alphabet which are not, at the critical moment, part of another person's mental content. Indeed, it should be noted that "good" percipients tend to score just as well under clairvoyant as under telepathic conditions. Some subjects piled up scores giving odds of several millions to one against chance under clairvoyant conditions.

The motor counterpart of these experiments is the attempt of a subject to influence the fall of dice thrown from a cup or to deflect their path as they roll down an incline (Rhine, 1943; Girden, Murphy, Beloff et al., 1969). Results in such PK experiments are less impressive statistically than those obtained in laboratory ESP tests, but some have reached critical ratios of 5.00 or better (Girden, Murphy, Beloff et al., 1969).

Well-documented instances of spontaneous PK incidents are few and far between. A notable exception are the semispontaneous phenomena of the Russian housewife, Nina Kulagina, whose ability to move such trivial objects as a pack of cigarettes, matches, or a piece of bread has been investigated by several Russian experimenters with impeccable scientific credentials, Professor L. L. Vasiliev (1963) among them. Several qualified Western observers have confirmed their observations. Films brought to this country likewise tend to bear out the genuineness of Kulagina's extraordinary feats of PK.

Thus PK need no longer be regarded as nothing but a cluster of freakish incidents or mere statistical artifacts. At the same time, the observations tend to give at least some support to such anecdotal accounts as Jung's "poltergeist" (1963) in Freud's bookcase and to stories of related phenomena usually attributed to disturbed children or adolescents.

Even more perplexing is the occurrence of apparent precognition, both spontaneous and experimental, reported in the literature of parapsychology. Nevertheless, it should be noted that the statistical evidence for precognition under laboratory conditions is in no way inferior to that for "simple" telepathy, clairvoyance, or PK. Yet, needless to say, in order to account for observations of this order, more than a mere extension of our traditional neurophysiological model of personality—functioning in the categories of classical Euclidian space and prerelativistic Einsteinian time—is required.

With this proviso, the extension hypothesis, as proposed here, is useful in several ways: First, it carries the basic dichotomy of our sensory-motor organization from the ego to the nonego; from the confines of individual personality structure to the universe at large. Secondly, it is suggestive of a striking structural similarity and clinical affinity of both ESP and PK to two major manifestations of conversion hysteria—hysterical anesthesia on the one hand and motor paralysis on the other. This is particularly important in the present context. The crucial point is that in conversion hysteria, a part of the body image is cut off from the whole, dissociated from conscious awareness, and inaccessible to volitional control: the anesthetic or paralyzed limb is turned into nonego as far as the patient's perceptions or motor behavior are concerned. By contrast, in telepathy, clairvoyance or PK, an ad hoc cathected segment or area of the nonego is temporarily turned into ego and becomes accessible to the subject's direct awareness or volitional control. In effect, both psi phenomena and conversion hysteria are marginal manifestations of our mental life. They are *grenzfalle,* borderline cases; one representing the mirror image of the other.

A third implication of the extension hypothesis is closely related to this state of affairs. In the late nineteenth century, Charcot, Janet, and their associates, puzzled by the discovery of glove- or stocking-shaped anesthetic zones in their hysterics or hypnotized subjects, were forced to the then revolutionary proposition that such disturbances cut across the familiar lines of neural distribution and must therefore be attributed to the power of the patient's ideas or imagination. This is how the new principle of functional disorders, of symbolic representation, of "organ language" transcending the familiar laws of cerebral localization was born. We shall see that the occurrence of psi phenomena forces upon us an even more revolutionary proposition—the proposition that the "power of ideas" may extend from what can be described as the autopsychic into the heteropsychic sphere, without the benefit of neural conduction or even anatomical contiguity. It is nevertheless in good keeping with this proposition that psi phenomena, though seemingly incompatible with causal laws, fully conform to familiar psychodynamic principles (Ehrenwald, 1955; Eisenbud, 1970).

A fourth implication is derived from further historical considerations. There is a vast body of evidence connecting psi phenomena with hypnosis, trance phenomena, and conversion hysteria. There is reason to believe that some of Mesmer's and de Puiségur's patients were indeed psychic. Janet's and Gibert's experiments with Léonie involving hypnosis at a distance are a matter of historical record. They were recently revived by Vasiliev (1963) and other Russian authors. On the other hand, many so-called physical mediums—from Eusapia Palladino and Rudi Schneider to Ted Serios—showed marked evidence of hysteria or other psychopathology. It should be noted, however, that such a clinical association is by no means unconditional. It is less apparent or altogether absent, in many mental mediums.

The Genetic Hypothesis

This hypothesis tries to account for the origin of the newly discovered continent of the mind discussed here. It is derived from a vast number of observations between mother and child at the symbiotic stage. I pointed out elsewhere that mother-child symbiosis can rightly be described as the cradle of ESP (Ehrenwald, 1971).

At the early symbiotic stage, communication is usually thought to be based on unconscious expressive movements, on body language; on mutual cuing, by intonation of voice, etc. However, in order to account for the flawless interaction and the delicately balanced regulatory functions operating within the mother-child unit, child psychiatrists and analysts have talked about empathy, intuition, or remnants of animal instincts lost to man (Mahler, 1968). Others suggest that "one unconscious" is able to communicate directly with "another unconscious." This, for instance, should account for the modus operandi of a symbiotic child acting out his mother's repressed antisocial impulses, as described by Szurek and Johnson (1952) and other child analysts. I have pointed to several cases in which strongly motivated mothers of mentally defective or otherwise handicapped children seemed capable of making up for their offsprings' shortcomings without the apparent aid of the usual channels of communication (1948).

How, then, in view of the limited repertoire of conventional signaling devices used by them, do mother and child succeed in functioning together in such a harmonious way? How does the mother know if baby cannot tell? How does baby respond to her cues if he doesn't understand? It is here that the telepathy hypothesis comes to our rescue. Telepathy, in this case, far from being a mere psychological curiosity without an apparent goal or discernible purpose, is well-suited to fill whatever communication gap exists between the two in the symbiotic phase. Introducing the telepathy hypothesis into the symbiotic model assigns a vitally important physiological function to an otherwise seemingly superfluous or redundant mode of communication. Indeed, mother-child symbiosis can well be described as the cradle of ESP. It is a means of preverbal communication gradually lost in the course of separation-individuation (Mahler, 1968).

Nevertheless, under pathological conditions—i.e., in prolonged symbiosis, in the REM state, or in the psychoanalytic situation—telepathic incidents may again make their appearance. They have frequently been reported between twins, lovers, marriage partners, or other persons tied together by intimate bonds (Stevenson, 1960). This is how we arrive at the concept of a symbiotic gradient ranging from the early symbiotic phase to ESP in the family and in society at large. In case of need, such a scheme can be extended to embrace inanimate objects and indeed the whole congeries of atoms, protons, and electrons from which both animate and inanimate matter has sprung. It would in effect amount to a vindication of some of the reports put forward by mystics of all ages and cultural backgrounds (See Figure 1).

Personality: Open or Closed?

Our third proposition is closely linked with the genetic hypothesis. It postulates an open, non-Euclidian, post-Freudian, versus the traditional closed, isolated, self-contained personality structure. It is paradoxical that more than half a century after the advent of relativistic physics and the formulation of quantum mechanics, current theories of personality are still steeped in the classical Judeo-Christian, Aristotelian, or Cartesian traditions. The classical personality structure, viewed in this light, is located in Euclidian space and prerelativistic time, subject to the ironclad laws of cause and effect. By contrast, the open, postclassical, post-Freudian, non-Euclidian model, as conceived here, is continuous with the nonego and with the rest of the world through the symbiotic gradient. It is potentially open to a virtually infinite range of impressions crowding in on the ego from outside. It is needless to say, however, that such an ego would instantly be swamped and disorganized by such a barrage of stimuli. It would suffer a breakdown comparable to that of an acute schizophrenic. It is to prevent such a contingency that our mental organization has erected diverse perceptual defenses or screening functions of the ego to protect it from sensory overload originating from both inside and outside—from the autopsychic and the heteropsychic sphere. This is why, except in diverse regressive states, the ego is relatively immune to psi experiences (Ehrenwald, 1948).

Be that as it may, the neurophysiological substratum of heteropsychic experiences is largely the same as in autopsychic experiences. The difference between the two lies in the fact that psi involves exclusively, or predominantly, cortical, cortico-thalamic, reticular, and limbic systems and no sensory input from outside. Psi phenomena are nonsensory or extrasensory in much the same way as dreams or hallucinations. Like dreams or hallucinations, they enter consciousness, or cortical plus subcortical centers, by the back door, as it were. Thus personality, functioning as an open system, is neither more nor less under the sway of an external, supernatural agency than when operating as a closed system. Even the laws of cerebral localization are roughly the same, subject to the principle of diminishing return of awareness and intentionality, characteristic of the symbiotic gradient.

Whether or not it is the right, supposedly intellectually inferior but more intuitive side of the brain, rather than the intellectually superior, dominant left hemisphere, that plays the leading role in the central processing of psi phenomena must remain a matter of conjecture at present.

The Psi Syndrome

Our fourth hypothesis should be mentioned in passing only. It suggests that the diverse modalities of psi phenomena form a syndrome of causal and spatio-temporal anomalies: they run together; they are mutually interchangeable, like time and space, or the particle versus the wave theory of light. By the same token, they include such perplexing occurrences as precognition in life and laboratory. It should be noted that in so doing they are apt to pull the rug out from under the feet of most purely physical theories of psi phenomena, including radiation, gravitational waves, bioplasma, or what not. A consistent theory of psi phenomena has to be a package deal: you have to take the whole syndrome on a lump-it-or-leave-it basis. To change the metaphor: if you give the devil the little finger, he will take the whole hand.

The fact is that telepathy and related phenomena tend to occur under virtually identical psychodynamic conditions. They are subject to the same laws of symbolic representation, isolation, reaction formation, as are postulated by psychoanalytic theory. At the same time, they conform to the same principles of compensation for an existing minus function as are characteristic of neuropathological or psychosomatic events in general. Still, they are equally incompatible with our standard time- and space-bound Euclidian personality structure. We must conclude that they have not been encouraged by the evolutionary process. This is why, apart from the early symbiotic stage, they have poor survival value for our species, especially for man of contemporary Western culture. This also accounts for their affinity to the dream or psychotic disorders; for their structural similarity to Freud's primary process functioning, as well as for our stubborn tendency to their scotomization, repression, and denial (Ehrenwald, 1971).

Psi Phenomena and the Existential Shift

The mental state conducive to telepathic or clairvoyant perception has been variously described as mental quietude, relaxation, as calm alertness, reminiscent of Freud's prescription for the psychoanalyst's free–floating attention in the therapeutic situation. Its original prototype was the mother-child symbiosis which in turn is duplicated in diverse other states of regression "in the service of the ego". So also is Zen or Yoga meditation and their attending alpha states. This is why attempts at producing alpha activity by diverse methods of biofeedback to promote ESP receptiveness are now being increasingly used by experimental parapsychologists (Honorton & Carbone, 1971). The same is true for Ullman's experiments in the REM stage of nocturnal sleep (Ullman & Krippner, 1970), and other "minus functions" of ego. Less information is available about the EEG concomitants of the agent's mental state, but suggestions concerning its psychodynamics go back to Freud himself (1953). He drew the picture of a mind in action, of a person motivated by unconscious or preconscious wishes, desires and impulses, even though he may be utterly unaware of his functioning as an agent.

A similar picture emerges from recent reports on the Russian housewife, Kulagina, the gifted physical medium. In her attempts to move by sheer "will power" such external objects as a match box, a top of a ballpoint pen, or a wine glass, she goes through a series of frantic body movements reflecting the physical effort involved in the process. Her whole behavior, as seen on the films, is strongly reminiscent of a patient's faltering attempt to move a paralyzed limb—that is, a part of his anatomy which has virtually turned into nonego.

Yet, needless to say, none of our conventional principles of cerebral localization, neural conduction, and so forth can account for perplexing feats of this order. We have to be ready for the literally mind-stretching conclusion that, given a proper set of beliefs, motivations, personality variables, interpersonal configurations, and otherwise favorable predisposing factors, even Western man is capable of shifting his attention, his set or *Einstellung,* his volitional posture, his outlook on the world from the standard, Euclidian level of adaptation to an altogether different level of functioning. This is what is here described as the existential shift. Yet the existential shift is by no means confined to the field proper of parapsychology. It can be effected by such widely divergent experiences and interventions as hypnosis, by catharsis in psychotherapy, by the transition from sleep to wakefulness, and last but not least, by electric shock treatment. Thus the existential shift, as it is conceived here, is far more inclusive than the narrower concept of altered states of consciousness.

Yet, despite differences, all these varieties of the existential shift have one thing in common—they consist of an abrupt, global reshuffling and reorganization of a person's physiological and psychological adaptations. In the ideal case, they affect all levels of his spiritual, cognitive, and perceptual orientation to the world and his whole repertoire of behavioral responses to the environment. If a physico-chemical agent is responsible for the shift, it is brought to bear on the raw nerve endings, synapses, or cortical chemo-receptors of the brain. On the other hand, such psychological influences as emotionally charged imagery, symbolic cues, incoming psi stimuli, and so forth may "home in" on the identical pharmacological or neurohumoral target areas of the brain, circumventing the familiar afferent pathways of the CNS. If so, they may be affected in much the same way as by a shot of norephedrin, a cortisone injection, or 200 mg. of LSD. In the last analysis, the final common pathway is the same in both instances—in response to both somatic and psychological stimuli. But whatever its modus operandi, the crucial point in the present context is the occurrence of a demonstrable shift from the standard Euclidian to the novel, non–Euclidian level of existence. It is existential shifts of this order, that is, a fundamental reorientation of our mode of experience towards a new, or rather age old, but culturally repressed, psychic reality, which give rise to psi phenomena.

References

Ehrenwald, J. Mother-child symbiosis: cradle of ESP. *Psychoanalytic Review,* 1971, **58.3**, 455–466.

_____. *New dimensions of deep analysis, a study of telepathy in interpersonal relationships.* New York: Grune and Stratton, 1955.

_____. *Telepathy and medical psychology.* New York: W. W. Norton, 1948.

Eisenbud, J. *Psi and psychoanalysis.* New York: Grune and Stratton, 1970.

Freud, S., in G. Devereux (Ed.), *Psychoanalysis and the Occult.* New York: International University Press, 1953.

Girden, E., Murphy G., Beloff, J., et al. A review of psychokinesis (PK). *International Journal of Parapsychology,* 1969, **6,** 27–37.

Honorton, C. & Carbone, M. A. A preliminary study of feedback augmented EEG alpha activity and ESP card-guessing performance. *Journal of the American Society for Psychical Research,* 1971, **63,** 66–74.

Johnson, A. M. & Szurek, S. A. The genesis of antisocial acting out in children and adults. *Psychoanalytical Quarterly,* 1952, **21,** 323–343.

Jung, C. G. *Memories, dreams, reflections.* New York: Pantheon Books, 1963.

Mahler, M. *On Human symbiosis and the vicissitudes of individuation.* New York: International University Press, 1968.

Rhine, J. B. Dice thrown by cup and machine in PK tests. *Journal of Parapsychology,* 1943, **7,** 207–217.

Sperling, J. Children's interpretation and reaction to the unconscious of their mothers. *International Journal of Psychoanalysis,* 1950, **31,** 36–41.

Stevenson, I. *Telepathic impressions, a review and report of 35 new cases.* Charlottesville: University of Virginia Press, 1960.

Ullman, M. & Krippner, S. *Dreams and telepathy: an experimental approach.* New York: Parapsychology Foundation, 1970.

Vasiliev, L. L. *Experiments in mental suggestion.* Church Crookham, Hampshire, England: Institute for the Study of Mental Images, 1963.

Berthold Eric Schwarz

Telepathic Humoresque

HUMOR CAN act as a safety valve. Humor sometimes prevents catastrophic detonations of unchecked hostility. It can tide us over rough spots and help make life bearable. It is one of the highest psychic functions and the sine qua non of the civilized man. Humor has its role in sexuality. Used tactfully and sparingly, humor can be an adjuvant in psychotherapy (Fodor, 1951; Poland, 1971). Bergler's excellent monograph (1956) reviews theories on the role of humor and wit in psychic development and in interpersonal relationships. There are many examples showing how humor is intimately related to the unconscious and how it is similar to dreams and mental mechanisms. Humor tells us about the individual: how he sees himself, how he believes others see him, and how he actually is.

The extraordinary paragnost Jacques Romano (Schwarz, 1968), who knew Mark Twain, once commented that many of Twain's humorous writings were really a defense against his being overwhelmed by melancholy. Incidentally, Mark Twain himself had many telepathic experiences (Ebon, 1971). In studies of such gifted paragnosts as Gerard Croiset (Tenhaeff, 1962; Pollack, 1964), who has employed his psychic abilities for the solution of various crimes; Joseph Dunninger (1944), world-renowned telepathist; Henry Gross (Schwarz, 1965), successful Maine dowser, and Jacques Romano, I noted that they all had a keen sense of humor. These sensitive, energetic, supremely self-confident gentlemen of proven psychic accomplishments all had delightful repertoires of humorous experiences and jokes, which seemingly provided them with a necessary respite from the serious, demanding nature of their work. Some of their most ridiculous examples also involved presumed telepathy.

For example, Thomas A. Edison once challenged Dunninger to tell him what was concealed under his dinner plate, and Dunninger promptly told Edison that it was hiding a hole in Mrs. Edison's new tablecloth—that Mr. Edison had burned the night before with one of his cigars (Dunninger, 1944). On another occasion Dunninger walked into a restaurant with a friend and called the waitress over and told her to think of her name and birthday. Dunninger was shocked to have the unperturbed waitress respond: "What are you telling me that for? I already know that!"

The purpose of this report is to show how telepathy and the paranormal (which is deeply rooted in the unconscious) might be allied to humor. Telepathic interaction and transactions are personal and truthful. By unmasking the unconscious and "telling it as it is," these telepathic occurrences reveal in sharp relief the realities and dynamics of interpersonal relations. The telepathic hypothesis in many instances makes an otherwise inexplicable communication intelligible and often humorous. Eisenbud (1972, 1970) has given examples involving humor and telepathy. His documented researches of "thoughtography" (1967) also provide a rich vein of weird and tragi-comic examples. Perhaps such techniques and insights could illuminate reported humorous classical paranormal events (Richet, 1923).

Three categories illustrate the possible role of telepathy—(1) humorous situations from early parent-child episodes; (2) physician-patient psychotherapeutic relationships; and (3) strictly personal anecdotes obtained from patients and my own life.

Humor in Parent-Child Telepathy

In more than 1520 possible parent-child telepathic episodes in my family (Schwarz, 1971), there were many examples of telepathy and humor[1] where the child frequently preempted his parent's attention by uncovering his parent's jealously guarded secrets; supplying the forgotten "key" word to a joke; complementing his parent's suppressed critical attitudes; supplying captions to his parent's mentally envisioned or actually seen cartoons; or in slapstick fashion acting out his parent's specific suppressed fantasies in relation to socially forbidden areas of sex, aggression, or body image. As with involuntary humor, telepathy gave added dimension to the unexpected—but always the naked truth.

---

[1]For examples see episodes 69, 538, 612, 793, 1116, 1210, 1269, 1297, 1324, and 1505.

The contagion and hypersuggestiveness of humor among children is self-evident. The credulous child, who looks upon his parents as omnipotent and omniscient, offers fertile soil for telepathic reactions. Compared to adult-to-adult presumed telepathic examples, the parent-child telepathic dynamics are simple and unsophisticated. Many of the later parent-child telepathic episodes completely resemble adult-to-adult exchanges and are so tragicomic and revealing that they cannot be published.

Example 1 —Just as I was going to phone my telepathist friend, Jacques Romano, in New York, I thought of a joke that our mutual friend Mr. Newton had told me. I intended to tell Mr. Romano that I had met Mr. Newton. However, I had had to see Mr. Newton in private because of some research I was doing on Mr. Romano, and I wondered if the latter would understand the reason for this and not be offended at my not including him. I thought Mr. Romano would be amused and matters smoothed over by the joke Mr. Newton had told me. While I was trying to recall the joke which concerned Pittsburgh (all I could then remember), four-year-old Lisa came up to me and shouted the word "Pittsburgh." The joke was about a shabby man in his fifties with an unkempt beard. The bum went to the Baptist church, but before he could enter the minister asked, "Where was Jesus Christ born?" The man answered, "Philadelphia," and the minister threw him out. The bum then went to the Presbyterian church. The minister asked the same question, and when the bum answered "Pittsburgh" he was again thrown out. Finally he went to an Episcopal church, but the minister didn't ask any questions—he invited the bum in. So the bum asked the minister where Jesus Christ was born. When the minister answered "Why, Bethlehem," the bum said, "I knew it was somewhere in Pennsylvania!" Lisa might have picked up her father's ambivalence toward Mr. Romano as epitomized in the joke he was trying to recall.

Example 2—Lisa, aged four, Eric, aged two, and Ardis, their mother, were walking down a street in Upper Montclair. Ardis intended to open a savings account for Lisa at the bank. Lisa was carrying her glass piggy bank when Ardis thought, "What would happen if Lisa dropped it?" At that exact moment Lisa did drop it, and it caused quite a commotion in front of the bank! Thirteen dollars in pennies and nickels! In this innocent and humorous act, there might exist the paradigm for the pathological relationship between a phobic mother and a subsequently phobic (or accident-prone) child. The charged fears in a state of intensified (mostly hostile or negative) rapport could be telepathically transmitted and acted upon, as well as in the more widely recognized and commendable state in which the parents think the best for the child and it is achieved.

Example 3—My wife, Ardis, and my nine-year old son, Eric, went into a stationery store to buy an evening paper. Eric went to the back of the store to look at magazines while Ardis, in the front, looked among the papers for the New York *Daily News.* A few weeks previously while at Lincoln Center in New York City with her girlfriend, Ardis had been interviewed by John Stapleton, the inquiring photographer from the *Daily News.* He also took her picture and said that it would shortly appear in his column. This was a secret she had kept from the whole family. She was embarrassed about the subject because she felt the reporter asked her a silly question, and perhaps on a deeper level she felt the picture would be uncomplimentary. While she was preoccupied with her surreptitious examination of the paper, Eric ran from the back of the store and thrust a magazine in his mother's face, saying, "Here is your picture, Mom." It was a picture of a woman who was half beautiful and half ugly. Eric had not done anything like this before, and his unexpected action could not have been more perfectly timed to embarrass his mother by divulging her secret, as if to say, on an unconscious level, that his mother could not fool him. The picture Eric showed might have reflected his mother's ambivalence concerning the article she had yet to see.

On a deeper level, Ardis probably had added reason to be concerned and embarrassed about her husband's possible response. When a friend sent her the clipping (February 27, 1967), I almost swallowed my tongue as I read the question: "Should women shoulder most of the blame for the decline of chivalry?" and the last sentence of Ardis's answer: "Children don't see chivalry at home, so they don't practice it." Ardis's girlfriend, who was single, was kinder to the male sex with her answer: ". . . You can't fault men for being less chivalrous. They're so intent and preoccupied with business."

Humor in Psychotherapeutic Relationships

During the course of psychotherapy, many patients spontaneously reported humorous situations that might best be explained by the telepathic hypothesis. The examples are analogous to the parent-child telepathic episodes but of course are more complex. The examples often pertain to emotionally polarized secrets, eroticism, various expressions of hostility, embarrassment, and "foot-in-mouth" disease

Example 4—In the course of psychotherapy of a young woman referred to me by a surgeon, she mentioned her strong attraction to him, and how on rare occasions she could not resist the impulse to telephone him at late hours and chat. But the woman did not know what the surgeon had confided to me when I saw him. On the rare occasions when she mustered the courage to phone him, he was, on one of the still rarer occasions in his life, cohabiting with his wife, from whom he had been estranged. When I offered the surgeon the telesomatic hypothesis, he blushed and said, "Why, of course!" This type of example is not unusual, and was mentioned by Stekel (Eisenbud, 1949). Another example is that of a colleague who was incorrectly convinced he was being framed by Cupid, because almost every random time he came to visit me the woman who interested him also came, without advance knowledge, to visit my wife. The colleague was being telepathically notified.

Example 5—A young college man was arrested for indecent exposure. Of this, he was very ashamed—it was his most jealously guarded secret—or so he thought. One day, several weeks after his arrest, he happened to meet one of his old high school friends. This was his first contact with someone from his past in a long time, and he was very concerned about his secret, although he knew that it was impossible that his friend or anyone else would know about it. However, his friend opened the conversation by saying: "Do you know they passed a new law in New Jersey that automobiles cannot be driven without hubcaps because their nuts would be exposed?"

Example 6—A middle-aged, rather hot-headed, phobic lady had a problem with her domineering, heavy-drinking husband. Furthermore, it was not generally known that their child was adopted because her husband was sterile. The patient had felt cheated because of this. Her husband was very sensitive about his problem, and his wife found it hard to restrain herself from reminding him of his "masculine deficiency." One hot summer day, the couple had to entertain a prominent visitor and his wife from India. This was an auspicious dinner engagement, and, if carried out successfully, could mean a promotion for her husband. The patient thought she would ingratiate herself with her guests by offering them for dessert, a choice of homemade American pumpkin pie or cherry pie. When she presented the desserts, the esteemed dinner guests started snickering. The patient's husband, who ordinarily preferred pumpkin pie, had chosen the cherry pie. The guests from India stated in jest that they appreciated their hostess's thoughtfulness but they, like her husband, could not take the pumpkin pie because in their section of India, it was a superstition that pumpkins were a cause of sterility. The patient's departure from her usual culinary routine—serving pumpkin pie in the summer—unwittingly made her the hit of the evening. She downgraded her downtrodden husband in more ways than she might ever have bargained for.

Example 7—A young businessman with many phobias had avoided most social contacts for years. One day in the course of his treatment, he said, "I'm a born loser. Last night I went to my first cocktail party in years. I knew only the hostess, whom I had met a few weeks ago. The party was on the thirty-ninth floor of a Manhattan apartment building. Of the fifty people in the room I picked one and started to talk to her. To make small talk, which is difficult, I said, "Those who read the *Reader's Digest* are idiots." She said that she worked for the *Reader's Digest!* I was flustered and didn't know what to say, so I continued, "I hope you are not in the editorial department." And she said, "Yes." This example of foot-in-mouth telepathy might illustrate a common event in the psychic dynamics of everyday life.

Example 8—Late one Sunday night, I checked my appointment book for the next day and, to my horror, discovered an error. Mr. S, a fragile schizophrenic, had been scheduled for seven in the morning by my secretary, who had automatically written Professor B's name, whom she knew came at 7:30. To avoid a conflict and to make the simplest adjustment in this case, I tried to contact Professor B, to tell him to come at eight o'clock, a half hour later than usual. Since I couldn't reach him on the telephone, I had to ask Mr. S to come at 6:30 a.m. When Professor B arrived at 7:30 a.m., he said: "It's a funny thing. I set the alarm for 7:30 instead of 6:30. This is the only time I've done that in two years of therapy. I had a dream about coming to your office a half hour later than usual." Furthermore, the professor identified his dream as being telepathic. Yet despite this urgent message, he decided that he could still come at 7:30 a.m. Thus in his dreams and conscious associations he correctly divined the situation and my confusion, and made the suitable adjustments. He even identified the telepathic nature of the event. Some of his telosomatic experiences are described elsewhere (Schwarz, 1967).

Example 9—Mr. J was invited to a formal banquet and went to the store he had used in the past to rent a tuxedo. Although the suit was wrapped in heavy paper, he felt uneasy about it. When he got home, despite his wife's joshing him for superstition, he insisted on unwrapping the suit then, and not a few hours before the banquet. His fears were confirmed when he discovered that one trouser leg was eight inches longer than the other. His hunch came in the nick of time and saved the day.

Example 10—During the noon hour, the day before the funeral of a close friend (January 21, 1966), while in my office, I expressed strong reservations to my wife about the religious services planned for the next day. I joked that I could better visualize the coffin in my consultation room, with the somber rites conducted there, than anticipate an unfeeling, cut and dried type of service elsewhere. This very private (and sacrilegious) wisecrack was linked to a family joke of long ago. A patient (seen in consultation for alcoholism) upon first entering my office had remarked, "Doctor, you have a very beautiful and spacious office!" I thanked her but then was floored by her next statement, "My husband would love to see your office. It would be just perfect for him. He's a funeral director!" It was a story that my late friend had heard and chuckled over.

On January 25, 1966, Tuesday, a phobic woman patient, whom I had not seen for two weeks, came to my office quite upset. She had recently returned to her job in a bank after an absence of many months. While out to lunch at noon on Friday, January 21, 1966, she had a most disquieting experience, the only one of its kind in her life.

It might be interjected that in her psychotherapeutic session, while she was describing another matter, I thought of my poor friend dying. I visualized the grim hospital reception room scene on Saturday before the death. In my mind's eye, I clearly saw myself talking to my friend's son and noted how the son's winter coat was on the couch beside me, and I was wearing my heavy leather overcoat. At that affect-laden, hovering, vivid complex of death and coats, the phobic patient said: "I went out to lunch with Frank (president of the bank and friend of her husband). We put our coats on a nearby chair. It was weird, almost as if a body were there. It was a man in a coffin. When you have a body next to you it's difficult—I'm nervous when I get inside a restaurant anyway—and it was disconcerting having *that* next to me. It resembled a body in a coffin! As I sat there, I could see this thing in the background. It was 12:30 in the afternoon. You'd better believe it. But I had to keep looking back at the coats. I kept telling myself it was ridiculous. There were just two coats on the chair. I can't account for these crazy things—I had one Rob Roy—the body was there before the cocktail and after it, but it finally went away. I kept saying to myself, 'I know they're just coats. This is ridiculous!'

But out of the corner of my eye, the side of my head, or whatever . . . that silly vision kept coming in. In minutes, it was over. I was very glad. It lasted five or ten minutes, but it seemed like hours."

The patient, who came from a city many miles away, was in a town more than ten miles away from my office when this episode occurred. She had no knowledge of any of the aforementioned events in my life.

The patient, whose own life was haunted by many tragic deaths when she was young, was a very dependent person. In her psychopathology she isolated herself from contacts with others. For these and many other specific reasons, it was conjectured that, like Professor Tenhaeff's paragnosts, (1960, 1962, 1965), she was poignantly sensitized for psychically apprehending such a tragic event in the life of her physician. She dramatically projected in her vivid telepathic hallucination her physician's grim joke. Her experience was in emotional resonance with her physician, to whom she was bound in transferring her dependent feelings and longings. Her experience might also be interpreted as a means of mastering the threatened separation of the future (death). Her projection could also be viewed as a repetition of her past tragedies. It condensed her underlying ambivalence of fear and dread of her repressed hostile wishes for what might happen. This was manifest in her anxiety over her new job and boss. This case was part of a psychic nexus and is more fully discussed elsewhere (Schwarz, 1971).

Other examples of the in-practice category include the combining of telepathic and telekinetic phenomena. These episodes, however, which are much rarer, seem to have a much greater repressed affective charge for the people involved and are, if possible, even more revealing and difficult to present (Schwarz, 1968, 1969).

Strictly Personal

These possible telepathic episodes of everyday life comprise husband-and-wife and adult-to-adult exchanges. These events are the most poignant and intimate. A. A. Brill (1956) once wrote how the favorite joke was an excellent way of understanding the patient in his life. He had many hilarious examples, but when people in the audience would ask him what *his* favorite joke was, he dodged their questions by saying he would give only his second-best joke. And so it is with what follows.

Example 11 —Once in the midst of trying times in my practice and personal life, I was upset because the Swedish mother's helper for our children, Britt-Marie, had insisted on going to New York and consorting with what I considered to be some wild-eyed playboys. After setting very strict limits on Britt-Marie to the effect that she either stayed home or we would send her back to Sweden, my wife and I went out to dinner and I told a colleague about this annoyance.

Although Britt-Marie was engaged to a boy in Sweden, she wanted to have fun with American boys. Feeling morally responsible for her, I tried to make light of a situation that could be dangerous for her (and myself) by jokingly telling my colleague: "I'd like to send Britt-Marie a dozen roses from Sweden and say they are from her boyfriend to remind her of her vows."

Later that evening, when I returned from the restaurant to my home and signed in with the answering service, I was stunned to learn that at the approximate time of my joke in reference to Britt-Marie, her fiancé had telephoned from Sweden, for no apparent reason. It was felt that this could have been a long-distance telepathic episode because of the specific psychodynamics which beautifully served the needs of Britt-Marie, her fiancé, myself, and my family.

This example occurred in the midst of some spectacular telepathic fireworks involving an unusual patient (Schwarz, 1966).

Example 12—During my studies of Joseph Dunninger, he once mentioned how he had heard about Mrs. Marie L. D'Alessio of New Jersey, who told him of her experience with a presumed phantom telephone call. Coming from Dunninger, one of the world's foremost telepathists, who had seen almost everything—legitimate and otherwise—in his investigations of psychic phenomena for more than sixty years, such a statement naturally made me curious. Dunninger would not be easily fooled with well-intentioned but unconsciously spurious examples, outright fraud, nonsense, and the like.

When we interviewed Mrs. D'Alessio, she confirmed her weird phantom-telephone-call experience. Mrs. D'Alessio told me that many years ago, she once dreamed of a girlhood friend Lorna, who sank into a pool of blood. Because this was similar to past dreams that symbolized something tragic, she told her husband, who suggested that she call her friend, whom she hadn't seen in a long time and who lived many miles away. The husband witnessed the call and learned that Lorna had gone into the hospital the previous week, but, "Because of a cold they sent me home, and I'm going in tomorrow."

"I [Mrs. D'Alessio] said I'd like to visit her, and she said she preferred that I didn't because she would contact me. When I didn't receive any call, or

Christmas card, I thought something was funny. I tried calling her, and, not receiving any response, I phoned a neighbor who said that Lorna had died. I thought, Lorna must have died in November (the time of the dream-prompted call)." The neighbor said that Lorna's husband was still away in Florida and that he would come and see me when he returned. When he visited us he said that everything I told him was true except for one thing— that I must have been mistaken about when I spoke to Lorna, because she had died on May 20th, some six months before I phoned her.

While listening to Mrs. D'Alessio's account of the grim alleged voice-after-death commentary, I wondered if she had had any humorous telepathic examples. She might have picked up my thoughts, for she laughed and gave me an amusing, possibly telepathic experience pertaining to her son, Arthur, who was in college in Georgia, more than 800 miles away. Mrs. D'Alessio dreamed: ". . . that our son Arthur was upset and couldn't find the key. I woke up my husband and told him. He said, 'What did you wake me up for?'—I always do that—my husband then said, 'Well, what could it be?' So the next morning I phoned Arthur, although I always hesitated calling him because he didn't like it; he wanted to be a man and show that he was on his own. However, Arthur laughed and said that at the time of my dream he was taking a shower, and the boys in the fraternity house locked him out of his room and took the key. He had to sleep on a couch in the hallway wrapped in a towel."

When I returned home from my visit to Dunninger, I dictated my notes of Mrs. D'Alessio's examples. I wondered about the weird, witnessed, alleged voice-after-death situation. In my mind this grim event seesawed with the more palatable locked-out-of-the-room situation, which was easier to understand. I told my secretary and members of my family about them. The locked-out-of-the-room example was similar to other reported humorous examples where a mother telepathically tuned in on her sons when they were away at college (Schwarz, 1965).

While still chuckling over the "slipped on the banana peel," missing-key example, and thereby denying the fascinating but frustrating case of the phantom-voice telephone conversation, I retired to my bedroom and closed the French doors. Since my wife had acute influenza, she was sleeping in a different room. When I awoke next morning, I had to dress in a hurry in order to see an early patient. I was shocked to discover that the doors to my bedroom were locked. Try hard as I could, the custom-made, gold-plated latch was immovable. Although we had lived in this house for sixteen years, this had never happened before. I naturally thought my wife had played a trick on me, carried away by the funny example I told her about before retiring. However,

I was puzzled about how she could lock the doors when there was no key. I still felt she must have done something and that it was in bad taste, since I was pressed for time. Finally, in desperation I phoned from the private line in the bedroom to the office phone, located in another part of the house, and my wife came to the rescue and opened the doors by releasing the top and bottom latches of the companion door. We both had a hearty laugh, for she was not responsible for this incident. To discover the difficulty and satisfy my curiosity, I removed the lock, which my wife took to a locksmith. When he opened it, he commented that one of the pieces of the mechanism had slipped down and jammed. We laughed again, but couldn't help wondering how this strange, bizarre coincidence could happen. It seemed that for indulging myself on the unfortunate plight of another, I received the horse laugh on myself, and thereby could not possibly deny the weird phantom-voice example and the difficulties in formulating an explanation.

Example 13—This highly personal example might be familiar to anyone who has had contact with the Internal Revenue Service. Once, my wife and I were having our annual income tax checked by a particularly redoubtable gentleman. Although he had little need to prove to us his expertise in mathematics, he seemed to insist on demonstrating his skills. At the conclusion of our session, he graciously accepted my invitation for lunch. While he and I resolved some of our tensions in a nearby restaurant, my wife, who was home alone, noted that the agent had left some papers in plain view, scattered on the desk. Although it undoubtedly was wrong, she could not resist the temptation to glance at the top papers, which were reports by a previous IRS examiner. When the agent and I returned to complete the task, he entered the room first and sat next to my wife. When I walked into the room, I don't know what madness seized me—for it could only have been that—but I put my hand to my chest, my hat to my heart, and started coughing. The agent blanched and in a very short while excused himself, saying he could readily finish the rest of the job in his office. Our ordeal was over. As soon as the agent left, my wife could hardly contain her laughter, for she told me the contents of the visually purloined former agent's notes. They were to the effect that the former agent was trying to justify to his supervisor my low income in previous years by stating that "The doctor, a psychiatrist, does not work as hard as the general practitioner who sees many more patients, because he had had pulmonary tuberculosis."

Possibly my wife had telepathically sent me the necessary information in this uncomfortable situation, which I had unconsciously acted out in our behalf, with a near-catastrophic effect on the IRS agent's psyche. If I had known what my wife knew, I could never have played such a ham role. My secret, which, was the agent's also, had boomeranged to my benefit. As a postscript, it might be added that the agent and I are both well and my wife and I even received a small refund that year.

Comments

What do all these examples have in common? Why might they be funny? What purpose does presumed telepathy serve in humor or vice versa? And how might telepathically tinged humor differ from other humor?

From these examples and others, it would seem that most of the telepathically-mediated humorous events occurred under keyed-up, or crisis, circumstances. One person was trying to suppress or repress a secret or information that would be embarrassing to him, while another person was unwittingly revealing the information. For both persons, the telepathic data symbolized an important part of their lives or their body image in relation to the other. Usually at the height of the polarized emotions, there was a telepathic crisscross between the two persons, and the forbidden or forgotten material suddenly exploded to the surface. Depending on the psychodynamics, this forbidden material telepathically catalyzed the data and usually signaled a change in the interpersonal relationships. Or perhaps it was analogous to Ehrenwald's description of *kairos* and the existential shift (1967). The whole process was, of course, on an unconscious level: a secret was divined or a situation uncovered without awareness of what either person had actually stumbled upon.

Telepathy in humor might be like some of the intuitive flashes of the genius or poet (Schwarz, 1967) and be akin to the folklore axioms of "love at first sight" or "first impressions are correct," for telepathy short-circuits social amenities, penetrates hypocrisy, and exposes redundant diplomacy. It can strike like lightning, have the pull of a magnet, and go to the heart of the matter. By catching us off guard, telepathy arouses our curiosity and has the ring of the uncanny. The combination of the sublime and ridiculous is akin to the unexpected or incongruous responses that are often seen in humor. The unconscious, which does not know the difference between fact and fantasy, magic and reality, provides the woof and warp of telepathy and humor. A situation which can be grimly suitable for shuddering or weeping can also paradoxically evoke laughter. Better to laugh than to cry.

Telepathy can serve a useful purpose in preparing us for emergencies and maintaining homeostasis. Like much ordinary humor, telepathically mediated or occasioned humor might not be funny to its participants at the time, but may indeed be so to outside observers. Later, when the participants have recovered from their bewilderment, they too can laugh. The observers' amusement is similar to the mirth of an audience watching a previously hypnotized subject carry out posthypnotic commands while offering ridiculous rationalizations for his actions. Such a situation is familiar to the astonished audiences who gleefully witness the fireworks between telepathic gladiators such as Dunninger or Romano and their willing or unwilling subjects.

As one cannot tell the same joke twice to an audience and get the same laughter the second time, telepathic events, like involuntary humor, are uncontrived and spontaneous.

Both telepathy and humor often display a high degree of inventiveness and creativity. Telepathy, occurring at a crisis point, almost always dovetails the needs of both parties. Telepathy is a two-way street. It is similar to jokes with a snappy punch line. The analysis of humorous telepathic events reveals sender-receiver roles not too dissimilar to the comedy team (e.g., Laurel and Hardy) with a buffoon and a straight man. One is as necessary as the other. Although some of the data in this study suggest that telepathically-mediated humor might act as regressive survival function, some of the material might also be interpreted as a progressive function, reaching out into new directions and trying to establish a more stable equilibrium.

Highly successful statistical ESP laboratory experiments are notoriously difficult to repeat. There might be good physiological and psychopathological reasons for this. Eisenbud (1972) has remarked that in such studies any success at all is unusual since the experiments seem to be designed to insure failure. Like involuntary humor, telepathy in the psychotherapeutic relationship is the quintessence of spontaneity and improvisation in the subtle nuances of ever-shifting and changing interpersonal relationships. By its very nature telepathy is hard to confine. The complex, humorous events, particularly the presumed telepathic ones, are stripped of much of their glamour and mirth when reduced to print.

Both telepathy and humor might have Scheherazade-like effects. It will be recalled how the Oriental heroine Scheherazade could only save herself from being strangled on the orders of her husband, the Sultan, by telling him a new story every night. Her 1001 Arabian tales had to be fascinating, creative, and spontaneous if she were to survive. In order to hold the Sultan's rapt attention, she undoubtedly had to be able to understand her own resistance to the unusual (telepathic-like situations) in order to be able to penetrate the Sultan's defenses. It was a transfer-countertransfer situation—a problem of understanding resistances with her life at stake (Eisenbud, 1963; Meerloo, 1968). Thus, like Scheherazade in a precarious predicament, telepathy and humor fundamentally have their serious aspects; yet, paradoxically, when they surface, they often appear to be trivial, insignificant, or coincidental.

Possibly a deeper exploration of the subject of telepathy and humor would yield many clues about this relatively neglected but important means of human communication.

References

Bergler, E. *Laughter and the sense of humor.* New York: Intercontinental Medical Book, 1956.

Brill, A. A. *Lectures on psychoanalytic psychiatry.* New York: Vantage, 1956.

Dunninger, J. *What's on your mind?* Cleveland: World, 1944.

Ebon, M. *They knew the unknown.* New York: World, 1971.

Ehrenwald, J. Hippocrates, kairos and the existential shift. *American Journal of Psychoanalysis,* 1967, **29,** 89–93.

Eisenbud, J. Psychiatric contributions to parapsychology: a review. *Journal of Parapsychology,* 1949, **13,** 251–252.

———. Psi and the nature of things. *International Journal of Parapsychology,* 1963, **5,** 245–272.

———. *The world of Ted Serios.* New York: Morrow, 1967.

———. *Psi and psychoanalysis.* New York: Grune & Stratton, 1970.

———. Some notes on the psychology of the paranormal. *Journal of the American Society for Psychical Research,* 1972, **66,** 27–41.

Fodor, N. *Telepathic dreams: telepathy in analysis, new approaches to dream interpretation.* New York: Citadel, 1951.

Meerloo, J. A. M. Sympathy and telepathy: a model for psychodynamic research in parapsychology. *International Journal of Parapsychology,* 1968, **10,** 57–83.

Poland, W. S. The place of humor in psychotherapy. *American Journal of Psychiatry,* 1971, **128,** (11), 5.

Pollack, J. H. *Croiset the clairvoyant.* Garden City, N.Y.: Doubleday, 1964.

Richet, C. *Thirty years of psychic research.* New York: Macmillan, 1923.

Schwarz, B. E. *Psychic-dynamics.* New York: Pageant Press, 1965.

———. Built-in controls and postulates for the telepathic event. *Corrective Psychiatry and Journal of Social Therapy,* 1966, **12,** 64–82.

———. The telepathic hypothesis and genius: a note on Thomas A. Edison. *Corrective Psychiatry and Journal of Social Therapy,* 1967, **13,** 7–19.

———. Possible telesomatic reactions. *Journal of the Medical Society of New Jersey,* 1967, **64,** 600–603.

———. *The Jacques Romano story.* New Hyde Park, N.Y.: University Books, 1968.

———. *A psychiatrist looks at ESP.* New York: New American Library, 1968.

———. Telepathy and pseudotelekinesis in psychotherapy. *Journal of the American Society of Psychosomatic Dentistry and Medicine,* 1968, **15,** 144–154.

———. Synchronicity and telepathy. *Psychoanalytical Review,* 1969, **56,** 44–56.

———. *Parent-child telepathy.* New York: Garrett, 1971.

———. Precognition and psychic nexus. *Journal of the American Society of Psychosomatic Dentistry and Medicine,* Part I, 1971, **18** (2), 52–59; Part II, 1971, **18** (3), 83–93.

Tenhaeff, W. H. C. Proceedings of the Parapsychological Institute of the State University of Utrecht. 1960, **1** (12); 1962, **2;** 1965, **3.**

Shafica Karagulla

Higher Sense Perception and New Dimensions of Creativity

TODAY, MAN IS pacing the outer perimeter of his five senses with an increasing awareness of limitations. Are there things to be sensed which his five senses do not encompass? Is a breakthrough occurring in the field of human perception? Is man breaking through the five–sense barrier into the realm of higher sense perception? Is a mutation in consciousness taking place?

My research in the last fourteen years has convinced me that there are many people today breaking through the five–sense barrier into higher octaves of awareness and perception. In 1967, I published a book entitled, *Breakthrough to Creativity—Your Higher Sense Perception* describing many of these HSP gifts and their application in the scientific community and in all walks of life (Karagulla, 1967). I found many individuals exhibiting a greater degree of creativity in their respective fields of work because of their gifts of higher sense perception.

Precognition and prophecy are actually a breaking of the time barrier. Individuals with this ability to break through the time barrier are able to see events in the future and to adjust their plans and activities accordingly. Sometimes they are able to take precautions to avoid an injury or adjust their activities to coming events. One sensitive with whom I worked twice avoided being in train wrecks because of her precognitive perceptions. Each time she got off the train before she reached her destination and before the wreck occurred. A physician, who is endowed with unusual precognitive ability which he uses in his practice, discussed his gifts with me. One incident will serve to illustrate his use of his abilities in his practice. While he was performing surgery on a patient with a blood clot in the right leg, he suddenly perceived a clot beginning to form in the left leg. He instructed his assistant to quickly prepare for an incision in the left leg. He was able to get to the blood clot in the left leg just as it was forming and in time to save the patient's life.

Telepathy breaks through the sound barrier. Many people are able to communicate across long distances on some kind of mental wave band. Many people do this a few times in their lives. There are a few who are able to do this more often under controlled scientific conditions. This ability has been recognized for hundreds of years, but today we are conducting scientific experiments to establish the validity of this kind of communication.

The dowser is breaking the touch barrier. He can sense or feel water flowing underground. Or he may be able to locate minerals, or discover archaeological sites, which lie underground. There are individuals who can feel the pain of a sick patient in their own bodies, and help to locate and diagnose the patient's problem. There are physicians with this ability, and they usually turn out to have a reputation for being very remarkable diagnosticians.

There are sensitives who insist that they can smell emotional or mental conditions. This is a type of breaking through the smell barrier. There are many individuals who will say that they "smell" something wrong with a situation. One politician insists that he can smell intrigue, and that it is actually a physical sensation to him.

Many people are able to break through the sight barrier to a greater or a lesser degree. I have worked with a few very gifted individuals who have the capacity of seeing into and through solid objects, including the human body. My data, collected over a period of fourteen years, as I have worked with these particular individuals, give valuable information about the constitution and condition of man. Orthodox medicine has now accepted the fact that electromagnetic energy emanates from man. However, the individuals who can see into and through the human body describe at least four other fields of energy, described below, that can be perceived independently, but not simultaneously. These fields are in addition to the electromagnetic field. These individuals can describe multiple energy fields and the changes which occur in them. The fields should be considered physical in nature with laws governing them just as physical laws govern the electromagnetic field.

The first described is the (E) field. It is also designated as the vital energy field or the etheric field. It is in this field that these sensitive persons discern the blueprint of the biological system. The (E) field penetrates every cell and molecule of the body, and extends for three to five centimeters beyond the body in a bluish grey haze.

The second field described by the sensitive is the (S) field, the sentient or emotional field. In this are seen the quality and the characteristics of the person's emotions and feelings. Emotional storms and stresses which disturb the individual can be perceived in this field much as a changing pattern of colors.

The third, the (M) field or mental field, exhibits the quality of the mind and thinking of the individual. It shows the changes in the mental response to environment.

These three fields each have within them seven major vortices of energy. These are interlocked and act as transformers from the mental to the emotional to the etheric and finally to the level of the physical body. These findings of the sensitive regarding his energy relationship give credence to our present-day concepts of psychosomatic medicine.

The fourth field is an integrating field which holds the first three fields in relationship and alignment. It is this fourth field that makes it possible for the individual to express the higher types of creativity.

The first field or (E) field has seven major vortices located in a straight line in the center of the body. These seven major vortices are related to the endocrine glands. Any changes from the normal in these vortices of energy are related to, and indicate changes in, specific endocrine glands and in the physical condition of the patient. I have made many case studies of these vortices in the (E) field evaluating the changes that take place in health and disease (Karagulla, 1967).

The energy vortex at the throat shows a harmonious rhythm and a pale blue violet color in the healthy individual. This vortex is related to the thyroid gland. It took several years of research with sensitives to establish this norm in the healthy individual. This was necessary in order to be able to evaluate the abnormal. If the rhythm is jerky, disharmonious, too slow or too fast, there is trouble in the throat area or in the thyroid gland. The appearance of red or orange color instead of the normal blue violet also indicates problems in this area or with this gland. Certain changes from the norm indicate tumor of the thyroid, which may be either benign or malignant. Early changes from the norm in this vortex appear before the actual disease appears in the physical body. Disturbance in this vortex will often appear many months before the actual disease can be diagnosed in the physical body. If we can devise sensors that can pick up what the sensitives perceive in this (E) field or in the (E) vortices, we could predict ahead of time what will happen in the physical body. This could make possible predictive and preventive measures in dealing with the disease processes.

Healers appear to be able to affect the (E) field of patients. However, there are many types of healers, and this kind of healing is more complicated than is immediately apparent. The so-called healers do show an (E) field greater in width and flexibility than that of other people. The hands and fingers of people with true healing ability show an extension of the (E) field to a far greater distance than the three to five centimeters observed in other people. Many healers appear to actually energize the patient and improve the energy level of the patient's field. Many individuals who do not show a definite pathology may show a weak or devitalized field. In this case a healer can achieve helpful results very quickly.

The (E) field itself may show a number of different deviations from the norm. It may appear devitalized or show fragmentation, it may appear droopy or too loose. All of these conditions indicate either present or eventual conditions in the physical body. It is interesting to note that in the case of trance-mediumship, the solar plexus vortex is disturbed and the etheric field appears loose and shows fragmentation. The trance medium is nearly always susceptible to diseases in the solar plexus area.

We are beginning to understand this whole realm of energy fields and their interaction, and this understanding is throwing new light on what we have already discovered in the fields of medicine and psychology. For the individual to be truly creative, his fields must be well-integrated. If he is too mentally or emotionally passive, he can be controlled by others. The highest type of creative work is accomplished when an individual is fully mentally alert and aware and in command of his own free will at all times. In any state of pacifity when someone else is controlling the mind of another person, there is loss of free will and there can be dangers to both parties concerned.

The most creative individuals are well-integrated and have a capacity for mental focus directed by their own free will. This state of awareness is the most favorable condition for that flash of inspiration which brings in new concepts and new ideas. Each individual has the capacity within himself to use his own creative potential. Human beings have always demonstrated this creative process, and today especially in the fields of medicine, geology, physics, chemistry, and the behavioral sciences.

Human society today is faced with a dilemma of a breakdown or a breakthrough within the human being himself. Our breakthrough in science and technology, coming with unbelievable rapidity, has precipitated a crisis within the consciousness of man himself. There must be a breakthrough in human consciousness to match the breakthrough in science and technology. As always, certain evolutionary developments begin with the few and gradually extend to the many.

A breakthrough in human consciousness gradually producing an increasing number of people with higher sense perception can reshape our world. Man must become aware of his superconscious and be able to tap this creative level with full awareness. Individuals receptive to the hitherto unperceived dimensions of environment can initiate the creative society.

So far, no society has ever had for its aim and purpose the discovery and development of the unlimited potentials of man himself.

Many societies have exploited man, conquered man, enslaved man, destroyed man. Our present society is on a collision course to destroy man. Whether before this happens or after a cataclysm, present development points to a Phoenix-like resurrection of the human spirit.

A new society will arise from the ashes of the old in which ever larger numbers of the human race will move forward into the exhilarating discovery of new dimensions of reality and experience. This truly creative society will seek to produce not the superman, but the supersane humanity, moving into new and higher dimensions of moral, mental, and spiritual perception and purpose.

References

Karagulla, Shafica, and Robertson, Elizabeth. Psychical phenomena in temporal lobe epilepsy and the psychoses. *British Medical Journal,* 1955 (4916); pp. 748–752.

Karagulla, Shafica. *Breakthrough to creativity—your higher sense perception.* Los Angeles: DeVorss, 1967.

Jule Eisenbud

Research in Precognition

PRECOGNITION IS generally defined as foreknowledge of a randomly-occurring future event not based upon inference from presently available data. Under roughly equivalent terms, such as "foreknowledge," "prevision," "prophecy," and the like, this phenomenon has been recorded in the dreams and visions of men since earliest times. And for almost as long—since the birth of civilization as we know it, at any rate—men have set themselves sternly against the very possibility of such a thing. In modern times this is one point on which the church and science are in perfect agreement.

The recalcitrant data, however, continue to pile up and to remain open to investigation. The four main types of data are: (1) documented reports of spontaneous precognitive occurrences in dreams, visions, premonitions, and so forth; (2) precognitive representations made by specially gifted psychics; (3) laboratory experiments, and (4) precognitive events observed in the psychotherapeutic situation.

There is little that need be said about the first category, which constitutes the largest part of the phenomenology of precognition. Several documented collections have been published (Lyttelton, 1937; Rhine, 1954; Saltmarsh, 1938; Sidgwick, 1888; Stevenson, 1970). A few of these have been subjected to various types of analysis, such as for content, form of occurrence (whether in dream, waking hallucination, etc.), degree of realism of representation, and so forth (Rhine, 1954; Stevenson, 1970). Case reports continue to appear in journals of psychical research and parapsychology in several languages and for the last few years there have been Central Premonitions Registries in England and in the United States to which persons may send dreams and premonitions felt to be prophetic.

It has been noted that events of common concern to large numbers of people, like the sinking of the liner *Titanic* some years ago (Stevenson, 1960) and the tragic engulfment of many school children by a mountain of slag in a Welch mining town, the Aberfan disaster (Baker, 1967), tend to be foreshadowed by multiple premonitory references in dreams and other types of experience on the part of many people. The largest share of spontaneous precognitive occurrences, however, appear to be isolated instances and, like ordinary dreams, tend to deal with trivial events.

The chief value of the second category of data, data supplied by specially gifted psychics, is the opportunity for precise registration of the prediction before its fulfillment, which is not often the case with purely spontaneous occurrences, unless a person happens to be so struck by his dream or vision that he makes special note of it in a diary or letter, or tells others of it. Thus, many recorded sessions with the noted medium Mrs. Leonard, to mention just one, contained material which turned out to be strikingly precognitive (Smith, 1964). However, one of the most extensively studied precognitive psychics of recent times, Gerard Croiset of Holland, does not operate within a mediumistic framework but employs the so-called "chair test," a format developed in the twenties by a French psychic. The essential idea of the chair test is that the sensitive makes a series of statements supposed to apply to a person or persons to be chosen at random (in the early tests it was the chairs to be occupied by these people which were chosen) from a number of people assembled in a hall or auditorium at a later date. Over the past twenty-five years, dozens of such tests have been carried out, with Croiset making the predictive statements, using different groups in Europe and America. Well over 50% have been attended with striking success according to the methods of evaluation of results available in the situation. In all tests, the predictive statements have been carefully recorded well in advance of the date of testing, and the methods used for ensuring a random selection of the target persons (or chairs) were scrutinized and carried out by experimenters other than Croiset or his mentor, Profesor W. H. C. Tenhaeff of the State University of Utrecht (Tenhaeff, 1960; Timm, 1966).

A transatlantic chair-test was done in 1969 with Croiset in Utrecht, Holland, and an audience assembled in Denver (Eisenbud, 1973). Among the statements made by Croiset on January 6, was that the person who would be selected for the second of two target persons would be a man about five feet nine inches in height, who brushed his black hair straight back, had a gold tooth in his lower jaw, a scar on his big toe, who worked in both science and industry and sometimes got his lab coat stained by a greenish chemical. With the exception of the item about the man's height (he turned out to be five feet nine and three-quarters), all of these statements and several others besides did apply to a man chosen by supervised random selection from among 24 persons who, from among 100 people present, volunteered as participants in the test given on January 23, two and one-half weeks after the predictive statements were made. The target person was a physicist at a large industrial concern doing classified work with a green chemical which did indeed stain his lab coat. Among eleven physicists in his department, he was the only one with a gold tooth.

The importance of formal, clear, and precise prior registration of the predictive statements of psychics claiming precognitive abilities cannot be too strongly emphasized. Several years ago I was party at second-hand to a series of extraordinary predictions made by a Chicago psychic, Mrs. Nora Sanders. These predictions came in the form of visions, which were communicated to Mrs. Pauline Oehler of Wilmette. Not long after Mrs. Oehler had adopted a system of putting these predictions on postcards and having them independently validated, postmarked, and sent to several witnesses in the scientific community, I received a card describing "a new star with a tail" approaching the earth. This was on January 11, 1965. On February 15th came the communication: "Has been seeing the new star again. . . . Thinks it has already been observed and recorded but the fact has not been announced." This was followed on February 16th by: "Sees a Chinaman looking at a star. Asks: Could there be a Chinaman, perhaps in a California observatory?" Eight months later, at the end of September, 1965, two Japanese astronomers announced the discovery of a new comet with a tail, which was subsequently named after them. At the time of the predictions in January and February, the comet was unsuspected by anyone.

A little more than a year later, Mrs. Sanders was awakened at 3:05 a.m. by a vision of a terrible explosion. She phoned Mrs. Oehler at 3:08 a.m. to give the details. She saw people jumping out of bed to investigate, gave the direction from her house, described a one-story factory building a block square with large multi-paned windows. Mrs. Oehler immediately took a report of this vision to the local police station, where it was witnessed and time-stamped by the lieutenant on duty at 3:59 a.m. Shortly after four, the report was put into the mail. At 6:19 a.m., three hours and fourteen minutes after the vision, an explosion of cyanide gas touched off a massive fire in a block-square factory about twenty-five miles from Mrs. Sanders' home in the direction given. The larger part of the plant, which was almost totally destroyed, had only one story and was banded on two sides by a continuous stretch of small-paned windows.

Since the explosion took place before its "prediction" could reach me through the mail, Mrs. Oehler phoned me several hours after its occurrence to tell me about the whole thing and informed me triumphantly that a victory call to the skeptical police would be next. "You needn't call them," I ventured, "they'll call you."

Unfortunately, the predictions made by this psychic are just vague enough to be discounted by the skeptical. For one thing, they are imbedded in great masses of predictive statements which have not panned out. Many of those that have, moreover, such as dramatic presentiments of danger to Martin Luther King, Jr., Moise Tshombe, and Robert Kennedy, were about of the same order of probability, even when made in 1965, as that a member of the Dallas Cowboys football team would suffer a sprained shoulder within a five-year period.

It was precisely because of the tantalizing ambiguity of data of this kind, and because of the impossibility or unfeasibility, even in the case of Croiset's chair tests, of successfully using conventional statistical methods to provide a more or less definite yes or no to the question of the chance factor, that investigators withdrew to the comparative simplicity of the laboratory. Here precognitive events could be trapped within a framework in which not only the time span involved could be precisely controlled but where, within a closed probability situation, the chance factor could be precisely defined. Moreover the question of exactly what constituted a hit could be made susceptible to either precise definition or great simplification.

A considerable variety of experimental formats have been used to entrap precognitive data within the statistical framework of the laboratory. For reasons of economy, I will give examples of only three types.

An extensive card-calling experiment was carried out in London during the grim war years of 1941 to 1943 (Soal & Goldney, 1943). The subject had already achieved some notoriety as a gifted prognosticator. In something like 11,000 trials the overall results were on the order of 10^{34} to 1 against chance. There were also internal evidences of a high degree of paranormality. For instance, when the rate of calling was approximately doubled from one call every two-and-one-half seconds to one call every second, the hits jumped the card next to be in the target position, the regular position for the precognitive effect, and piled up on the card *two* yet to come. Moreover, the scoring rates varied with the particular agents (whose task was to view the target cards) so that when individual agents were switched without the subject's knowledge, the scoring rates went from highly significant to chance level and back again, according to the agent used.

In a second type of experiment the spontaneous decay of Strontium 90 was used as a randomizing system. Subjects were asked to guess the arrival time of the next electron hitting a Geiger-Mueller tube registering an average of 10 electrons per second, as determined by a 4-position electronic switch rotating at the rate of 4 million steps per second. According to the fundamental axiom stating that quantum processes are unpredictable, most people are expected to obtain only chance scores. But three subjects culled from preliminary trials to weed out all but high scorers together obtained a scoring rate on approximately 63,000 trials which would be expected by chance only once in 500 million trials (Schmidt, 1969a, 1969b).

In a third experiment done recently by two French biologists (Duval & Montredon, 1968), mice were the subjects in a cage divided by a low central partition across which they could jump. A random selector directed an electric current to one or the other half of the cage in a normally unpredictable sequence. The idea was to see if the mice would act as if they knew what was coming by managing to be in the nonshocking side of the cage more than they would be expected to by chance. In order to minimize human influence, all recording was automatic. What amounted to animal precognition was inferred from the highly significant results of two extensive series of tests. A repetition of this experiment by American investigators yielded an only moderately significant result (Levy et al., 1971), and it is not yet clear whether the French mice were psychically more gifted or any of several other hypotheses could best account for the discrepant results.

A study by an American investigator (Cox, 1956) some years ago, however, showed that American railroad travelers, at least, were as good as the French mice which jumped from the wrong to the right side of the tracks. Cox's study showed that fewer than the normally expected number of passengers tended to show up on trains which were about to have a mishap.

From the standpoint of demonstrating simply that the phenomenon of precognition (as defined) exists, the statistical experimental method is as objection free as any known method of arriving at reliable inference. From the standpoint of telling us what precognition is all about, however, this method suffers from certain limitations. These limitations are the same as those that plague just about all parapsychological experiments contrived to isolate and manipulate selected variables. They arise from the fact that when capacities for which there are no known barriers are being dealt with, it is impossible to shield the subjects from influences not called for in the design of the experiment. Thus, one cannot eliminate the possible influence of the unconscious attitudes, biases, and hopes of everyone connected with the experiment, not least of all the experimenters themselves. It may very well be for this reason that most first-shot experiments, the brain children of very much involved experimenters plumping for one hypothesis or another, give results that, however marginal (if they pan out at all), fail to be confirmed in subsequent replications. And if the results do manage to get confirmed at the first attempted replication, they are apt to fail at the second hurdle, and so on until results wash out altogether. The one reliable inference that can be drawn from this state of affairs is that despite the many fancy twists that have emerged in breakdowns of statistically processed experiments, only the fact that psi can be observed to show up in a variety of ways is demonstrable. This applies to experiments in precognition. Nothing like a reliable correlation between a given condition and a specified result has been shown to stick after repeated attempts at replication. Indeed, it might well be asked how worthwhile it is to go on contriving elaborate laboratory set-ups merely to show that psychic capacities, like fluids and gases, can be poured into containers of an infinite variety of shapes.

One of the containers into which precognitive occurrences now and again find their way is the dyadic psychotherapeutic relationship. What this framework for observation lacks in simplicity and rigor is counterbalanced by the opportunity it provides for more or less continuous study of the multi-dimensional life context in which the precognitive event occurs. It also enables observers to make proper note of such events, for example, in dreams, prior to any fulfillment.

Only a handful of psychiatrists and analysts have reported precognitive dreams (Ehrenwald, 1954; Eisenbud, 1954, 1956, 1969; Fodor, 1948, 1955; Greenbank, 1966; Servadio, 1955), which may indeed be because of the comparative rarity of this type of event in the clinical situation. I myself have observed only three dozen instances of what I would call truly precognitive dreams in almost as many years. The investigation of these comparatively rare events, however, can yield data of considerable interest and importance.

What emerges from the study of precognitive events within the clinical setting, particularly dreams, is that such events are not simply random flashes of some supernatural spark, or the meaningless lifting of a veil to reveal an ordinarily inscrutable future, but an adaptive maneuver on the part of a personality striving toward the fulfillment of its needs. But while most dreams accomplish their wishful alterations of reality by fantasied situational manipulations, the precognitive dream in its very nature allows the ultimate transcendence of reality by escaping from the domination of the one thing governing all else in nature, time, which more than anything else signifies hard and seemingly unalterable fate. It is thus particularly where time and fate are virtually identical, such as in the loss of one's biological powers or of loved ones, that the precognitive dream can be seen to set the stage for an unconscious syllogism to the effect that, "If one miracle, why not another?" If time can be reversed, why cannot the dreamer regain a lost fertility, or a waning virility, or a loved one, or even annihilate the generation gap that puts a secretly desired parent a fixed time span ahead and forever out of reach? The evidence for the relationship of the precognitive dream to this last, described under the heading of "Time and the Oedipus" (Eisenbud, 1956), continues to mount.

Other psychological problems, too, can be seen to be dealt with in the precognitive dream, problems covering the full scale of human involvements. Let me give an example. On leaving my office one day, I became aware of a certain lightheadedness. I started down the corridor to the elevator, and just as I came abreast of the adjoining apartment, my next-door neighbor came out. After the usual salutation, she began to complain (I being a doctor) that she could not rid herself of a distressing bronchitis, despite three weeks of steaming. After giving her some advice, mainly to discontinue the steaming—I found that she had kept the nozzle of the steamer about one foot from her head—I put my arm around her in a friendly fashion as we continued down the corridor together. From the very first moment I did this, however, I became aware that this was a displacement of my feelings for a woman patient who had just left my office a few minutes before. The lightheadedness disappeared at once. The next day a male patient reported the following dream, which he had had about fifteen to eighteen hours *before* the episode just described. *"I was observing you in your office. You were stripped to the waist and were putting your arm around some woman patient. I thought, 'This is a kind of communication to facilitate therapy.' "*

Note the emphasis on observing in the manifest content of this dream, and on a kind of communication. If this latter was, as the dream had it, "to facilitate therapy," it succeeded. The patient had spent his hour before the dream trying to get into his terrible feelings of rage against the female breast, which he had fantasies of clawing and tearing off, an attitude that was not very popular with his women friends, as well as being responsible for certain somatic symptoms with which he was currently bothered. As it happened, my next-door neighbor, who could be construed, on the precognitive hypothesis, as having figured by displacement in the patient's dream, just as she had in my acting out of some hours after the dream, had had a bilateral mastectomy some months before, so there was not much there the patient could have torn off. Nor was there on me, stripped to the waist as the patient had me in his dream. What the dream did was not only highlight the specific area under discussion, which stunned the patient when I told him about the events in reality corresponding to it, but it also highlighted my own reaction formation against the kind of infantile aggressions involved. This, no doubt, had led to my acting out with the neighbor and was no doubt responsible for my exaggerated protective feelings for the patient for whom she was a stand-in.

The night after I told the patient about my part in this, he dreamed that *he was sitting in an outhouse so full of what outhouses are usually full of that the stuff came right up under his seat. Even though this gave him a nice warm feeling, it was somewhat uncomfortable. He tried to move only to find that he was unable to.* In this dream, the patient was obviously stating that what I had been telling him was a pile of crap. As so frequently happens in resistance dreams, however, the patient's very denial turned out to be an affirmation. On the night following the dream, the patient went to a party where one woman, out of the blue, told of an incident in her childhood when she fell into the muck below the outhouse seat while fishing for a ring that had fallen through, and how her mother had to strip and scour her before letting her back into the house. This story inspired the recollection by someone else at the party of an obese man in his hometown who fell into the outhouse muck when the seat gave under his weight, and of his having to be fished out by the fire department.

As you can see, the precognitive dream sometimes concerns itself with far more trivial events than the things which occupied Teiresias, Cassandra, and the prophets of old. However, it may yet turn out that as more and more instances are investigated, the unconscious will be seen as far less in awe of the sanctity of time than we are in our conscious waking lives, and that if it needs a tool to make a point in a dream, the day after tomorrow's "residues" are as good as any other "day's residues."

If this is so, certain questions immediately demand answering, such as why, if precognition is a faculty so easily available on demand, the acculturated ego in the civilized society has developed the illusion that the future is necessarily hidden except through rational prediction. It would also be in order to try to understand the nature and strength of the societal forces, including the institution of science, aimed at fostering and buttressing this illusion.

The psychiatric approach to precognition is peculiarly suited to investigate these and other problems surrounding this number one enigma of life and science. It is also advantageously equipped to make some contribution to the seemingly unanswerable problem of mechanism, not simply by providing original insights into the nature of time, a mystery which has occupied thinkers from the day the sun first rose, but by the painstaking and carefully annotated observations of phenomena which might go far toward providing important threads in a view of precognition that does not necessarily demand the ultimate of time and causality reversing themselves. Such phenomena as telepathic influence and psychokinetic effects at a distance, which might provide these threads, are also observable in the psychotherapeutic relationship where, like precognitive phenomena themselves, they are for the most part cultured products rather than purely spontaneous occurrences. It is, however, by very virtue of the fact that these cultured events are stimulated into actuality by the irritant of the transference relationship that we are able, as in the case of all other derivatives of the transference, to gain the insights we have into the nature of what is transpiring. The transference relationship is our laboratory. It is one in which objectivity and subjectivity play complementary roles. And it is a laboratory which will hopefully play an increasingly important part in research in precognition.

References

Barker, J. C. Premonitions of the Aberfan disaster. *Journal of Society of Psychological Research,* 1967, **44,** 169–181.

Cox, W. E. Precognition: an analysis II. *Journal of American Society of Psychological Research,* 1956, **60,** 99–109.

Duval, P. & Montredon, E. (pseudonyms). ESP experiments with mice. *Journal of Parapsychology,* 1968, **32,** 153–166.

Ehrenwald, J. Precognition in dreams? *Psychoanalytical Review,* 1951, **38,** 17–38.

Eisenbud, J. Behavioral correspondences to normally unpredictable future events. *Psychoanalytical Quarterly,* 1954, **23,** 205–233, 355–389.

———. Time and the Oedipus. *Psychoanalytical Quarterly,* 1956, **25,** 363–384.

———. Chronologically extraordinary psi correspondences in the psychoanalytic setting. *Psychoanalytic Review,* 1969, **56,** 9–27.

———. A transatlantic experiment in precognition with Gerard Croiset. *Journal of American Society of Psychological Research,* 1973, 67, 1–25.

Fodor, N. A precognitive diagnostic dream. *American Journal of Psychotherapy,* 1948, **2,** 658.

_____. Through the gate of horn: a clinical approach to precognitive dreams. *American Journal of Psychotherapy,* 1955, 9, 283–294.

Greenbank, R. K. A prophetic dream. *Corr. Psychiatry and Journal of Soc. Ther.,* 1966, 12, 213–218.

Levy, W. J., et al. Repetition of the French precognition experiments with mice. *Journal of Parapsychology,* 1971, 35, 1–17.

Lyttelton, E. *Some cases of prediction.* London: Bell, 1937.

Rhine, L. E. Frequency of types of experience in spontaneous precognition. *Journal of Parapsychology,* 1954, 18, 93–123.

Saltmarsh, H. F. *Foreknowledge.* London: Bell, 1938.

Schmidt, H. Precognition of a quantum process. *Journal of Parapsychology,* 1969a, 33, 99–108.

_____. Quantum processes predicted? *New Scientist,* 1969b, Oct. 16.

Servadio, E. A presumptively telepathic precognitive dream during analysis. *International Journal of Psychoanalysis,* 1955, 36, 27–30.

Sidgwick, E. On the evidence for premonitions. *Proceedings of the Society for Psychical Research,* 1888, 5, 288–354.

Smith S. *The mediumship of Mrs. Leonard.* New Hyde Park, N.Y.: University Books, 1964.

Soal, S. G., & Goldney, K. M. Experiments in precognitive telepathy. *Proc. Soc. Psych. Research,* 1943, 47, 21–150.

Stevenson, I. A review and analysis of paranormal experiences connected with the sinking of the *Titanic. Journal of American Society for Psych. Research,* 1960, 54, 153–171.

_____. Precognition of disasters. *Journal of American Society for Psych. Research,* 1970, 64, 187–210.

Tenhaeff, W. H. C. Seat experiments with Gerard Croiset. *Proc. Parapsychology.* Institute of the State University of Utrecht, 1960, 1, 53–65.

Timm, U. Neue experimente mit dem sensitiven Gerard Croiset. *Z. F. Parapsychologia und Grezgeb. dem Psychologia,* 1966, 9, 30–59.

J. B. Rhine

Security Versus Deception in Parapsychology

FROM THE SIMPLEST beginning in any science, precautions have to be taken to insure the product of the field against errors of observation, recording, logic, evaluation, reporting, and other uncertainties. In parapsychology this general concern over the basic security or reliability of the results divides conveniently into four major questions.

First: Have the experiments been firmly controlled against counterhypotheses (mainly *sensorimotor leakage*)?

Second: Have the *statistics* been appropriate?

Third: Would the problem *logically* permit a definitive conclusion if significant results were obtained?

Fourth (the topic of this paper): Has the research been adequately secure against *experimenter deception*?

The first and second of these major areas of insecurity were the leading counterissues to ESP in the 1930's. For example, the early test results at Duke were first suspected by their critics mainly of being produced either by sensory leakage or by improper handling of the statistical evaluation of the data. These were the main topics in the critical attacks made at the APA roundtable at Columbus in 1938. There, however (along with the informal meeting of the American Institute for Mathematics at Indianapolis the year before), the concern about statistics was largely quelled, and by 1940, with *ESP After Sixty Years* (Rhine, Pratt, Smith, Stuart, & Greenwood, 1940) in print, the issue over sensory cues was fairly well resolved; the successful tests for precognition that followed definitely ruled out that problem.

By 1955, another of these areas of insecurity received major attention when Dr. George Price's critique of ESP appeared in *Science* (Price, 1955). His critical attack by-passed the first two issues and moved on to number four on the list, the reliability of the research personnel. Curiously enough, however, the reason Price gave for going all-out on the issue of experimenter fraud was the number three issue on the above list—that the problem of the occurrence of ESP was not a scientific one. It simply could not qualify as he saw it. (Nevertheless, with perfect inconsistency, he did propose a test design himself, an "adequate" one.)

But in the meantime, the questionnaire studies by Dr. Lucien Warner (1952, 1955) and by Warner and C. C. Clark (1938) were bringing out strong indications that American psychologists were not rejecting the ESP hypothesis as unscientific. In large majorities they were accepting the problem (that is, as distinct from the *answer*) as a legitimate one for psychology, but they were still hung up on the first two major questions, cues and chance.

Finally question number three has now been given its day. Parapsychologists themselves are at last beginning to re-examine critically in advance of actual research the scientific testability of their hypotheses in order to avoid the wasteful frustrations of the past (I discuss this number three type of problem, with telepathy as an example, in an article to appear in this journal in June.)

The General Deception Problem

In turning now exclusively to the question of deception, I am aware that it may seem late in the day to open up a general discussion of this problem. But the late timing is not so surprising. Students of parapsychology will recall Professor Henry Sidgwick's classic prediction that questions of the honesty of investigators would arise when all other counterexplanations had failed; he expected it to be a late issue. However, it is not because of any such desperate last-ditch status of the case for the occurrence of psi phenomena that the deception problem is being opened up here now.

Rather, the stimulus for making this review came from realizing how comparatively slow the recognition of parapsychology has been, and from reflecting over the possible factors responsible for this. It occurred to me that doubts may still exist in many minds which are too unclear and unsupported to be actually expressed, but sufficient to deter a more positive interest and reaction. As I thought of the more explicit attention that has been given to the other three major questions of research reliability listed above, it appeared quite possible that this more subtle, slightly distasteful, and sometimes embarrassing issue of fraud might need more frank and forthright recognition and response.

It seemed, therefore, worth the effort to review the grounds for concern over this fourth major problem area, to outline what has already been done to cope with it, and then to show where the psi research field stands today with regard to it.

Subject Deception

To avoid confusion I will pass over the problem of deception by the test subject as belonging to question number one. In the early days when mediums and stage performers composed a large percentage of the participants in tests and demonstrations, the question of trickery applied mainly to the performers rather than to experimenters. Even as psychical research became more experimental, beginning in the 1870's, and the testing of subjects came under better control, one of the main purposes of the experimenter, of course, was to exclude all the possible deceptive (and other) practices of the subjects that would permit sensory cues. But as indicated, this exclusion of sensorimotor leakage comes under question number one. The more elementary problem of subject deception had to come first, and it has long since ceased to be a major issue.

Self-deception

Another order of deception, this one involving the experimenter himself, can also be passed over briefly here although it, too, has been an important one. This is self-deception, an expression that actually covers a range of relatively innocent mistakes. However, it parallels many of the types of deliberate trickery and is an important element in every science. I have personally seen more of this "fooling one's self" type than I have of conscious fraud. A few examples will suffice here.

Innocent, so-called "self-deception" is, of course, most likely in inexperienced observers, but it is possible even in highly trained individuals, especially those approaching parapsychology from some other field in which problems and controls are different. Even some experienced psychical researchers have been deceived for a time because of an excessive and disarming trust in, and attachment to, a test or overconfidence in a research assistant. Again, lack of experience with the dangers of defective test cards (or other test materials) or loose test conditions may mislead the honest researcher, especially one who is working in isolation. But he can also innocently misuse his records, take liberties with his statistics, and, most easily of all, make unwarranted interpretations of his results.

But let us pass over this nonfraudulent section of the experimenter-deception aspect of psi research because, first, it will be partly covered incidentally in the discussion of deliberate deception. Second, unintended errors of this kind are not likely to get by the editors of today without being detected, since they result mainly in weaknesses covered by the first and second questions. They are in any case likely to occur in the work of comparative beginners; and even with the slightly improved chances of training that are possible today, the subspecies of unprepared experimenters may soon be approaching extinction.

What About Deliberate Deception by Experimenters

Those psi researchers who have been at least suspected of being really crooked are all that are left for discussion; and in the final analysis, it can be said that this small but untrustworthy group is today all but threatened with extermination also. The known case histories go back somewhat to certain earlier stages of the research (or out to those that still need instruction in the elements of safeguarding). Let us see in brief review how reasonable this optimism appears.

Background

It is not necessary to look all the way back to the founding stages for untrustworthy psi researchers, since the weaker characters involved are not the kind to "rough it" over the first strenuous stretches of a rugged research road. They do not often appear on the scene until there is something else than the actual research results to be gained (something like easy notoriety). Also, I will stay within the more active *experimental* psi testing era that began in the 1930's, since, as I have said, the trickery in the heyday of mediumistic demonstrations almost entirely involved the subjects instead of the experimenters.

Even after my monograph, *Extra-sensory Perception* (1934), it was some years before the ugly hand of fraud began to appear among the experimenters who followed up on the ESP work. There were, incidentally, numerous and various innocent errors that were more typical of the period. For example, one well-known mathematician came to my laboratory to try to convince me that my results were meaningless (as he put it, they were close to mean chance expectation). This, he said, was about 7.5 hits for a run of 25 trials with five target symbols; but when I saw his analysis it was possible to show him his misinterpretation of the conditions of the method. (He wrongly assumed feedback on each trial.) Another visitor, one of the leading psychologists of the day (1935), reported a negative (i.e., below-chance average) deviation of approximately 2.5 hits per run on 500 runs in which he tested himself. But he refused to submit a paper for publication, and I could only infer that he made the same mistake with reference to the expected chance average that the mathematician had made, but that he was trying to *avoid* making hits. These men were perhaps a bit overeager to disprove the new claim, but I see nothing dishonest in these diligent efforts to "expose the error."

Perhaps there is a shade of difference in parallel cases of some individuals and departments of the great universities. One of these well-known departments of psychology invited me to give a report on the ESP work. A staff member there had conducted some successful ESP tests (unknown to me), but he did not mention them at all during my visit. When asked later by a fellow staff member why he had remained silent about them, he replied, "Do you think I wanted Rhine to be able to go around saying our university had confirmed him?"

As a matter of fact, during the late 1930's there were many academic people, both staff and students, who independently confirmed the ESP tests of clairvoyance I had reported in 1934. (There were also many who, for one reason or another, failed in their attempts to repeat the tests, a fact that means little because there are so many wrong ways to do it.) Because of the hesitation on the part of many of the successful experimenters to publish their results, the mass of confirmation we might have been able to claim was never normally reported. A small part did come out anonymously; some was given restricted circulation by mail; and some of the best records (one described only orally by a well-known professor of psychology) were deliberately destroyed to insure non-publication. Is not this a kind of deception-by-omission?

A Sampling of the Worst Stage

A certain change occurred, however, after World War II. Parapsychology had to some degree prevailed over its critics and had become almost excessively popular, sufficiently so to attract a number of band-wagon type of "pioneers." In fact some of these enthusiasts claimed they had done research in the psi field and presented papers, either for publication or for a convention program.

From these adventurers I have selected a dozen cases to illustrate fairly typically the problem of experimenter unreliability prevalent in the 1940's and 1950's. These twelve individuals themselves are all rather hard to classify. As it was, however, four of them were caught "redhanded" in having falsified their results; four others did not contest (i.e., tacitly admitted) the implications that something was wrong with their reports that seemed hard to explain and they did not try. In the case of the remaining four the evidence was more circumstantial, but it seemed to our staff they were in much the same doubtful category as the other eight.

What sort of people were these more obvious tricksters on the border or at least near the border of the field for a time? They ranged widely in many ways. Seven did not have the doctorate, although all were eager to get graduate degrees. Three of the seven were found to have claimed a degree fraudulently. Several were persons of evident ability but were located (some of them abroad) where research in parapsychology was extremely hard to manage but not nearly so hard to fake.

With all the worldwide publicity ESP research received so freely at that stage, it doubtless seemed easy to many weaker minds to concoct an experimental report based partly on their own imagination. In all the cases I knew personally, however, there was indication of some actual testing having been done. But this reaction was, with most of those who tried it (and were caught), shockingly crude and shameful. Perhaps a quarter to a third of them were able, clever people who need not have used trickery at all; they could surely have learned to do careful, effective testing. Odd as it may appear to some people, the ablest among this little collection of weak characters seemed to be the most irresponsible. This observation, plus the fact that we could obviously not run a character-rehabilitation clinic, led us to discourage further contact at once.

Fortunately the culprits have thus far been caught (at least in our "known" cases) before serious damage has been done. Then, too, as time has passed our progress had aided us in avoiding the admission of such risky personnel even for a short term. As a result, the last twenty years have seen little of this cruder type of chicanery. Best of all, we have reached a stage at which we can actually look for and to a degree choose the people we want in the field. Finally, as will be seen in a few more pages, we have been able to do quite a lot to insure that it is impossible for dishonesty to be implemented inside the well-organized psi laboratory today. So after one further step into the background of the deception problem, I will be ready for the search for solutions.

Fine Points in Developing Methods

What makes this next step difficult is the fact that the indication of trickery described in this section is not nearly so definite in all cases as in the preceding one. (As a matter of fact, I shall even cite one case in which someone else claims evidence of fraud—a judgment with which I disagree. I shall use it partly because it is already in print, but mainly because it will illustrate my point no matter who is right about the charge of fraud.) We must deal firmly with all *possible* deception in parapsychology to make this problem the negligible consideration it has become in most other sciences.

One other qualification is needed. Some of the breaches of faith (suggested or proved as the case may be) in this further group of examples are so minor that I can be justified in making them out to be probable cases of culpable malpractice (as I aim to do only in principle) simply because this is science and because this particular science is in an inordinately sensitive stage.

The members of this second group were all better qualified for psi research than those of the preceding selection (the "dozen"). They all knew the rules and standards that had been developed through the years, standards which compared favorably with those of the neighboring sciences. In fact, it was these more advanced test procedures that had largely ruled out the earlier types of fraud discussed above. Thus the kind of deception left as at least a possibility at this more sophisticated stage mainly consisted of ways of somehow lowering or somewhere skirting these precautionary bars in some slight degree and thereby leaving the safeguarding doors ajar by as much as a tiny crack or more. This borders in some cases on little more than a reasonable suspicion by someone of intent to cheat, leaving in most instances a possible alternative explanation. However, psi is so important and so revolutionary that it seems reasonable to aim at allowing no possible opportunity for an experimenter to mislead even a little.

Example No. 1. One of the most frustrating weaknesses among research workers has been the difficulty one experimenter has in actually exercising the precautions against dishonesty when collaborating with his trusted friends (and most of all, with close relatives). This difficulty is more acute among people inexperienced with regard to experimental deception, especially when dealing with colleagues whose relationship has been friendly and of long standing. In example No. 1, two mature experimenters had undertaken to do a well-designed double-blind experiment in which psi test data were to be correlated with another series of non-psi measurements. The main control over experimenter insecurity lay in avoidance of any inter-experimenter leakage of the individual scores until the final well-guarded checkup. However, the two experimenters in this case were discovered to be covertly exchanging tips with each other whenever outstanding subjects turned up in the series. These experimenters doubtless believed they were sufficiently objective not to need stringent rules. They were, of course, too interested in the results to wait until the series was finished.

Was this really cheating? Perhaps a sufficient answer can be found in the fact that it was done surreptitiously. I do not need to say (or wish to imply) that they actually *were* biased by this leaked information in their final analyses, but at least the results were not approved for publication and the individuals were not encouraged to continue work at the center.

Example No. 2. This case is essentially similar except that only one of the two experimenters was suspect. The experimental design again was of the double-blind type, and again analyses were to be made of the correlation of ESP test data with another set of measurements of a non-psi type. In principle the double-blind design could be perfected to a high degree because of the distinctiveness of the two types of measures used. These two sets of data were both meant to be analyzable on wholly objective (double-blind) lines. One experimenter (E-1) was responsible for the psi records and the other (E-2), for the non-psi recordings. The results of the correlations were quite significant throughout a number of confirmatory repetitions and with several E-2's as well as with a variety of subjects. E-1, however, was the single common factor throughout.

The point of interest is that when the exchange of recordings was made there was a short gap in the double-blind coverage in which E-1 briefly had sole possession of both sets of records (before delivery to the analyst doing the blind checking). Also, there were some adjustments of timing between the two series of data that could with inspection somewhat influence the evaluation. Here was a gap that needed to be closed to prevent any possible manipulation of the timing.

When it was arranged that E-2 would leave no time lag at all for E-1 to have unwitnessed possession of both records, the successful performance discontinued. It resumed, however, when the original conditions were restored; then it stopped when the time gap was closed again by E-2—with all else kept the same.

What was wrong here? Everyone urged going on to see what emerged with further patient variation, everyone but E-1 himself; he left, and fortunately the experimental results had not been published so that no one was misled by this particular instance.

Example No. 3. One of the better controlled psi test methods consists of the guessing of card (or symbol) order as a way of predicting future events, i.e., precognition. In checking these guesses against the future random targets, two experimenters can safely use double-blind conditions to insure against error. Much of the best psi work has been done with this method, with two responsible experimenters and with independent records to be matched jointly (or better still, matched independently with the use of duplicate records). But unfortunately it has not always been done in the way the design requires. Example No. 3 is a case in point.

In this experiment E-1 supervised the test performance of the subject and arranged for E-2 to be ready to prepare the future target series of symbols independently as soon as the subject's records were completed. The method thus in principle provided strong protection against any possible cheating by the subject. When properly conducted, it also guaranteed two sets of independent records that neither experimenter could interfere with by trickery.

In the editing of a report of this experiment special analyses were made of the data that showed an interesting hit distribution on the record sheets; this in turn suggested a further investigation of the actual test conditions, and this revealed a rather simple trick. A few spaces on E-1's hand copy of the subject's calls were left blank (as though by accident) until the actual checkup when they could be filled in as hits by E-1 himself. The use of duplicate sets of records to be exchanged by E-1 and E-2 at the checkup time had been omitted, evidently by E-1's intention. Completely mutual vigilance in the joint checking procedure was also obviated. With a well-trained and more watchful E-2 on the job, this cheating could not have occurred.

Example No. 4. Some of the best test methods in the ESP researches have been the gamelike card-matching techniques. They went through several forms, one of them eventually taking shape as STM or Screened Touch Matching. It was used most often in clairvoyance tests and finally evolved into a procedure in which the five key cards were hung on the subject's side of an opaque screen with a one-way opening which afforded visibility on E-2's side. By using a pointer visible to E-2 through the opening, the subject could indicate his guesses for the target cards being laid down one-by-one. Thus the subject could not see the test cards in E-2's hands. and E-2 could not tell what the key-card order was; that is, the keys were to be rearranged as randomly as possible by the subject before each run, under the continual observation and collaboration of E-1. On the opposite side of the screen, E-2 shuffled the target deck for each run.

The best known work with STM was the Pratt and Woodruff experiments (1939). Since the question of experimenter deception regarding this work has already been raised in publication by C. E. M. Hansel (1961), I can use it as case No. 4, and do so without accepting the theory of fraud; this interpretation was definitely not proved by Hansel. However, the mere fact that the actual conduct of the experiment was such that trickery was a conceivable possibility qualifies it for discussion here. There is some virtue in considering the possible weakness of the method whether or not any advantage was taken of it (a policy I also follow in case No. 1).

To support his charge of fraud in the Pratt-Woodruff tests, Hansel presented the results of analyses of the records of the highest-scoring subject in the experiment and claimed that E-2 could sometimes have partially identified one or more of the five key cards (partly because of inadequate rearrangement of them by the subject) and also that the records of the hit distribution of this one subject supported the hypothesis that E-2 could intentionally have taken advantage of this knowledge in laying down the test cards opposite the key cards (to some extent known to him). This was not proof that E-2 necessarily did this, and Pratt and Woodruff (1961) pointed out serious errors in Hansel's argument for his fraud hypothesis. A further round of the analyses begun by Hansel has been extended by George Medhurst and Christopher Scott to a large group of subjects in this experiment and is awaiting publication in the *Journal of Parapsychology*. The argument will then be continued with a further rejoinder by Pratt. This research can serve meanwhile to illustrate a step in the long and tenuous effort at improving experimenter security through developing experimental design.

The point that is specifically relevant to the present issue is that what was in 1939 considered a strong test design, i.e., the two-experimenter, double-blind technique, was not as secure as it could be made. It was a clear advance over general psychological test conditions and had not at that stage met with criticism either in or outside of the laboratory. Nevertheless, modifications followed, even in the next year's research, that tightened the precautions further; for example, in precognitive matching tests (Rhine, 1941 a).

Other Points Needing Attention

I will end this section with a few added generalizations about these finer points of experimenter security. Cases could be drawn, for example, from projects in which a too free abuse of statistics has lent itself to deceptive conclusions. While the help of statistical editors on the *Journal of Parapsychology* has been a most important service against this hazard, one gap that has been hard to keep closed is the omission (on improper grounds) of data that might legitimately belong in a report. Such cases are often impossible to rate because of the lack of full records or because of a question as to the completeness of the reporting; but whenever the decision is found to have been a secret one (that is, without an objective sharing with colleagues qualified to judge) that makes a serious difference. If there were need (and space for more illustration) there would be an example of this type. The subtle, private judgments about what data to "declare" in reporting constitute an area that needs the fullest possible safeguarding.

A final risk to be listed will surprise most of those accustomed to the justly exuberant confidence inspired by the reassuring words "automated," "electronically recorded," "computer analyzed," and the like. While great benefits are already being contributed by the advanced technology now available (or at least borrowable) in some laboratories, and the hopes of almost endless further gains are high, some caution definitely needs to be extended here too, even though on a slender basis of judgment as yet. An early experience of my own with fraud (in the case of Margery, the Boston medium) showed me rather convincingly that apparatus can sometimes also be used as a screen to conceal the trickery it was intended to prevent. Some of the suspected instances of intentional selection of data already mentioned were not necessarily insured against just because they had been more easily or automatically recorded. Perhaps the main thing to keep in mind is that the increased reliance on the equipment (which makes double-blind methods based on two experimenters appear less necessary, almost a luxury at first thought) does not necessarily mean that the need of the two-experimenter design is in any way supplanted; the experimenter-machine team is not at all the same as the two-experimenter plan. It would be a real retreat to think it ever could be. Machines will not lie, but. . . .

The general point of this section is that in a developing research field, the methods themselves are always on trial from the first. *If we have to argue* over the adequacy of the design or the trustworthiness of the experimenter (or the subject) it is wise to back up and improve the method before advancing further or expecting really firm credence from fellow scientists. The emphasis has to be on the tightening of security.

Safety Measures Against Deception

What can now be said (in outline) of the way to judge whether or not a psi experimenter has been reliable? The primary effort, of course, has been directed into seeing that dishonesty would be impossible if significant results were obtained by the experimenter under the prescribed conditions.

One of the earlier steps taken was the use of two sets of independent records (the record of the targets by the experimenter and the record of the calls by the subject), both to be handed to a second experimenter before checking was begun. This method was used in our laboratory at Duke in 1933 in the Pearce-Pratt series of clairvoyance card-guessing tests (Rhine, 1934). In addition, the two-experimenter practice began shortly thereafter in a later subseries of the same experiment. This meant double witnessing at the experimenter's end of the test, with the subject being sent to another building. Another precautionary step reported by Pratt and M. M. Price (1938) was to have two experimenters testing individual subjects for clairvoyance, with one experimenter handling the screened cards and the other recording the subject's guesses; the two experimenters then checked the results together. By 1939 the two-experimenter STM method was developed, as described above in the Pratt and Woodruff (1939) experiment. A further advance of the double-blind card matching method was reported in the 1941 *Journal of Parapsychology*. For example, completely independent (double-blind) checking of records was introduced in both of my reports of that year, one on clairvoyance with the target cards in sealed boxes (Rhine, 1941 *b*) and the other in precognition matching tests (Rhine, 1941 *a*). In addition, the latter report was done with the two experimenters operating completely double-blind, one handling the target records in one room; the other, those of the subjects in a second room. As conducted and reported, these conditions were, I think, very secure; and I know of no criticism of them thus far.

Still other variations of two-experimenter and double-blind techniques were introduced in the years that followed, especially with the precognition tests. The latter became the best controlled of all the types of psi known and tested up to that time. For example, with two trained experimenters adhering to the rules, neither experimenter could deceive the other; that is to say, it looked as if deception would have to involve *collusion between the two*—a rare situation indeed. (My No. 1 example of two-experimenter deception, or at least dishonest breaking of the rules, is the only case in my memory.) But, as I have aleady indicated, a good method itself is no guarantee that it will always be faithfully carried out. One over-tolerant experimenter alone can innocently allow another to get around the barriers that have been set up to insure the reliability of both. What must be kept in mind is the possibility of the method itself being less than cautiously applied and the necessity of preventing that from occurring unnoticed. These few examples will perhaps illustrate the need to continue to reinforce experimental design in parapsychology still further against possible experimenter unreliability even after all the controls developed thus far have been taken fully into account.

Incidental Evidence: The "Signs of Psi"

Yet, even with all I have said, let us remember, for balance on this difficulty, that most other branches of science have already matured to the point where the problem of experimenter trickery causes no great concern. That is partly because deliberate fraud would be too quickly spotted and exposed at their present stage. Also, in the more advanced sciences the research personnel are increasingly well selected through a long program of university training. But it was not always thus; I recall that fifty or more years ago, there were notorious cases of experimenter fraud in physics, biology, and medicine, among other fields. Obviously the possibility of easy repetition of tests as a way to check up on a new claim offers the best protection against trickery in research. Parapsychology has only in very recent years been coming into the stage of a reasonable likelihood of confirmation in other laboratories. Such repetition naturally requires first of all that these other laboratories exist, and again that they have staff members qualified and equipped to repeat the new findings. This period in parapsychology is only beginning, and is coming along slowly at that.

However, we have at least got past the older phase of having to use detectives and magicians to discover or prevent trickery by the subjects. The psi laboratory's experimental precautions of early years were (and had to be) mainly countertrickery measures (directed especially against subject fraud), although they had to safeguard against innocent mistakes as well. All of these devices were defensive in character and were quite necessary until enough knowledge was acquired to bring parapsychic phenomena into good laboratory test conditions. Then it became possible to look beyond the mere evidence for more *positive* "signs of psi," incidental earmarks of a more distinctive and peculiar nature. A few representative selections of these signs will be reviewed as an important part of the answer to the deception question reached thus far.

Decline Curves

One of the first of these "signs" came from the work of my first graduate student in parapsychology, H. L. Frick (Rhine, 1934). In his exploratory experiments in clairvoyance for the A.M. thesis he made a series of daily runs of 100 guesses of playing-card suits. The pooled results were close to the expected chance average, but later examination showed a continuous decline of the average scores over the five 20-trial segments of the run. The fifth (or last) segment averaged about as far below the expected chance mean as the first one did above, and the two were significantly different. When this type of decline was found to recur frequently in later analyses of comparable test data in other researches, it began to acquire some useful identification value. In fact, it was sometimes the only safe evidence of psi to be found in a given experiment.

This decline in the run thus became a "sign of psi"; it could serve as evidence against experimenter deception when it was discovered later by another analyst. Such a finding can be about as objective a type of evidence as fingerprints. In forming my own judgment about the reliability of psi research, I have leaned most heavily on such hidden evidence, mainly based on significant internal differences. The analysis usually has the great merit of being completely repeatable. To appreciate it fully, however, one needs to understand the evidence and nature of the various other position effects, as well as the related psi-missing effect. I have already reviewed elsewhere the main evidence that has accumulated on these effects (Rhine, 1969 *a*, 1969 *b*).

The decline curves reached their greatest value for security to date in the quarter-distribution (QD) analyses of the PK research data resulting from tests with dice. In these studies more than 30 years ago, Dr. Betty M. Humphrey and I made QD analyses of hit distributions over the record page (Rhine and Humphrey, 1944 *a*) in all the available PK test records for the preceding nine-year period. None of the 18 experiments available had been conducted with a decline of scoring rate in mind; yet, taken as a block, this great mass of research data showed a highly significant diagonal decline in the right-and-downward direction. This diagonal decline was conclusively confirmed by a further internal consistency test made on smaller record units (sets) within the page (Rhine and Humphrey, 1944 *b*). Moreover, an independent recheck was conducted by Dr. J. G. Pratt (1944), and this, too, produced almost perfect confirmation. To cap it all, a published invitation for still another analysis was made; it has thus far, after a period of three decades, received no takers. It appears to me to be the firmest block of evidence yet offered in a behavioral science in support of a new hypothetical principle.

The U-curve

If this were a book, I would go on next to develop chapters on the various other signs of psi to be derived from position effects as definitive types of evidence against experimenter deception (and error in general). One of these would be devoted to the U-curve effects. The U-curve was produced as another incidental sign of psi which came out of the use of one of the early card-guessing tests, the one called DT (down through) (Rhine, 1934). In these tests the subject made 25 responses (usually written) to guess the card order *down through* the undisturbed deck. By the time of my study of comparative test techniques (Rhine, 1941 *b*) it was well known that it was the *subject's response to the structure of the record sheet* that produced the U-curve. The sheet which he used had 25 spaces, in segments of 5 each. The hits tended to fall into U-shaped curves of frequency in a lawful way that could be statistically evaluated. A "salience ratio" statistic was devised by Dr. J. A. Greenwood (1941). The U-curve, like the decline curve, was a good antifraud feature when it emerged in the second stage of analysis, especially from test data of an experiment in which such curves had not been anticipated by the researcher.

Psi-missing

The psi-missing effect has furnished some of the surest signs of psi, evidence that meets the highest standards of objective science. To give this topic a better starting point I would go back to my precognition article (Rhine, 1941 *a*). The subjects in these card-matching tests were kept in separate groups of children and adults. The adult results gave deviations that were *below* chance to almost the same extent that the deviations of the children were *above* chance; both gave larger deviations in reward sessions, and smaller ones (about half as big) in sessions when no rewards were given. The experimenters had no basis then for anticipating such lawful distinctions as these (and other) breakdowns in this two-experimenter, two-room, double-blind experiment. The point is that natural lawful psychological effects occurring to the adults in these negative deviations paralleled the opposite (positive) results in children, and this fact goes far toward carrying the rational mind beyond the point of doubt about the trustworthiness of the experimenters.

It would require many chapters to round up the peculiar but lawful effects of psi-missing, some of them even more intricate than the differential signs of deviation shown by adults and children in the research just cited. These complex findings have often been completely unanticipated by the experimenters and thus have allowed no possible opportunity for deception by them.

For my own part, I have most effectively reduced my own skepticism by watching decades of these signs of psi emerge, often with such surprise as to make the experimenter himself an obviously "innocent bystander." Those who are not familiar with this most solid of psi evidence can follow it up through the past records or in its ongoing development. No critic, so far as I know, has tried to do this yet. But the historians are coming!

And yet, hard as it is to say it, I am not entirely satisfied today with all these many objectively factual and repeated signs of psi with their various types of internal verification, appealing as they are to my own rational scientific judgment. They do most forcefully reassure me personally; and yet, for many more than myself I think something more is needed for the field. For one thing, such extensive, involved analyses as those of the QD studies cannot be made by just anyone and could not be made so well again without that decade of accumulated records of PK data which were on hand in 1944.

Then, too, these signs of psi are puzzling in themselves. We can easily use them as effective empirical test devices and very often have done so. More than that, they pose challenging ideas about how psi functions. But for security purposes the signs have had their best safeguarding value when completely unexpected as effects by the experimenter, and thus not possibly attributable to his own intentions, conscious or unconscious. Therefore, as evidence against fraud, they lose some of their potency as they acquire familiarity.

Rather, there ought to be ways of so well embedding adequate safeguards against experimenter deception in psi research methodology that no reasonable question of the honesty of the researcher will ever arise. I think these safeguards can be provided along the lines suggested in the section to follow.

A Program for Experimenter Security

First, let us recall why there is concern about fraud in parapsychology, as compared, for example, to fraud in chemistry. As already stated, it is because in psi research it is still harder to test a new claim than it is in most sciences, and there are fewer researchers in a position to do it. This suggests, then, an obvious need, not only to encourage more widespread effort at repetition, but also (as a new emphasis) to encourage every psi researcher to make his experiment as easy to repeat as possible. If from the start he recognizes independent confirmation to be an essential part of his own goal, he will be able to do much to aid and insure such replication. Exchange of information and even visits with other research workers, loans of equipment, subjects, and the like are all advantageous in extending research into other laboratories for duplication by other experimenters. Logically enough, for parapsychology's present stage these *independent confirmations take on a value rating above that* of the original work itself simply because of the assurance they give on the security problem. Because of this current situation in parapsychology, any new piece of work should be taken as almost a sort of pilot research. In order to give it the proper status of acceptability it is more than ordinarily important for another laboratory to repeat it with adequate success. This then will complete the project as a sufficiently effective research contribution. Is that too high a standard to set for our field? Not for a science that is still so obviously fighting its way to the acceptance required to render it useful and meaningful.

The greatest difficulty will be in obtaining the cooperation necessary for the large-scale repetition needed. As it is, there is far too little "will to repeat" in this field at present; most researchers want to be innovators, since it looks more creative. But those who want the field to be taken seriously beyond its own small group will in time see the basic need of this reinforcement of security through repeating each other's experiments. Obviously we are all in it together.

Second, a similar step toward reinforcing the reliability of the individual experimenter's role in the research would be to include one or more coworkers as early in a research series as is feasible. This would also give further assurance of success when the transfer of the project to another center is undertaken; i.e., to show that the experiment is not dependent on one experimenter alone is best managed right "at home," and as early as possible. In principle, the more teamwork the better, with the idea in mind of extending the number of experimenters who can share in the responsibility for the reliability of the conclusions reached.

At the same time, this idea of teamwork in research needs careful study, planning, and, of course, the necessary facilities. It is a painful fact that few places are ready yet for *all* these needed advantages. Also, individual initiative needs to have its place in a research field that is to retain its fertility. No one's personal enthusiasm must be dampened by an overspreading of responsibility.

However, I have seen in several fields and in more than one center enough examples of successful research-group life to make it reasonable to hope that parapsychology can achieve the full benefits of teamwork, security among them. The idea largely reduces to this: a good psi research worker can multiply (not merely increase) the value of his contribution by use of a well-developed, suitably staged partnership. Such a partnership can be one that shares concern and responsibility for basic precautions and makes the eventual transfer of independent replication to other experimenters easier and much more likely to succeed.

Third, another strong fence against personal unreliability can be built by developing the best possible system for the exchange, the registration, and the safe preservation of research data. It is recognized that the research worker must be assured reasonable independence in order to cultivate and shelter his own ideas at the sensitive stage of innovation. He should be free to do his own preliminary explorations within the field more or less as he prefers; but when he has performed a promising pilot experiment and wants to set up a confirmatory project, he then needs to go on record with his group and to try openly to share his project with one or more of his colleagues. The research should go through one round of experimental confirmation after another with the *center's review system keeping the complete records.* This is an easier matter today with modern equipment; but it can always be done in any set-up, and it is necessary in order to avoid risk of omissions and improper selection of reportable data. With frequent reviews at staff meetings, and (as the work grows) at suitable conventions, the step-by-step developments will be shared and welcomed with growing interest beyond the original laboratory. All this sharing of progress (as well as failures) can do something not only to sustain morale but also to keep the data record straight, complete, and always ready for review and re-examination.

Fourth, in order to be taken seriously, the research of an experienced worker should be aimed well beyond a single initial experiment. When the immediate experiment is a recognized start on a long-view objective, it carries added assurance, security, and magnitude of purpose *because of* this larger perspective. The greater the problem to which the experiment makes a relevant approach, the more conviction the results are likely to carry. Moreover, the more closely the immediate project relates to already established territory, either within parapsychology itself or other branches of science, the more substantial and well-based it appears and the more trust it inspires in the credibility of the experimenter. The growing interrelations in the emergent picture of the nature of psi rank high in the building of a requisite overall confidence. This, of course, is the long-view answer to all the doubts about the field of parapsychology.

Finally, the really best clincher of all can well come with the finding of linkages between a new result and one or more of the identifying signs of psi, especially when the linkage is such that it could not possibly have been anticipated and "planted" by the original experimenter. These linkages will always be prime evidence, even if only incidental to the more adaptable program I have outlined.

As we proceed now to close in on this experimenter-deception problem by combining these added safeguards with those already in use, I do think it should be possible almost immediately, if a resolute move is made, to put an end to the long-lingering anxiety that I think has sapped the confidence our field has needed for its effective recognition.

As distrust of experimenter security diminishes and the concern over personnel unreliability reduces to the level of the older sciences, the findings of the psi research field should, after having waited for too many generations, come to be accepted on their actual objective merits. That is enough to ask, but nothing less than that should any longer be considered acceptable.

A Final Reflection

Parapsychology appears to those who know its history to have come a rather long way in its advances in methods, even if it has taken a long, long time to do it. It has come far in ferreting out all the many far-ranging doubts and questions and counterhypotheses both its friends and foes could identify or even merely suspect. It has stretched out its patient pursuit of an ever more conclusively tight experimental design and statistical evaluation until the growing burden on the research field is almost frustratingly depressing to much of its personnel. If now there is still a latent last-ditch sort of holdout against it, this may be due in large part to a residue of suspicious, half-concealed distrust of the human researcher that keeps parapsychology in a state of futile unacceptability—a state in which scientists distrust their own best methods.

If this uneasiness over unreliable personnel (no matter how rare it is) is indeed what has largely been sustaining the existing hesitancy over parapsychology so long after it has had twice the normal period of trial, by all means let us firmly insist on a fuller sharing, controlling, and accounting of the entire research operation. This added vigilance need not impose any undue burden on research when it becomes adopted practice. Rather, it should relieve the active concern one often feels—but always hesitates to express—when impressive results occur, especially in some other laboratory. In other words, now that we have found out how to verify the occurrence of psi, let us try in the way we do the research to make it completely convincing.

References

Greenwood, J. A. "The statistics of salience ratios." *Journal of Parapsychology,* 1941, 5, 245–49.

Hansel, C. E. M. "A critical analysis of the Pratt-Woodruff experiment." *Journal of Parapsychology,* 1961, 25, 99–113.

Pratt, J. G. "A reinvestigation of the quarter distribution of the (PK) page." *Journal of Parapsychology,* 1944, 8, 61–63.

Pratt, J. G., & Price, M. M. "The experimenter-subject relationship in tests for ESP." *Journal of Parapsychology,* 1938, 2, 84–94.

Pratt, J. G., & Woodruff, J. L. "Size of stimulus symbols in extrasensory perception." *Journal of Parapsychology,* 1939, 3, 121–59.

Pratt, J. G., & Woodruff, J. L. "Refutation of Hansel's allegation concerning the Pratt-Woodruff series." *Journal of Parapsychology,* 1961, 25, 114–29.

Price, G. R. "Science and the supernatural." *Science,* August 26, 1955.

Rhine, J. B. *Extra-sensory Perception.* Boston Society for Psychic Research, 1934. (Republished: Bruce Humphries, Branden Press, 1973.)

Rhine, J. B. "Experiments bearing upon the precognition hypothesis. III. Mechanically selected cards." *Journal of Parapsychology,* 1941, 5, 1–57. (a)

Rhine, J. B. "Terminal salience in ESP performance." *Journal of Parapsychology,* 1941, 5, 183–244. (b)

Rhine, J. B. "Position effects in psi test results." *Journal of Parapsychology,* 1969, 33, 136–57. (a)

Rhine, J. B. "Psi-missing re-examined." *Journal of Parapsychology,* 1969, 33, 1–38. (b)

Rhine, J. B., & Humphrey, B. M. "The PK effect: special evidence from hit patterns. I. Quarter distributions of the page." *Journal of Parapsychology,* 1944, 8, 18–60. (a)

Rhine, J. B., & Humphrey, B. M. "The PK effect: special evidence from hit patterns. II. Quarter distributions of the set." *Journal of Parapsychology,* 1944, 8, 254–71. (b)

Rhine, J. B.; Pratt, J. G.; Smith, B. M.; Stuart, C. E.; & Greenwood, J. A. *Extra-sensory Perception After Sixty Years.* New York: Henry Holt, 1940. (Republished, Boston: Bruce Humphries, 1966.)

Warner, L. "A second survey of psychological opinion on ESP." *Journal of Parapsychology,* 1952, 16, 284–95.

Warner, L. "What the younger psychologists think about ESP." *Journal of Parapsychology,* 1955, 19, 228–35.

Warner, L., & Clark, C. C. "A survey of psychological opinion on ESP." *Journal of Parapsychology,* 1938, 2, 296–307.

J. N. Emerson

Intuitive Archaeology: The Argillite Carving

THIS PAPER holds that intuitive or psychic knowledge stands as a viable alternative to the knowledge obtained by the more traditional methods of science.

I stated in a paper (*Midden,* 1973) to the Canadian Archaeological Association that "it was my conviction that I had received knowledge about archaeological artifacts and archaeological sites from a psychic informant who related this information to me without any evidence of the conscious use of reasoning [pp. 16–20]." It was argued that learning, mind-reading, and mental telepathy were not involved.

The most helpful evaluation of my paper was received from J. B. Rhine, founder of American parapsychology. Dr. Rhine has long been associated with Duke University and, although retired, is the very active director of the Foundation for Research on the Nature of Man at Durham, North Carolina. In a personal communication from Rhine on August 6, 1971, he says:

> The value of this paper, in my judgment, depends upon what it does to the author, and those who hear or read it, in the way of further action. It has evidently led you to a decision to take the possibility of a parapsychic function seriously in George's performance. If it suffices for that, it has had an acceptable value. Conclusions and more important valuations can be left to the kind of thing you will be led to do by this paper. It is a pilot finding and that is one of the links in the chain of the search for truth.

Upon hearing the 1973 paper, Jack Miller, a nonprofessional archaeologist, of Port Clements, B.C., was immediately stimulated to further action. He presented to me a black, carved argillite stone artifact to be studied psychically.

Mr. Miller did not reveal to us what he knew about the artifact. He secretly believed that it represented a Sasquatch. The Sasquatch is the legendary or real counterpart of the European "Abominable Snowman." Footprints, sightings, photographs, and filmstrips have been accumulated but so far "establishment" archaeologists and anthropologists have chosen to ignore them. Others had speculated that it was an unfinished pipe blank. The time and location of the find were known, but there was no significant archaeological context.

My psychic informant, George, when presented with the artifact at the annual banquet of the Canadian Archaeological Association, stated that it was carved by a Negro from Port-au-Prince. I, too, was moved to action. I was appalled! I was convinced that George was patently wrong; for to me as an archaeologist the material was British Columbian black argillite. Any suggestion that it was carved by a black man from the Caribbean seemed to me to be the wildest flight of fancy. I suggested to George that the study be deferred until we returned home to Ontario.

After our return George studied the carving further and presented me with an even more fantastic story, namely: The carver was a Negro born and raised in Africa. He was taken as a slave to the New World where he worked in the Caribbean. He was later taken to British Columbia on an English ship. He escaped, met the natives, was accepted, married, lived, and died there. A fantastic story to me in April, 1973, but not so fantastic by March, 1974.

I was stimulated to further positive action. The idea of a "psychic team" to carry out a comparative study of this artifact evolved. Independently, with no knowledge of what anyone else had said, and with no information about where it had been found or under what circumstances, the black carved argillite stone artifact was given to seven additional intuitive or psychic persons for study. I stress that for each of them, confronted cold with the carving, it would have been easy to assume that it came from any place or any time in the world.

This study has occupied nearly a year; several hundred pages of transcribed, tape-recorded texts have been accumulated. Amazingly, the story related by George in April, 1973, has been confirmed and reconfirmed by new members as they were added to the psychic team and they, in turn, have added information and confirmed each other's statements.

The material presented in this paper is only the briefest abstraction of the available texts, and represents only the tip of an analytical iceberg. It seeks to document the feasibility and credibility of the psychic team approach and addresses itself to confirming three salient points:

1.   The carver was from Africa.

2. He was brought to the New World as a slave.
3. He came to British Columbia.

On the topic of African origins, let us now consider excerpts from the tape-recorded statements of our psychic informants, Jim, George, Sandy, and Sheila:

Jim: He came from Africa, as I said before, about half way down the west coast of Africa and about thirty miles inland. . . .

George: There was a certain amount of water where he came from . . . there's waterfalls, quite high waterfalls . . . the central . . . west central, it seems to me. It was very heavy, very thick jungle . . . it was very heavy, very dense, very wet, very damp.

Sandy: He was from the interior of North Africa. . . . Getting back to North Africa . . . now there was a lot of French influence in North Africa, but he wasn't in that area, directly involved with the French. He was more in a jungle area going from the desert area into the savannah area of North Africa, savannah land.

Sheila: Somebody who handled this at one time was a black man. . . . The jungle is behind me here. . . . It's not really jungle country, though. It's hot. I feel as though I'm up on a big plateau—high up, and the ocean is miles down below. It is a very big plateau and lots of dried grassland, lots of bush, and there are lots of trees; but you know there is lots of space and grassland in between the trees. So it is not jungle.

Jim stated that the carver came from Africa. George clearly described the damp, wet jungle country. Sandy confirmed the jungle environment but also saw savannah land. Sheila saw the jungle behind her but described the dried grassland and brush of the savannah country before her. There could be little doubt that our psychics saw the homeland of the carver located in northwest Africa, perhaps the Gold Coast area.

On the second point—that he was brought to the New World as a slave, we first hear from George:

George: I don't know whether he was picked up in a group or whether he was sold by other people. Anyway he ended up in slavery; he came over in a slave ship.

Sandy: And he was the victim of a massive, sweeping slave trade insofar as people went into the interior because they needed men to come to the New World to work for them.

Jim: They were raided by a renegade African and his cohorts who captured quite a few of his village, including his own family, to sell them as slaves to the English or the Americans.

The psychic evidence that the carver was brought to the New World as a slave appears to be confirmed. For point three—that he came to British Columbia:

Jim: He made the carving out of the black rock from the mountains there nearby . . . in the west part of the North American continent. Canada comes to mind, but the United States has some connotation in there and so I can't say whether it is the American or the Canadian side.

George: Anyway, he got on a boat and got over to the Pacific anyway. That was up in B.C. that he did that . . . around Bella Coola and Bella Bella, Bella Walla—up there in that area, that general direction up there, south of Prince Rupert.

Sheila: Kind of looks like the kind of stuff that comes from the Queen Charlotte Islands—what is a black man doing in the Queen Charlotte Islands?

It was a good question: "What was a black man doing in the Queen Charlotte Islands?" But there seemed little doubt about it in the minds of our psychics. With the whole world to choose from, Jim located him in northwestern North America. George saw him in B.C. around Bella Coola, Bella Bella, and Prince Rupert. The artifact was actually found at Skidgate on the Queen Charlotte Islands located 200 miles northwest of Bella Coola and Bella Bella and 100 miles southwest of Prince Rupert. And then, Sheila actually saw the material as having come from the Queen Charlotte Islands. The artifact was found one-fourth mile south of Skidgate!

The members of my psychic team were not professional registered psychics, with the possible exception of Sheila, who does give formal lectures and college courses on parapsychology. Sandra gives classes in awareness development upon a less formal basis. For the rest of the group, with the exception of George, the exposure to the argillite carving was almost their first attempt at psychometry.

As I mentioned, the material presented here is only the tip of an iceberg of information. However, it does seem patently evident that at least three statements about this artifact were psychically confirmed:
1. The carver *was* born and raised in Africa.
2. He *was* brought to the New World as a slave.
3. He *did* come to British Columbia.

I am now convinced that it can be argued that intuitive or psychic knowledge does stand as a viable alternative to knowledge obtained by the more traditional methods of science. By utilizing a psychic team, and by cross-analysis of their independent statements, which reveal an amazing degree of correspondence and concurrence, I am convinced that we have been able to abstract intuitive truth about man's past. In the study of this one item we have gone far beyond the limits of chance and coincidence as an explanation.

In my previous paper I stated that by means of the intuitive and the parapsychological, a whole new vista of man and his past stands ready to be grasped. By this kind of research I have been able to recover three major events in the life of this African carver. The texts available will allow me to recover much more with a wealth of detail about this man who was otherwise unknown or obscured in traditional history. If the life of this black man is available, why not the life of all men? As it has been said, "By their works ye shall know them." It is a mind-boggling thought.

I do not wish to convey the idea that I am so enamored of the psychic or psychic team approach that I am prepared to ignore the findings and resources of traditional science. Rather, I consider that progress will only be made by a melding and an integration of the two—intuition and science.

At this point I offer an illustration. On April 25, 1973, I was fortunate enough to obtain the following diagnosis of the argillite carving from Allen Tyyska, a graduate anthropologist who, because of his experience as a cataloger of African art specimens at the Royal Ontario Museum, was well-equipped to provide the following statement for me:

Allen: While I was cataloging at the Royal Ontario Museum, we had a large collection come in from West Africa. Mr. Rayfield, who lives just west of Toronto, goes on trips and he bought the things. And, well, there was a large number of sculptures and little passport masks and things that all came from the upper Volta, the Niger, and generally that area of West Africa between Sierra Leone and the Cameroons, along the coast; you know, Nigeria, Gold Coast, Ghana. . . .

J.N.E.: I was going to say, that is what they call the Gold Coast.

Allen: Yes. So this little piece of argillite looks like it fits into those art styles; and there are a number of things about it that would belong somewhere in that general area—maybe more precisely along the upper reaches of the Volta. You see how thin it is, relative to how long it is? That's a pretty good characteristic of that art style. . . . When you look at the face—just the face on its own—you see that the nose is sort of triangular in its section there. That's the way they used to break the face down into planes, on the passport masks of the Dan. For example, the face would be a series of planes— geometric planes that came together to block out the features; and this is about the way they did it—that deep notch below the eyes—sort of the way that that eyebrow is one kind of plane and there is a notch cut out for the eyes that leads to the triangular nose with a notch below it for the mouth. And the chin being in a different plane—that little groove above the eyebrows—all those things are just right for that art style.

Mr. Tyyska felt that the art styles manifested to him by the carving are to be found specifically in the Gold Coast area of West Africa and perhaps "more precisely, the upper reaches of the Volta." This certainly coincided with the statements of our psychic informants, although environmental statements needed to be checked out in detail. But it has been encouraging and salutary to have the ideas of the psychics apparently confirmed by evidence drawn from a knowledge of native African art.

In a similar vein I am well aware that a host of topics can be abstracted from the text material which can be tested by the accumulated knowledge of anthropology, ethnology, ethnohistory, geology, history, musicology, primatology, and a wide variety of other sciences.

George has given me detailed information about native behavior that can only be the "potlatch." The potlatch is a major social mechanism of Northwest Coast Indians generally interpreted as a gift-giving ceremony by which prominent people gain prestige. Sandy has given me information on how the carver produced the throwing element in the Spanish or Mexican Jai Alai game. Sheila gave me the name of a ship to be searched out. She also gave me a detailed description of the British Columbia shoreline where the carver and his brother had lived. Maureen, George, and Sheila were conscious of the presence of Russian sailing ships, and Sheila described them. George said that the carver came to B.C. on an English ship, and Maureen wondered why she could hear old English sea chanteys being sung. Tom, both in word and by body movements, provided me with a description of a native African dance. Sheila heard the shrieks of monkeys and baboons swinging through the trees just as the sun went down. Is this typical primate behavior? These are all questions to be studied and researched. Such a program could lead to the integration of intuitive and scientific knowledge.

I assure you that I approached these studies with an open-minded skepticism. It is also useful, however, to maintain a sense of humor. The fantastic story which George told me in April, 1973, I now find not so fantastic in March, 1974. I offer in conclusion two other statements from our psychic, Sandy:

Sandy: The individual I see as being reddish—yellow-red . . . red . . . red-brown . . . big, hairy. . . . Because I keep getting this picture of this ape-man, going about his business.

And so there it is: reddish, red-brown, big, hairy—an ape man going about his business. Doesn't it sound rather like the legendary descriptions of the

Sasquatch? Mr. Jack Miller seems to have been vindicated and perhaps rewarded for the day that he handed his argillite carving to George and me for intuitive study; or, in the words of the editor of the *Queen Charlotte Observer*, September 6, 1973:

> So . . . although authorities may yet make a gorilla out of a Sasquatch, they'll never make a monkey out of Jack Miller of Port Clements, Q.C.I.

Reference

Emerson, J. N. Intuitive Archaeology: a psychic approach. *The Midden,* Archaeological Society of British Columbia, 1973, **V** (3), 16–20.

Section II

CURRENT PSYCHIC research is more than a rehash of such veteran standbys as ESP, telepathy, clairvoyance, psychokinesis, poltergeists, and reincarnation, important as they may be. Current psychic research is a new ball game, augmented by an impressive, sophisticated, scientifically credible lineup, whose names somehow have a robust, unesoteric sound: biofeedback, Kirlian photography, energy fields, biorhythm, biocycles, voluntary control of internal bodily functions, alterations of consciousness, biological effects of meditation, transfer of energy in psychic healing, atmospheric and electronic effects on behavior, and electroencephalographic mind training. Studying that roster is almost like observing a metamorphosis of science fiction into science fact.

The Kirlian photographic technique, developed in Russia more than three decades ago, is one of the most eerie and fascinating, yet still controversial discoveries in psychic research. If the emanations (called bioplasma by the Soviets) that it pictures are authentic rather than artifacts, it will not only help explain many religio-psychic beliefs, but might become as important for medical diagnosis as electrocardiograms and X-rays. *Medical World News* (October 26, 1973, 197:43–48) has provided an excellent review of the debate as to whether the auras are merely an induced form of corona discharge or actual biological emanations.[1]

Another source of widespread interest is biofeedback, a method of modifying or controlling a range of bodily functions once considered to be entirely automatic. Essentially this is done by a variety of instruments that emit visual

---

[1]The reader is also referred to a very recent book, *The Kirlian Aura*, edited by S. Krippner and D. Rubin, Garden City, New York: Anchor Books, 1974

or auditory signals in monitoring muscles, skin, temperature, circulation, brain waves, and several other bodily functions and organs. Though still in its infancy, it is claimed by its proponents to be especially effective in treating psychosomatic conditions and even organic dysfunction and pain. Like Kirlian photography and meditation, biofeedback offers potential promise for enhancing medical practice.

Businessmen, scientists, physicians, and people in all walks of life are becoming more and more receptive to such practical developments. The increasingly popular practice of meditation has convinced many that the human mind possesses a great untapped potential, and that everyone is endowed with latent psychic powers that can be developed. *Business Week* has reported that the Institute of Electrical and Electronic Engineers recently presented a panel on parapsychology; the National Science Foundation is interested in psychic research; the National Institute of Mental Health has granted Maimonides Medical Center in Brooklyn funds for research on dream telepathy; the National Aeronautics and Space Administration has financed a Stanford Research Institute program to teach ESP skills to NASA personnel; the Pentagon's Advanced Research Projects Agency (ARPA) is closely monitoring developments in psychic research; the Central Intelligence Agency has interviewed some scientists conducting ESP experiments; Bell Telephone Laboratories have briefed their scientists on telepathy and clairvoyance; Hoffmann-La Roche and other drug companies are exploring ways to train the mind to control stress; and various professional consultants are advising clients to test potential executives for ESP abilities (*Business Week,* January 26, 1974, "Why scientists take psychic research seriously," pp. 76–78).

One of the greatest obstacles to the scientific acceptance of psychic healing is the insistence by healers that they are special agents of God, and that's that—we need go no further.

But it isn't that simple. The potentialities of medical science are far from being exhausted. Granted that everything, if you will, is the work of God, nevertheless He is not a magician who merely waves a magic wand and commands something to happen by some secret legerdemain. He works through painstaking laws and mechanisms that are intended for mankind to unveil. Healing is not only a matter of antibodies and leucocytes and DNA and surgery and vaccines and antibiotics, but also involves other factors as yet unknown. One of these may well be an invisible transfer of energy from healer to patient, which though God-given, can still be scientifically investigated, discovered, developed, improved and used along with other healing procedures in a methodical, rational, controlled, responsible manner.

Two thousand years ago, a gifted poetess of India, Saint Avvaiyar, wrote:

> What we have learnt, is like a handful of Earth,
> While what we have yet to learn, is like the whole World.

That verse holds true even now, for the knowledge that we have today is only an infinitesimal part of what we yet must learn.

John C. Pierrakos

Psychiatric Implications of Energy Fields in Man and Nature

Historical Perspective

THE PHENOMENA of the energy fields of man are to be found recorded over thousands of years in the history of humanity. They were first mentioned by the Chinese approximately 3000 B.C., as the principle of *yin* and *yang*. There is a strong relationship between Chinese cosmology and the philosophy of the Egyptians as indicated by the duality of Osiris and Isis, the numerological conception of Pythagoras, Plato's dualism, and the Chrimus–Ahriman of Zoroaster.

In Greek culture, Hippocrates mentioned the influence of weather rhythms on distempers. He also pointed out that "nature heals and not the physician." The specific energy force in the Greek body of knowledge was called the *speira*. However, it was Paracelsus who applied the principle of the *archeus*, or healing force, in his practice of medicine.

In the modern era, Isaac Newton, in his paper on light and color, spoke of an electromagnetic light, ". . . subtle, vibrating, electric and elastic medium." Newton's concept in many ways anticipates the electromagnetic field of Faraday. In 1704, Mead theorized that atmospheric tides act as "external assistance" to "inward causes" present in animal bodies. He spoke about a "nervous fluid with electricity." About that time, Nollet and Fredke published related theories and experiments on the "nervous fluid." Mesmer in 1779, called the force "animal gravitation," and later, "animal magnetism." In 1783 Bertholon published work on the influence of atmospheric electricity on plants. The well-known German chemist, Baron von Reichenbach, made a detailed study of the energy fields of crystals, animals and plants in 1851 and named that field "odyl." Mesmer's work deeply influenced Bernheim and Charcot, who used the principles of hypnotism and suggestion for therapy in their respective schools.

The theory of the unconscious mind, upon which psychoanalytic knowledge is based, came into existence through the use of hypnotic techniques, since Freud was Charcot's pupil and a coworker with Bernheim. His concept of the libido was, at the beginning, purely that of an energetic principle similar to the principles of animal magnetism described by Mesmer in 1779. Freud's concepts of the libido were also based on his understanding of the vital energy process of the organism.

The physical investigation of the energy field, however, followed very slowly. Dr. Kilner, of London (1917) objectively investigated the visual appearance of the energy field, which he called "the human atmosphere." In 1925, and for a period of approximately twenty-five years thereafter, Wilhelm Reich (1949) conducted a systematic and detailed study of the phenomena of energy fields in man and nature. Reich named the specific energy of the vital processes, orgone. His work in both psychoanalytic and biological fields is slowly being recognized by many as of great importance in the understanding of the energetic nature of man.

In the United States, since 1930, Burr and Northrop conducted detailed studies in the biological domain (1932). Their work led them to conclude that there must be a force field helping the living organism to conduct the complex chemical interchanges that accompany biological processes. Their research was facilitated by developing specific instruments measuring minute voltage differences. Leonard Ravitz (1953), using Burr's instrumentation, conducted extensive experiments indicating that significant changes occurred in the electromagnetic field of man during states of sleep, hypnosis, and drug ingestion. In England, George de la Warr, whose work was based upon discoveries made by two American physicians, Carl Abrams and George Star White, developed specific apparatus demonstrating the effect that the conscious mind has over plants and biological processes.

It would take many pages merely to list the references of the numerous investigators in this field who have been working on the fringes of scientific investigation. Here, for example, belong the parapsychological investigations of the theosophists, the phenomenon of radiaesthesia, psychic healing, and the techniques of Yoga.

Recently (1965) Dr. Bernard Grad of McGill University demonstrated the marked effect of the healer's *hand* on enhancing the growth process of experimental barley seedlings. At the present time, in the United States as well as Russia, there is extensive work relating to the study of the energetic functions of man, including Kirlian photography and the study of the "fourth bio-plasmatic dimension." In the laboratory of the Institute for Bioenergetic Analysis, in New York City, work has been conducted for many years in defining the characteristics of the energy field of man as described below.

Description of the Nature of the Field

In nature there are several groups of unicellular organisms such as bacteria, and multicellular structures such as flagellates, sponges, fish, and fireflies that are able to emit light and luminate as a result of their inner biological processes. In higher organisms it is known that vital processes such as cell mitosis, oxidation, and other metabolic reactions are accompanied by luminescence. Living organisms are able to emit light through the entire surface of their bodies. They have not lost their ability to illuminate. These emissions belong in a part of the spectrum that is almost invisible, being very close to the ultraviolet. They constitute the visual manifestation of the field or aura, which is, in effect, a luminous cast of many bioenergetic processes occurring within the organism. These energy field phenomena are closely correlated with metabolic process—emotional excitement, physical activity, and rest. They are also affected by atmospheric conditions such as relative humidity, polarity of charges in the air, and many other unknown factors.

Subjectively, the energy field can be perceived with the naked eye by rare individuals as a luminous, pulsating envelope around the body, which extends far beyond the surface of the skin. Human beings seem to swim in a sea of fluid, tinged rhythmically with brilliant colors which constantly change hues, shimmer, and vibrate. In truth, to be alive is to be colorful and vibrant. The field may also be seen with the aid of certain filters as an envelope, blue-gray in color and extending two to four feet away from the periphery. It is pulsating in nature, and swells slowly for one to two seconds, forming roughly an overall oval shape with fringed edges.

The field is roughly divided into three layers. (See Figures 1 and 2.) The inner layer is one-fifth to one-eighth of an inch and is composed of a dark blue layer. The intermediate layer is a blue-gray hue extending 3 to 4 inches. The third outer layer has a light blue color extending 6 to 8 inches.

Attempting to describe the exact features is difficult because of their variability. Some general characteristics, however, can be pointed out in the average

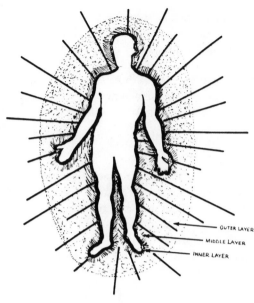

Figure 1

OUTER LAYER
MIDDLE LAYER
INNER LAYER

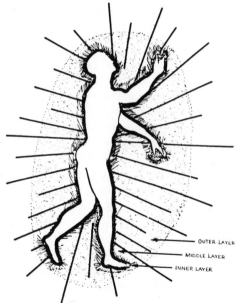

Figure 2

OUTER LAYER
MIDDLE LAYER
INNER LAYER

person. The inner layer is transparent and gives the appearance of an empty dark space. It closely follows the outline of the skin. The second, or intermediary layer, is more complex, and has a blue-gray color, except around the head, where it tends to be yellow. It is made up of three basic patterns. There is a ripple-like movement like the waves created by throwing a stone into a still lake. The second is a corpuscular movement similar to the Brownian movement, and the third, is a linear movement that travels extensively away from the body. Its overall appearance is that of a blue shimmering liquid, extremely rarefied and brilliant. The raylike movement is dominant over the head, forming a fringe-like effect. In painting, it is represented as a halo around the heads of saints. The outer layer extends several feet away. The principal movement of the three layers can be described as a wave moving away from the body. However, there is also a longitudinal movement alternating in the two halves of the body, giving the appearance of an up and down motion.

I consider the field to be primarily an expression of all aspects of man—physical, emotional, mental, and spiritual. The aura itself is only a small fragment of the entire range of the energy field. There seem to be infinite extensions and interactions in the energy field as a whole.

In illness I have seen various changes. Fear causes a dulling of the color, and a slowing down of vibratory movements. The result is dirty, dull, and not glowing. A schizophrenic patient shows severe disturbances in the energy field in that the contour of the three layers is broken. The color is converted into brownish yellow and the pulsatory rate is considerably diminished. Patients with a pyknic habitus, having masochistic characteristics, show severe interruptions in the neck and pelvis. Patients with specific areas of tension show corresponding changes in the energy field over these areas.

In physically debilitated individuals, the field is diminished, the pulsatory rate is below 15 per minute, the width of the three layers is thinned out, and the overall color is dull gray. In pregnancy, the intermediary layer loses its defined structure. It fuses with the outer layer and both expand to double size. In infants, the field has practically no structure—all three layers are fused together, and the color is light blue and extremely brilliant. As the child grows, the field slowly forms three layers and becomes organized. In general, it can be said that the field shows great sensitivity to the physical changes in the organism relating to illness and health.

Having studied these phenomena for years with the aid of filters, a group of basic scientists in the Institute for Bioenergetic Analysis organized the Energy Research Group, of which I am a member, and developed an objective method for defining the phenomenon of the aura. Our group observed that extremely low light levels were radiated as components of the human energy field, and these could be studied with objective instrumentation. We found that this radiated light fell within the wave lengths of the near ultraviolet spectrum (3000 to 4000 angstroms). A photomultiplier tube was used with a peak sensitivity in this range, and with extremely low external noise. A ventilated light-tight darkroom was constructed. A subject was placed in front of the tube. Any light signals radiated were converted by the tube to highly magnified electric currents which could be measured by various methods. A permanent record of signals was made, using a graph-like recorder. It was found that a subject with a high energy level showed a light level in the millilumen range. Medium energy subjects showed a lesser magnitude. By developing this technique, it has become possible to define the components of the energy field in man.

Work is continuing to increase further the sensitivity of our instruments so that clinical studies can be undertaken with different pathological conditions for medical and psychiatric disturbances.

Energy phenomena, through subjective and objective research, can provide a new dimension in further understanding the basic characteristics of illness and health. They seem to belong to a class which constitutes the interphase level between energy and matter. They are also closely related to the dimension of perception and consciousness, and have their own laws of pulsatory movement and vibration not yet fully understood.

Note: More detailed descriptions of instruments and techniques are beyond the scope of this chapter. They are described in my monograph, "The Energy Field in Man and Nature" (1971).

References

Burr, H. S. An electro-dynamic theory of development suggested by studies of proliferation rates in brain of Amblystoma. *Journal of Comparative Neurology,* 1932, **56,** 347–371.

Energy Research Group, Institute for Bioenergetic Analysis. Physical measurement of human radiation, 1973, unpublished report.

Grad, B. Some biological effects of "the laying on of hands": a review of experiments with animals and plants. *Journal of the American Society for Psychical Research,* 1965, **59,** 95–127.

Kilner. *The human aura or atmosphere.* London: Keejan Press, 1917.

Pierrakos, J. C. *The rhythm of life.* New York: Institute for Bioenergetic Analysis, Fall, 1966, Lecture Series.

———. *The energy field in man and nature.* New York: Institute for Bioenergetic Analysis, 1971.

Ravitz, L. J. Periodic changes in electromagnetic field. *Annals of New York Academy of Sciences,* 1953, **46,** 650–660.

Reich, W. The function of the organism. In *The discovery of the orgone.* Vol. 1. Rangeley, Me.: Orgone Institute Press, 1949.

———. *Character analysis* (3rd ed.). Rangeley, Me.: Orgone Institute Press, 1949.

James B. Beal

The Synthesis between Psychiatry, Biology, Technology, and Mysticism

> There is a principle which is proof
> against all argument, and which cannot
> fail to keep a person in everlasting
> ignorance. That principle is—
> Condemnation Before Investigation. . . .
>
> Herbert Spencer

DURING THE RISE and fall of various cultures throughout history, the reliance on experiential, subjective beliefs (inner feelings) and problems in communicating these beliefs have prevented the overall view of life system interactions and subsequent consequences; negative cultural conditioning (it can't be done) has prevented true scientific inquiry into natural laws. Today, with the multitude of ecological, sociological, psychological, and physiological interactions which occur, due to the primarily unplanned actions of humanity, it is clear that the broadest possible overview of effects on the environment, environmental effects on the human being, and the mental-physical results, is needed as a basis for the self-insight and self-control necessary to realize optimum self-potential. The total effect of the interacting systems on and within a person is greater than the sum of the effects of the individual systems. The end effect cannot be ascertained by a study of the discrete components— thus the need for a synergistic or total systems approach to the study of the nature of the human being (Beal, 1974).

It is interesting that in the autobiographical accounts of the great breakthroughs in our understanding of the universe, the role of intuition, or some mysterious comprehension, led to the breakthrough rather than any systematic analytic process. "I didn't arrive at my understanding of the fundamental laws of the universe through my rational mind."—Albert Einstein (Alpert, 1971).

Most of the breakthroughs in knowledge have resulted from unpredictable people working in unconventional ways. Many important ideas and concepts have had their origins in nonrational, nonlinear, intuitive thoughts that have burst unexpectedly from the imaginative depths of the personality who "danced to a different drummer" or looked at the pattern from a different angle—the try-angle? (Krippner, 1968).

With all our scientific knowledge of the physical universe, we still know virtually nothing about our subjective nature and how to live in harmony with our environment, technology, and each other. Indeed, the information available on the subjective nature of the mind is usually highly speculative, misleading, contradictory, inconclusive, loaded with creative overbelief, and, at best, qualitative. Despite heroic efforts of early psychical researchers, only within the past decade has technology advanced to the point where both environment and individual could be monitored (with a minimum of disturbance) as a symbiotic interrelated system, and the mind–body interactions studied quantitatively (Beal, 1972)! Within the past three years, the results and implications for the future have just about outstripped science-fiction. The extension of scientific method to the essential phenomena of altered states of consciousness (ASC) is now underway; the results will prove to be mind-boggling, literally and figuratively.

I would like to postulate here, for consideration, that psychic energy is a higher synergistic form of regular energies in some unique pattern-holding configuration determined by the nature of living systems and associated complex electrochemical bioenergies. There appear to be intriguing comparisons between the nature of memory storage and the three-dimensionality storage of the hologram. Also, if we may place any credibility on recent and detailed accounts of psychokinetic (PK) effects used to move and affect objects, there seems to exist energy beam collimation, focusing, and energy exchange (temperature differences). The PK phenomenon is a rare event and will not be understood by studying the individual sensing systems, conscious and unconscious, i.e., putting each body input in its own little black box. The *total human being* must be considered. It's how the inputs are combined that counts, and how the combinations act in symbiosis with the environment (Beal, 1972).

The advent of computers and solid state electronics has made the study of complex systems more accessible. Thus an interdisciplinary evolvement of the "hyphenated sciences" and "scientific generalists" has occurred to apply the systems engineering concepts basic to aerospace developments. Interdisciplinary efforts can now be applied to question basic life processes and the electrochemical, rhythmical patterns which can be combined in a hierarchy of systems toward increasing stages of complexity, awareness, and higher-order effects.

The Situation Today

Much of what goes on in space, especially in the earth-sun relationship, and cosmic rays from deep space, affects our environment, ecology, and biology. It is wise and prudent to learn the mechanism of these relationships and radiations, and what trends they may be causing in the earth's evolution, climate, and ourselves (Beal, 1971).

The scientists of the Renaissance gave man an impetus toward total awareness that has carried him beyond the earth as well as toward the center of life. We are beginning to understand the structure of mind.

The human brain is the most complicated structure in the known universe, but as practically nothing of the universe is known, it is probably fairly low in the scale of organic computers. Nevertheless, it contains powers and potentialities still largely untapped, and perhaps unguessed at. Probably 99% of human ability has been wholly wasted; even today, those of us who consider ourselves cultured and educated operate for most of our time as automatic machines, and glimpse the profounder resources of our minds only once or twice in a lifetime.

Until comparatively recently, the 1950s, biologists regarded a cell as a minute bag of fluid that was relatively simple in structure. But under the electron-scanning microscope, cells were seen to be exceedingly complex. What earlier seemed to be a simple cell wall was likely to be folded and convoluted—precisely the right kind of structure to serve as a semiconductor (Cope, 1971). And components of the cell are likely to include organic semiconductors such as liquid crystals, a material that is hypersensitive to temperature changes, magnetic and electric fields, stress, radiation, and trace contamination. To complicate matters even more, many cells have a double outer membrane; electrically, such a membrane functions as a capacitor with the characteristics of a leaky dielectric (Garrison, 1969). It should be mentioned here that recently superconducting fluctuations have been observed experimentally in organic molecular crystals at transition temperatures of 60

K (*Machine Design,* 1973). A number of investigators feel that a strong possibility exists for superconduction in special circumstances at room temperature within living systems (Puharich, 1971).

The mind, as a product of brain, body, and environmental stimuli, may be the highest form of synergistic pattern now known to exist. The phenomenon of consciousness (and learning processes) needs more objective study; however, this may prove a tough objective, since the consciousness or mind has only itself to study itself with! It may be worthwhile to start with simpler systems and work our way up. Perhaps the emerging use of biosensors such as plants, tissue cultures, and single–cell organisms will give us the necessary amplification and selectivity for specific quantitative data of value. Remember also the use of "biosensor" canaries by miners to detect poisonous gases before electronic sensors were available.

There is quite a bit of work going on in Russia and Europe on the effects of EM (electromagnetic) and ES (electrostatic) fields on the central nervous system; also EM and ES effects (and amplification of these effects) around the human body during certain types of paranormal phenomena. The Russian research in parapsychology and paraphysics appears in proper modern semantics as "biological radio communication," "the problem of information transmission," "perception of space effects," "meteorological feeling," "generic memory," "bioenergotherapy," "bioenergetics", and so forth.

We should be concerned that the work in Russia and Eastern Europe will result in some sort of most useful technological surprise, at the very least in some worthwhile biomedical breakthroughs. Instead of heaping scorn on an unexplainable phenomenon, they accept it as a natural, spontaneous, rare event characteristic of mind and proceed to investigate it, though perhaps not as thoroughly as required here. Frankly, they don't have to prove it to themselves as much as we in the Western world have to! There are not as many built-in cultural biases and mental blocks to overcome (Beal, 1973).

To digress briefly, it seems that serendipity, hunches, and creativity are borderline cases similar to psychic phenomena and just as difficult to analyze logically. So much of what goes on in the mind is experiential and not subject to experimental analysis. Did you ever try to describe an emotion to someone? Or a rainbow to a blind person? How does a mango taste? (like a peach with a hint of turpentine!). Usually, the best you get is an analogy to something else, which is poor communication and extremely subject to distortion.

Creative processes, like psychic processes, can be stimulated by strong emotion and prolonged concentration; creativity is also commonly accompanied by neurotic symptoms and personality, because of a different **way of** looking at things and resultant interpersonal and cultural conflicts. However, if we recall that the profound basis of creativity is a free flow of ideas from the subconscious to the conscious mind, we see that this is similar to other psychic phenomena; that although messages may register on the receiver's subconscious mind, there are so many stronger and more dynamic mental functions to restrict the registration of these messages on the conscious level, that more frequently than not, the message will be repressed. J. B. Rhine (1953) noted the close association of para–psi phenomena and creativity as early as 1934, when he indicated that the highly creative skills of the composer, the inventor, the poet, the reflective scientist, required the highest integration of the nervous system for their best creation. Not only do skepticism ("snicker effect") and low motivation preclude good test results, but so do physical fatigue, and depressant drugs.

The way to learn something is to try and see if it exists. When someone theorizes a new nuclear particle, gigavolt particle accelerators are fired up, massive hydrogen bubble chambers are activated, and 100,000 photographs are taken. Computers are programmed to search all the plates seeking the proposed behavior pattern. The physicists say, in effect, "If such a particle exists, then it should have these properties . . ." and then they make a test to check the proposed model. Now the psychic researchers are starting to do the same thing on psi phenomena, using some of the ultrasensitive testing equipment now available for application as detectors, enhancers, suppressors, and biofeedback training aids (Campbell, 1967).

Specific Examples

Recent brain–wave experiments indicate that ES fields can influence the rate of spontaneous electrical impulse generation by the nerves. Other recent tests have demonstrated that brightness discrimination and alertness improves under the influence of a ($+$) ES field, and the visual critical flicker frequency is affected (Presman, 1970; Carson, 1967; Mizusawa, 1969; Sugiyama, 1973). Overall beneficial effects of ($+$) ES field applications are caused by the following (Schaffranke, 1972): (1) *Reduction of the viscosity-index* of blood and lymph fluid, discovered in 1745. This produces an antifatigue effect and acceleration of growth factors. It should be noted that the earth's ($+$) potential gradient reaches a maximum during full moon to third quarter; the metabolic processes of life increase, as does oxygen consumption (Brown, 1959; Mill, 1826). Traditionally, crops are planted at this time for optimum germination. In addition, it is wise to avoid surgery at this time to prevent problems with "bleeders"; (2) *Electrophoresis Effect* causes microbes, virus, and bacteria to travel to the anode (+) of an ES field because their net surface charge is (−). This produces germicides and clean room conditions. In larger cells, the internal charges create (+) surface charges. The surface charges are very important to all living processes and can be demonstrated by electrophoresis; and (3) *Ion-regeneration of the body cells.* Cell renewal happens through ion exchange. Waste products are partially expelled through the skin, and partially through the excretory tract. The electric field attracts these surplus ions away from the body surface, permitting rapid and unhampered renewal of all cells. This effect contributes to the general well-being of man.

The beneficial effects of electrical fields are apparently the results of the combined action of the positive field and the suspended (−) ions in the air. The electric field is the force of motion and the ions are the carriers of electrical charge. This may be the explanation of why effects of (+) and (−) ions on living systems, without the proper ES field present, have shown erratic or contradictory results. Tests have been conducted under the proper conditions with qualitative results indicating (−) ions (oxygen molecules with a surplus of electrons looking for electrochemical processes to enhance) produced improved performance, disposition, equilibrium, burn recovery and healing, and relieved pain and allergic disorders; (+) ions decreased performance and depressed disposition or had no effect. Dr. Puharich (1973) and others have noted the improved results for biological radio communication (telepathy) experiments where the receiver was exposed to a (−) ion environment inside a Faraday Cage.

Feasibility tests were performed by this researcher to determine the effects of a 2000 volt ES (+) field, located 2.5 cm from the top of his head, on the "down-through" clairvoyance test, guessing the order of the cards in the standard 25-card, five symbol ESP card deck. The proximity of the (+) direct current field generator to the head (normally placed 1.0–1.5 meters above head) evidently caused suppression of any clairvoyance ability, i.e., all results during exposure to the intense field were of zero statistical significance (100 card decks = 2500 guesses). With equipment inactive, the result for one curve obtained with 50 decks (10 decks per plotted point) was a probability = .007; another run of the same type produced a $p = .001$. Based on statements made in Dr. Presman's famous book *Electromagnetic Fields and Life* (1970), the effects of high intensity fields on brainwave activity are definite; when near the head an increase in frequency is usually noted, at a distance the opposite effect is noted. It may be that a suppression of natural, spontaneously occurring alpha rhythm resulted from the field exposure, thus reducing the number of hits when equipment was on during the test (assuming that low frequency 7–14 Hz alpha may be an indicator present during better ESP scores). These tests were performed in 1969 with no monitoring of mind, body, and environment; further investigations must be made under more controlled conditions (Beal, 1973).

All bodies of our known physical universe above absolute zero are characterized by the emission of electromagnetic (EM) radiation. On theoretical grounds (corroborated extensively by experiment), a reasonable amount of energy is emitted in the X-band (9 GHz) microwave region, which falls within the detection capabilities of conventional microwave radiometry. Experiments were performed with an X-band microwave radiometer of the correlation type. The microwave emission showed a large increase from the body relative to the background. Other interesting features have been observed, such as information about emotional, pathological, and physiological states of the system. The radiation emissivity in the microwave region changes with electrical and dielectric activity of the living system. Communication, for transfer of complex information between biological systems, seems plausible. More study of emission and absorption spectra in microwave regions is advised (Bigu del Blanco & Romero-Sierra, Feb., June, 1973). There appears to be a possibility for exchange of information over long distances by temporal summation of signals until a threshold is attained and the message gets through; the information may be exchanged through some type of sensitive, coupled oscillator phenomena of life (Franklin, 1973).

The recent advent of solid state physics and field effect transistors (FET) has made possible inexpensive, portable instruments, such as ES field intensity meters (or scanners), which can monitor living system biofields as well as the local environment (McInnis, 1972). The availability of these instruments should lead to some interesting applications for mind–body–environment research in the near future. The equipment output can be fed into an area scanning system (or video presentation), which with suitable electronics of multiple fixed detectors and multiplexing, can produce a two-dimensional plan view of the ES field potentials around the object or person and the way these potentially change patterns. Selective electronic "gating" can be used to produce shades of grey (or color, if color enhancement is used) on the recording display to indicate field intensity ranges of interest (Beal, 1973). Feasibility will be established for development of rapid imaging and recording equipment, similar to present infrared medical scanner systems. Results may show that this phenomenon is an ES analogue of what is known as human "aura."

At least the ability to observe mind–body–environment interactions would be improved and we could become more aware of how the mind affects the body through emotional effects on the electrochemical balance. We now know that acupuncture points differ considerably in resistance from the rest of the body, and these values change during treatment. It would be interesting to see what information patterns we could obtain from dynamic viewing of more than one point at a time. One potential approach for a more rapid and dynamic imaging system (utilizing hints from reported work on Kirlian effects in Russia) would be to investigate the ultraviolet components of high frequency, high intensity, low current electrical corona discharge. The subject under test could be coated selectively with a conductive material, if necessary, and the high-intensity field applied to a potential just below the arcing point. Ultraviolet corona characteristics can then be observed by a low-light-level-image vidicon television camera tube of high sensitivity, using ultraviolet transmission filters to replace the glass tube front (Strong et al., 1970). Sophisticated electronic color enhancement can be used to provide a color readout of changes in applied field, caused by amplification of electrochemical and dielectric biosystem changes (modulation of applied field).

Preliminary investigations into body field variations (since 1920) indicate that the natural body field is $(+)$, while certain types of malignancies are $(-)$; other pathologies produce drastic changes in body potential of an identifying nature (Crile et al., 1922; Burr & Langman, 1949; Cone & Tongier, 1971). Further work remains to be done toward interpretation of the received data, and development of suitable equipment. Consideration of many factors is required so the very minute signals of interest can be sifted from all the internal, external, and emotional background "noise" present, i.e., a standardized series of conditions is required that must consider environmental, geophysical, and astrophysical factors, as well as control of psychological attitudes and physiological factors. Studies are now underway to determine which of the multitude of variables are most important to replication of experiments.

The magnetic field of the earth averages about 0.5 Gauss and has continuous pulsations of low magnitude at frequencies ranging from 0.1 to 100 Hz, *peaking around 10 Hz;* this is known as the Schumann resonance (1952), where the earth-ionosphere cavity acts as a natural resonator; this was much more powerful during primitive earth development and may have played an important part in the origin and evolvement of life (Graf & Cole, 1967; Cole & Graf, 1973). The typical 7–14 Hz alpha brainwave pattern for sleep and dreaming falls precisely in this range, and a relationship between these phenomena has been suggested by many investigators. This is known as biological entrainment of the human brain by low frequency radiation (Konig, 1971). Note that similar frequencies of light and sound pulses can trigger epileptic attacks, induce altered states of consciousness, and cause nausea. The step from external sensory stimuli to subconscious EM stimuli in entraining cerebral rhythms is not a radical concept (Graf & Cole, 1967; Cole & Graf, 1973; Konig, 1971; Hamer, 1965). For example, approaching storm fronts appear to have a local E-field variation of 3–5 Hz: the ion balance of the atmosphere and the ES field polarity are also affected by the storm front; in addition to reaction time reductions, headaches, general depression, and lethargy occur in weather-sensitive individuals; paranormal abilities and events decrease. Accident rates of automobiles and aircraft may also be associated with these effects.

The possibilities of bioentrainment (for enhancement, training, or suppression of psychic ability) are already with us when you consider that medical equipment for treatment of hearing loss is now available for inducing sound into the cochlea electrically and noncontact, by use of audio signal modulation of the 100 kHz carrier frequency. Although those in the vicinity hear nothing, the subject near the antenna perceives sound as if through earphones.[1] The ability of many individuals to "hear" radar microwave as a "buzzing like bees," is well-documented, as are sporadic reports of "hearing" aurora displays and meteors passing overhead (Halacy, 1967). As one might expect, these reports have, until recently, been dismissed as unfounded; after all, the effects were subjective and not everyone "heard" them. Nurses who work in mental institutions describe patients who are always trying to get away from the terrible noise. Certain rooms or areas seem to be more quiet for them (electrical field null points?). How many people are now in mental institutions or psychologically afflicted because of hypersensitivity to electric fields (Wioske, 1963)? Russian investigators report that changes in hypothalamus activity can increase the sensitivity to EM fields many times (Kholodov, 1967).

A magnet at 60 Hz and 8700 Gauss held to the temple gives rise to a visual light sensation known as the "phosphene" effect. This effect can also be induced by electrical frequencies and chemicals (Knoll et al., 1963), fasting, meditation, fatigue, or light flicker (with eyes closed) techniques (Van Someren, 1973). It is not known why, but a person under hypnosis or in a state of mescaline intoxication can often perceive a static magnetic field—through modification of visual images. A flicker effect is associated with a varying field.

---

[1] Laser Sound System in Glendale, California, and Intelecton in New York City are conducting research in electrical stimulation of hearing.

This is confirmation of Reichenbach's research with ill psychic sensitives in Europe about 1850. Their. extreme sensitivity to magnetic fields—pain and visual effects (in a dark room)—was well-documented. It appears there may be some potential clues for electronic stimulation (or simulation) of vision in the above areas for aid to the blind (Garrison, 1969).

Of particular environmental interest to those in the Middle East (with possible political and emotional interest, also) is the *khamsin* or *sharav* wind which moves up out of the desert each spring and fall for approximately 150 days out of the year. It picks up hot air and dust as it sweeps across Africa and the Sinai Peninsula, bringing a variety of afflictions in its northerly thrust. The moistureless air causes feet to swell painfully, noses and eyes to itch, and asthmatics to gasp for breath. Automobile accidents, crime rates, and mental cases increase. Other countries suffer from such hot dry winds containing an excess of positive ions. Italy has the sirocco, Southern Europe has the *foehn,* France has the *mistral,* and the United States has the chinook and Santa Ana winds. Young people become tense, irritable, and occasionally violent; older persons become fatigued, apathetic, depressed, and sometimes faint. Professor Felix Gad Sulman of the Hebrew University's Department of Applied Pharmacology in Jerusalem has conducted a nine-year study involving 500 people using drugs such as monoamine oxidase (MAO), and negative ion generators, which readily bring relief to *khamsin* victims. In the bloodstream, thrombocytes react to the positive ions by releasing their neurohormone, serotonin, which reduces breathing capacity by about 30%, causes headache or dizziness, sore throat, and nasal obstructions. MAO and negative ions prevent the release of serotonin (Sulman, 1971). A. P. Krueger of the University of California in Berkeley has performed similar work which verifies Dr. Sulman's studies (1969). Tests made on animals 80 years ago showed that a negative electric field markedly reduced vitality and fertility of animals, whereas a positive field stimulated respiration, digestion, and metabolism in general. Forty years ago, European research revealed the effect of a positive field on plant growth and on human performance. (*Time,* 1971). This author also performed some experiments with bean seedlings using a simple dc power supply radiating a 2000 volt (+) potential electrostatic field from a metal plate parallel to and 15 cm above the soil surface. A four-day earlier germination resulted for the exposed plants compared to the control group. Both subject and control plants were grown in screened and grounded enclosures under the same conditions, except the control group had an inactive plate above it. The same equipment was used on a child of fourteen months, who had recurrent monthly bronchial asthma attacks requiring hospitalization. In the four months last year with the metal plate installed 1.5 cm over his bed, there were no further attacks. On removal of the equipment for shipment to Israel (for World Institute evaluation with Dr. Sulman of Hebrew University), there were subsequent mild attacks which could be controlled with routine medication.

It is recognized that there may be more psychological factors associated with asthmatic pathologies than almost any other body condition, but there seem to be some possible field effect tie-ins to the old wive's tale that can be called the Chihuahua or Dachshund Effect! Basically, the idea is to give a child with severe asthma a small dog (assuming the child is not allergic to animals). The dog must be near the child as much of the time as possible and must sleep with the child. I remember that there was much controversy about this type of therapy when I read about it over twenty years ago; the only possible answers at that time were the psychological benefits of a child having a small, lovable animal to play with. When I started to collect information on EM field effects associated with living systems, the beneficial effects of the positive field–negative ion interrelationship began to accumulate. In addition, information on the positive field around plants, animals, humans, and the earth supplied interesting potential tie-ins. Equipment became available (electrostatic field meters) to easily check out these conditions, and what do you know? Small dogs, such as dachshunds and chihuahuas, have up to 400 volts/meter (+) potential! This is due to their short hair and high metabolic rate. The potential generated is about twice that found in the Huntsville, Alabama, area. Of course, we can now replace the dog with a dc power supply and save a lot of possible mess and bother.

This example reminds us of other similar cases, such as tempering the Damascus sword blade, which required running the red-hot blade through the body of a surplus slave. When slaves became expensive, it was found that oil would do the job as well; it was also once thought necessary to throw a virgin into the molten metal for casting a suitable peal of temple bells in ancient Japan; the body supplied the potassium required, but eventually they found out that any old bones would do. Perhaps these examples are a bit drastic, but they serve to illustrate that science usually evolves out of empirical observations of nature, and the quest for causes to explain the effects observed.

Viewed as a minute, but extremely elaborate electrochemical system, the living cell is subject to the influence of EM fields both static and dynamic, as indicated herein. And these fields may induce not just one but a complex system of currents, as well as act as indicators of environmental conditions. Small wonder, therefore, that reported field effects at the cellular level (and psychic phenomena at mind level) are diverse and debatable; the effects will depend upon the field orientation, components of the system, its organization, its energy, and other variable factors. Indeed, effects are often more apparent in living systems that are not healthy! Schizophrenia may be an example of this, and Familial Periodic Disease, a type of periodic paralysis (with preponderant 4–6 Hz EEG waves), shows evidence of psychic ability in a large number of cases.[2]

The bioelectric field effects, described briefly and inadequately herein, are not to be construed as the cause behind psychic phenomena. They may only serve, at best, as weak indicators, precursors, or second derivitive effects of higher system interactions basic to life processes. As indicated by Julius Stulman, president of World Institute (1972), "Suffice it to say that we are dealing in a new science, the Methodology of Pattern, which, as we have indicated, should be the direction of our search. We must learn its laws and relationships as it exists in irregular pulsating reference frames in integrated systems so that we may emerge to new understandings in all our concerns." Thus, as a product of the cosmos, we are all tuned in, and our biorhythms react accordingly to EM and ES fields, low frequency radiation, ions and other unknown factors (Luce, 1970).

Important Considerations

There is a lack of detailed information on environmental effects: Psychic and biological phenomena unique to unusual geophysical environments should be investigated. The existence of special cases due to natural causes has a high probability. The changing or absence of common factors are good indicators.

It must be clearly established whether or not there are psychic and–or biological effects which can be enhanced or suppressed by the application of our science and technology on the natural environment. We don't exist in our environments, we exist by means of our environments (McInnis, 1972). The technological age of the twentieth century finally presents an opportunity to control or change our immediate internal and external surroundings. Up to now we have only had the natural ES and EM field to which we are adapted to contend with, largely undetectable by the senses, but affecting mind and body in subtle ways.

It seems obvious we should be studying how to evaluate and enhance psychic abilities in a controlled geophysical environment, complementing the

---

[2]Correspondence with Neil Terhune, March, 1973 and discussion with Jules Eisenbud in February, 1973.

internal body environment by the proper ties with the nerve network, blood chemistry, glandular chemistry, and body time. For example, possibilities seem to exist for effects on brainwave frequency and bioentrainment of brainwave rhythms with light, sound, and EM fields; visual phosphene effects and sound can also be induced with suitable power and frequencies.

There is a lot of qualitative data, going back to the beginning of history, about psychic phenomena effects on living processes, people, domestic animals, plants, and inanimate things, but little background data in terms of astrophysical, geophysical, psychological, and physiological conditions required to develop the effects. Such evidence as exists in arcane and ancient literature is clouded by dogma, ritual, theology, semantics, and secrecy. However, empirical evidence does exist that a number of ancient cultures knew about the vectorial relationship existing between the EM field direction and the neuraxis, and that the geomagnetic field appeared to affect the functioning of higher neuronal centers. The magnetic field orientation in tests of living systems is often overlooked in our present culture, but was considered most important by the Chinese, for example, who felt that beneficial health, mental, and spiritual qualities could be obtained by proper geophysical orientation of homes and religious shrines—in relation to the earth's magnetic poles, subterranean streams, geology, and topology. Thus, reappraisal of the historical and ancient literature in myths, legends, religious systems, and philosophies, where applicable in the field of psychic phenomena, is warranted.

Complex interacting variables will require development of models and standards: We need to start developing specifications for producing and monitoring the optimum laboratory and field environments. The suitability of specific living systems as experimental models for best effects response must be more thoroughly established. Physiological rhythm effects must be considered and we must look for patterns, implicit and explicit. It may be possible that certain pathological conditions serve as amplifiers of effects, as mentioned previously. Quite a few species of animals, plants, insects, and aquatic organisms have already been investigated in some detail and may serve as suitable experimental subjects. We should also keep in mind that we can't separate a living system from its environment; the environment is not an external entity.

Safety standards for mind and body are of the utmost importance and must be observed and developed relative to electrical shock hazards, radiation exposure, dosimetry, and intrusive equipment applications into the living system. The use of selected biosensors should be considered here as insurance against unknown quantities.

Education and communication needs in psychic research: Expansion of choices in curriculum for college students in order to encourage interdisciplinary interests is needed. It is encouraging to see a steadily rising number of higher educational institutions offering courses of study and experimentation with altered states of consciousness and subjective experience. These usually start out in the free schools adjacent to the college, and prove so popular with the students that courses are added to the regular curriculum.

Apprenticeship and–or intensive short courses in productive areas, programmed autogenic training, and self-instruction meditation methods are often useful with proper guidance and follow-up with practical applications. A primary motivation of learning is the need to discover and understand what makes us possible. We must value, in order to care for, whatever makes us possible. We can best be moved to care about and for our environments when we see how they make us possible. (McInnis, 1972).

Application of existing technology must be made as soon as possible. Get the new developments into circulation and to the other investigators so that optimum results are obtained and "reinvention of the wheel" is kept to a minimum. It is important to remember that information about what can't be done, mistakes commonly made, research blind alleys, and equipment limitations are very important information factors in any developing area of scientific inquiry.

It seems that there are at present too many specialists in some areas; not enough persons skilled in interdisciplinary work involving physics, electrical engineering, biology, behavior, and general systems. There is a need for interpreters or application teams of individuals who can interface as generalists between disciplines. This would be a means by which a scientist or student in one discipline could obtain information in another discipline and understand it. It is always worthwhile to learn the other person's point of view and terminology, preferably before he learns yours.

Implications for Science, Technology, Philosophy, and Culture

We are a world with the greatest total awareness potential ever known. We have reached goals formerly considered unattainable—in spirit and in fact—new worlds! Unfortunately, people seldom relate science and technology to the everyday business of living, fighting the daily traffic, getting the kids off to school, and buying the groceries. If they do, they are apt to curse it, particularly when it comes to new ideas to improve knowledge of self, or change quality, quantity, or environment. Far too many do not understand or care little about the need for research into the subjective nature of man (except when the kids bring it home to threaten parental authority with a little "future shock" item that upsets the family status quo).

We can point in vain to biofeedback, control of autonomic processes, meditation benefits, Russian advances in bioenergetics. People simply yawn, since it doesn't confront them directly. So, who needs any more science and technology? We've got too much already—look at the shape the world is in! (as seen on their new solid-state color TV, by satellite transmission—of predominantly negative news coverage—from 10,000 miles away!) Unfortunately, we live in a culture where a large portion of our information and emotional inputs are of a negative nature. It appears we need some "negative attention-getting" statements to reach the man on the street and get his interest, then expand his awareness with the useful, positive possibilities (as applied to himself, of course) of inner space research.

Based on recent evaluations of psychic phenomena associated with Uri Geller, Ingo Swann, Nelya Mikhailova, and Alla Vinogradova, the Heisenberg uncertainty principle assumes a formidable importance! The instruments science trusts cannot be trusted under some circumstances; the human mind can affect them. Catalytic reactions may be enhanced or suppressed occasionally, the whole basis of modern measurements is jeopardized. This may be why we get such adverse reactions from people in the scientific establishment. It's difficult to entertain such a concept until you are personally affected by unexplained phenomena. Talk about implications for the future and threats to the sense of security for scientists!

Few seem to realize that civilized man (whatever that means) cannot long survive on this planet without the creation of new knowledge and its enlightened use to handle the fantastically complex, interrelated, and synergistic challenges of the future. Unfortunately, altruistic individuals with funding for exploratory research are scarce.

Our difficulty is that as a world of short-term pragmatists, most persons are not geared mentally to long-range planning and some of the cultural changes and benefits that result from advanced scientific and technological programs, not to mention inner space research effects.

Concepts of man and the universe, and man in the universe, motivate our thinking and actions on earth. Are contributions to such concepts unimportant to the quality of life we strive for today? On the contrary, they are basic to the definition of what we mean about quality in life. Without a growing precision of our definition of the universe, external and internal, objective and subjective, material and spiritual, and the elements involved, we cannot hope to improve more than the physical aspects of day-to-day living.

A. *Goals to Consider*
1. Collection, correlation, validation of the enormous mass of subjective effects data that exist.
2. Systems research with existing data combined in new patterns to provide greater insights into the complex facets of subjective experience (noetics).
3. Integration of the knowledge obtained into existing knowledge of the physical universe and therefrom to construct a more complete paradigm of the total extent and functioning of the human organism.
4. Communication and coordination with the mainstream of human thought, through the various multisensory methods and educational media.
5. Implementation of knowledge for the benefit of humanity. It is recognized that "bare" knowledge without action or application is sterile, and misapplication of knowledge—action without wisdom —is dangerous!

B. *Methods Development*
1. Suitable equipment, evaluation techniques, and facilities (fixed and mobile) should be developed as first priority. As equipment is developed, the range of spatial and temporal variations of electrical, ionic, magnetic, gravitic, and other influence fields generated by the geophysical environment and–or man, animals, and plants, must be established. Development of a standard environment for psychophysiological enhancement in the laboratory and in the field is recommended. Mechanisms by which biological fields are generated and influenced must be studied.
2. The types of equipment to be considered would be the environmental and EM/ES field monitors, detectors, and recorders, plus EM- and ES-shielded rooms, sensory stimulation and deprivation devices, environmental control or simulation equipment, and safety monitors; biofeedback equipment is needed also, and as much psychophysiological monitoring (preferably nonintrusive) as is comfortable to the subject. Biosensors of environmental changes, emotional states, and living system hazards of unknown origin

should be considered. Placebo devices can serve as training aids by the psychological transfer mechanism. In these days of science and gadget-worship it is easy to blame something not understood on a machine because such talents are impossible from human beings due to negative cultural conditioning.

3. During the evaluation or training of the subject, certain factors are recommended for consideration, such as facility environment; attitudes toward equipment used; the experiment conductor and any other subjects; emotional, mental, and health state of subject; other factors such as subject's biological rhythm schedule, personal values, cultural conditioning, situation safety. In man, animals, fish, and birds, we must look for behavior changes (individual and group, learned and instinctual), psychophysiological effects, biorhythm alterations, and navigation or homing errors. In plants we must consider effects on growth rate, biological rhythms, germination, mutation, orientation, and electrochemical changes. For unicellular organisms, mobility, growth, mitotic effects, mutations, orientation, and rhythms may be affected.

C. *Applications Development—Enhancement/Enrichment of Human Resources*

1. Training of mind, for optimum control and awareness of body field conditions and internal and external influences, is recommended. Use of simple monitoring or enhancement electronic aids would be likely, combined with meditation and–or autogenic techniques, and perhaps audio-visual-EM field bioentrainment methods to stimulate a particular type of altered state for a particular application (chanting, mandala patterns, and selected geophysical locations were used for this purpose in the past). Training for personal self-development and guidance for others should be stressed, and a background in psychology is essential, of course.

2. It is recommended that field effects on and from empathic groups experienced in bioentrainment, awareness, and ASC projection techniques be investigated.

3. Counselors with psychology background for human resources enhancement-enrichment training toward positive attitudes and realization of creative self-potential, should be provided for education of the public, and as scouts for exceptional individuals with psychic talents.

Conclusions

As more data are gathered in fundamental studies involving the nature of subjective awareness, the how and why of psychic field effects and other patterns should emerge. We will have to apply more systems engineering, electronics of complex nature, and computers than ever before in seeking the proper patterns. Toward this end the fine arts, as expressed in creative combinations of sensory inputs (audio, visual, kinesthetics, etc.) must also be considered for training and enhancement of human resources to eliminate considerable external, internal, and emotional "noise" present.

Individuals with considerable psychic ability are known and are under intensive evaluation by serious researchers; the extension of scientific method in investigation of these people and the essential phenomena of ASC is now underway. As the awareness for the need of a synergistic, total systems approach to the study of the nature of the human being (mind-body-environment), becomes more generally known, far-reaching and rapid changes now beginning in the sciences and social order will accelerate and a new cultural paradigm may emerge. It seems that the threshold point has about arrived, but this may be a biased feeling.

As indicated herein, we're getting the tools and techniques to start a concerted research effort into inner space. Is anybody ready to indulge in "constraint removal analysis" to extend the limits of the possible? Possibilities of bioentrainment of living system rhythms, by external audio-visual-EM field fluctuations and–or ASC for training and enhancement of psychic and creative ability, are already under investigation; results will be most worthwhile and applicable to medical, psychological, and educational areas.

Reappraisal of historical and ancient literature is beginning, especially environmental and group effects, in the search for qualitative clues to the nature of consciousness and formation of new test paradigms.

As the public is becoming more knowledgeable (not necessarily correctly informed) about possibilities of altered states of consciousness and psychic phenomena, we can see the rapid expansion of educational media, both good and bad. We must do all we can to keep the quality of the information and training at a high level; there are enough mental problems already in the culture. Unfortunately, distorted acceptance by the public will be in direct proportion to personal application in areas concerning, 1) health and comfort —mental and physical; 2) ego benefits (hope, confidence, power, status); 3) stimulation (emotional-sexual excitement); and, 4) income-wealth-energy to obtain desired elements of all three. The movie, *The Exorcist,* fulfills item 3, above, in a most negative way, so we can expect a tremendous increase in mental cases of possession by another personality, already publicized in the papers. How are you planning to treat these cases? We can't sweep them under the rug and they may not respond to standard treatment. Is your exorcism kit ready? We are going to have to try to counter some of the negative distortions with positive, useful applications, and this is where the confluence of psychiatry, biology, technology, and mysticism will provide some answers.

Man used to say that man the scientist brought order out of chaos.

The scientists are rapidly discovering that all that was chaotic was in man's illiterate and bewildered imagination and fearful ignorance.

Our knowledge of the universe, at the present, is only measurable in dimensional units of energy, time, and space. These are mostly above or below the narrow dimensions which man is accustomed to detecting by direct sensing and by consciousness awareness (Fuller, 1963). Recent extension of our perceptions to other areas, objective and subjective, has shown that new information is gained wherever we look, without bias, whether it be in inner or outer space.

"A new world is only a new mind!"

William Carlos Williams

References

Alpert, R. *Be here now.* San Cristobal, N.M.: Lama Foundation, 1971.

Beal, J. B. The emergence of paraphysics: research and applications. In J. White (Ed.) *Psychic exploration—a challenge for science.* New York: Putnam, 1974.

_____. Electrostatic fields, electromagnetic fields and ions—mind-body-environment interrelationships. Paper presented at the Neuroelectric Society Symposium and Workshop, Snowmass-at-Aspen, Colorado, February, 1973.

_____. Paraphysics and parapsychology. *Analog Science Fiction/Science Fact.* 1973, **XCII**(4) 68–83.

_____. Kent State Inner Space Research Center prospectus outline. Unpublished report, 1972.

———. Methodology of pattern in awareness. Fields within fields within fields. *The World Institute Council,* 1972, **5**, 42–48.

———. The new bio-technology—potential applications to the educational environment. Paper presented at the International Symposium, Evaluation in Science Education and the Uses of Educational Technology. Jerusalem, Israel, August, 1972.

———. Space—for all. Paper presented at Mankind in the Universe Conference, Southern Illinois University, April, 1971.

Bigu del Blanco, J. & Romero-Sierra, C. Microwave radiometry techniques and means to explore the possibility of communication in biological systems. Paper presented at Neuroelectric Society Symposium and Workshop, Snowmass-at-Aspen, Colorado, February, 1973.

———. Radiofrequency fields: a new ecological factor. Institute of Electrical and Electronic Engineers. Symposium on Electromagnetic Compatibilities, New York City, June, 1973.

Brown, F. A. Living clocks. *Science,* 1959, **130**, 1535.

Burr, H. S. & Langman, L. A technique to aid in the detection of malignancy of the female genital tract. *American Journal of Obstetrics and Gynecology,* 1949, **57**(2), 274–281.

Campbell, J. W. Sense of security. *Analog Science Fiction/Science Fact,* 1967, **LXXVIII**(2), 5–7, 170–177.

Carson, R. W. Anti-fatigue device works by creating electric field. *Product Engineering,* 1967, Feb. 13, 52–54.

Cole, F. E. & Graf, E. R. Extra low frequency electromagnetic radiation as a biocommunications medium: a protein transreceiver system. Paper presented at Neuroelectric Society Symposium and Workshop, Snowmass-at-Aspen, Colorado, February, 1973.

Cone, C. D. & Tongier, M. Control of somatic cell mitosis by simulated changes in the transmembrane potential level. *Oncology,* 1971, **25**, 168–182.

Cope, F. W. Biological interfaces behave like electrode surfaces. Summary of discussion at Workshop in Bioelectrochemistry, Princeton, N.J., October, 1971.

Crile, G. W. et al. The electrical conductivity of animal tissues under normal and pathological conditions. *American Journal of Physiology,* 1922, **60**, 59–106.

Curing an ill wind. *Time,* June 14, 1971, p. 73.

Dewan, E. M. Rhythms. *Science & Technology,* 1969, 20–28.

Franklin, W. Teleneural physics. *Physics Today,* 1973, (8), 11.

Fuller, R. B. *No more second-hand God.* Carbondale, Ill.: Southern Illinois University Press, 1963.

Garrison, W. Magnets and human life. *Science & Electronics,* 1969, Aug.-Sept., 29–33.

Graf, E. R. & Cole, F. C. Radiation noise energy and human physiology in deep space. *American Astronautical Society,* 1967, Document AAS67–322(EN-2) –1.

Hamer, J. R. Biological entrainment of the human brain by low frequency radiation. Technical memo 532–65–45, Northrup Space Lab, Jan., 1965.

Halacy, D. Biological radio—ESP. *Popular Electronics,* 1967, April, 53–58.

Hardy, J. D. *Physiological Problems in Space Exploration.* Springfield, Ill.: C. C. Thomas, 1964.

Kholodov, Y. A. Effect of electromagnetic and magnetic fields on the central nervous system. NASA Technical Translation, TTF-465, June, 1967.

Knoll, M. et al. Effects of chemical stimulation of electrically induced phosphenes on their bandwidth, shape, number and intensity. *Confinia Neurologica,* 1963, **23,** 201–226.

Konig, H. Biological effects of extremely low frequency electrical phenomena in the atmosphere. *Journal of Interdisciplinary Cycle Research,* 1971, 2(3), 317–323.

Krippner, S. & Meacham, W. Consciousness and the creative process. *The Gifted Child Quarterly,* 1968, Autumn, 141–159.

Krueger, A. P. Preliminary consideration of the biological significance of air ions. *Scintia,* 1969, **104,** 460–476.

Luce, G. Biological rhythms in psychiatry and medicine. NIMH Public Health Service Publication, 1970, 2088.

McInnis, N. You are an environment—teaching-learning environmental attitudes. The Center for Curriculum Design, Evanston, Illinois, 1972.

Mill, N. Influences of the moon on animal and vegetable economy. *The Franklin Journal-American Mechanics' Magazine,* 1826, **1,** 237–239.

Mizusawa, K. The effects of atmospheric ions on visual parameters. Paper presented at Space-Optics Seminar at University of California, Santa Barbara, September, 1969.

Presmau, A. S. *Electromagnetic Fields and Life.* New York: Plenum, 1970.

Puharich, A. Protocommunication. Paper presented at annual conference of the Parapsychology Foundation, Le Piol, St. Paul de Vence, France, August, 1971.

————. *Beyond telepathy.* Garden City, N.Y.: Anchor Press, 1973.

Rhine, J. B. *New world of the mind.* New York: Wm. Sloane, 1953.

Shuman, W. O. Uber die strahlungslosen eigenschwingungen einer leitenden Kugel, die von einer Luftschicht und einer ionospharenhulle embeden ist. Z. Z. Naturf. 1952, 7A, 149–154.

Speeth, S. D. Alpha wave synchronizing and ESP. Parapsychology Laboratory, Duke University, Durham, N.C., 1954.

Schaffranke, R. Summary of information on the basic causes of the overall beneficial effects of biological dc field applications. Personal communication.

Strong, N. G. et al. Visual, ultraviolet, and ultrasonic display of corona fields in air. *Proceedings, Institute of Electrical Engineering.* 1970, 117, 1453.

Stulman, J. The methodology of pattern. Fields within fields within fields. *World Institute Council,* 1972, 5, 36.

Sugiyama, S. A study on cycling of the critical flicker frequency by the application of electric fields. Paper presented at Neuroelectric Society symposium and workshop, Snowmass-at-Aspen, Colorado, February, 1973.

Sulman, F. G. Serotonin-migraine in climatic heat stress, its prophylaxsis and treatment. *Proceedings of the International Headache Symposium,* Elsinore, Denmark, May, 1971.

Superconductivity observed at 60 K. *Machine Design,* April 19, 1973.

Van Somereu, L. Dream machine. *Mensa Bulletin,* 1973, 171 (II), 11.

Wioske, C. W. Human sensitivity to electric fields. Laboratory for the Study of Sensory Systems. Tucson, Arizona, 1963.

Thelma Moss, John Hubacher, Frances Saba

Kirlian Photography: Visual Evidence of Bioenergetic Interactions Between People?

OVER THE PAST few years there has been increasing interest and controversy over a particular kind of electrical photography developed by the Soviet scientists, Semyon and Valentina Kirlian (1961). This photography, which requires neither camera nor lens, obtains a picture by placing an object in direct contact with a piece of film, and pulsing an electrical current through it. The resulting picture reveals both internal and external characteristics not visible to the eye; and the nature of those characteristics remains a puzzle, for which several hypotheses have been offered (Inyushin, 1969; Adamenko, 1970; Krippner & Krippner, 1974.)

Differences Between Organic and Inorganic Materials

Before discussing these hypotheses, let us first examine a few typical Kirlian photographs (1961). Here is one, obtained in the Soviet Union, of a Russian two kopek coin (Figure 1), which reveals not only surface details of the coin, which are visible to the eye, but an external corona which of course is not visible to the eye. And here, in color, is a United States penny (Figure 2) also showing in a patriotic red, white, and blue, the representational surface detail, as well as external corona. It is remarkable that with inorganic objects such as coins, stones, and metals, the external corona seems never to change.

This constancy does not occur with organic substances. Take, for example, this photograph of a leaf, freshly plucked from a plant (Figure 3). Here we do not find a representational surface as with the coins. Instead, we see a complex pattern of "bubbles" which, according to plant physiologists, are not related to the plant's anatomical or physiological structure; nor, of course, is the corona which surrounds it. If a leaf such as this one is left for several hours and photographed again (Figure 4), it loses much of its interior detail, and the corona becomes less pronounced. And, typically, after two or three days, the leaf—although still green and intact—is no longer able to be photographed (Figure 5).

Photographs of Human Finger Pads

Like the leaves of plants, human beings, too, demonstrate changes in both internal and external characteristics, with much more lability, and, frequently, much more emphasis. In our laboratory (1972) we have concentrated on photographing the finger pads of many people, under a variety of emotional and physiological conditions. And we have learned that there generally seems to be a continuum within each person, ranging from high arousal to deep relaxation. Here, on black-and-white film, are seen what we believe to be typical of a state of deep relaxation (Figure 6); there can be observed a large, bright corona and vivid fingerprints. This same subject, with less relaxation, shows a narrower corona, and his fingerprints have disappeared (Figure 7). In a state of tension, the subject's corona becomes, as can be clearly seen, thin and sketchy (Figure 8). And with strong emotion, such as anger or anxiety, his picture changes dramatically: instead of the corona, there is revealed a strange–looking cloud-like effect (Figure 9), which extends far beyond the finger pad. In color this cloudy emanation is invariably represented by a brilliant red blotch (Figure 10), whereas the corona typical of relaxation is almost always a vivid blue/white combination (Figure 11). Occasionally we find that the subject will give a combination of blotch-and-corona (Figure 12). And on a few very rare occasions we have found persons who do not seem to change at all, no matter how aroused or relaxed they appear to be.

Drug Studies

With this basic background, we began to examine what happens to individuals under deliberately contrived conditions, with one particular variable. For example, a medical student at U.C.L.A. volunteered to come to the lab one evening and get thoroughly drunk. We offered him as much of his favorite drink (bourbon) as he could hold, with only two conditions stipulated: (1) he had to drink one ounce of whiskey every fifteen minutes until he wished to stop, and (2) he would permit us to photograph his right index finger tip after each drink. This is how his finger tip looked when he first arrived in the lab, before he had had anything at all to drink (Figure 13). From this narrow, sketchy corona, we inferred that he was tense or nervous about the ensuing experiment. After just one drink, his finger pad looked like this (Figure 14); after 7 ounces, he had begun to get a "rosy glow" (Figure 15); after 14 ounces, he had a very rosy glow indeed (Figure 16), and after 17 ounces, he was "all lit up" (Figure 17). In fact, immediately after this picture was taken, he got very sick. Unfortunately we were not scientists enough to take his picture under that condition; we were too busy trying to alleviate his misery, and cleaning up the lab.

Marijuana intoxication has also revealed dramatic changes. In this photograph we can see two finger pads of a subject before taking the drug (Figure 18); and here they are during the height of the intoxication (Figure 19).

Exploring These Emanations in Terms of Bioenergy

We had observed so many interesting changes in emanations that we began to wonder if we were obtaining visual representation of bioenergy, and the energy fields (or life fields) described by Harold Saxton Burr (1972). We reasoned that if we were, in fact, obtaining pictures of bioenergy, then we might expect to see a transfer, or interaction of energy between objects.

Our first foray into the possibility of bioenergetic interactions involved the phenomenon (or mythology) of the "green thumb" claimed by some expert gardeners. We asked volunteer subjects, who believed they were successful with plants, to perform what we called the "leaf healing" experiment. An experimenter would pluck a leaf from a plant and photograph it in its healthy, intact condition (Figure 20). Then he would mutilate the leaf by gashing it, and punching holes in it (Figure 21). After obtaining a picture of the mutilated leaf, he would ask the subject to hold his hand about two inches *above* the leaf, and keep it there as long as he felt it necessary in order to "heal" the leaf (generally a procedure lasting no more than two minutes). After that, the leaf was photographed a third time (Figure 22). In a majority of the 40 "leaf healing" studies, this was the result—the leaf showed a greatly increased luminescence after the "treatment." But occasionally, unexpectedly, we obtained a radically different result. Here, in color, is a freshly plucked leaf (Figure 23); here it is after mutilation (Figure 24); and here it is again after the subject had held his hand above the leaf for about 90 seconds (Figure 25).

The leaf has all but disappeared. We have called this the "brown-thumb effect," and have obtained it several times. There were several occasions, too, when there was no visible difference in the leaf after "treatment."

If, in fact, we are photographing a kind of bioenergy which is transmitted between person and leaf, it would seem that the bioenergy has a bipolar quality, similar perhaps to the positive and negative polarity of electricity. Clearly, from this photographic evidence, it appears as if the subject either sends energy *into,* or takes it *out of,* the leaf.

Human Interactions

After those studies, we began to concentrate our efforts on a possible bioenergetic exchange between *people.* Our first study in that direction was one involving a treatment modality called, from Biblical times to today, the "laying on of hands" (a subject which has received rigorously controlled laboratory investigation from biochemists Grad (1965) and Smith (1972). A healer who claimed success with this unorthodox method of treatment volunteered to give his services to a special study, done in collaboration with a kidney specialist, Dr. Marshall Barshay, who brought into the lab 12 patients who were on dialysis. It was our vain hope that just one of those patients might be freed from the tyranny of the dialysis machine. None were. However, again and again, we were able to observe in the photographs an apparent transfer of energy from healer to patient. Here is a typical picture of a patient *before* treatment (Figure 26); and here is that same patient's finger pad after fifteen minutes of the "laying on of hands." (Figure 27). By contrast, here is the healer's finger pad before treatment (Figure 28), and here it is after treatment (Figure 29). In a composite slide, showing those four photographs (Figure 30), it seems clear that the patient's finger pad shows an increased luminescence after treatment, while the healer shows a decreased luminescence. Has there been a transfer of bioenergy from healer to patient? If this is a transfer of bioenergy between people, would there be other occasions in which this exchange might be manifested?

Interactions Between People

Along about this time, our lab had acquired several different Kirlian devices, each with its special electrical parameters, and each producing pictures unique to the instrument. Obviously the lack of a standard apparatus creates difficul-

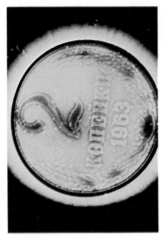

Figure 1

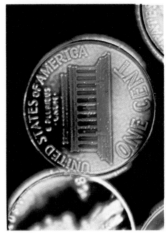

Figure 2

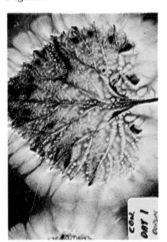

Figure 3

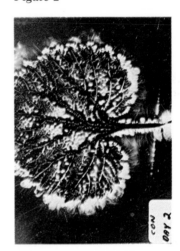

Figure 4

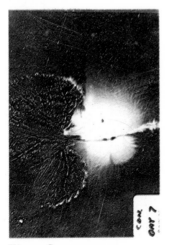

Figure 5

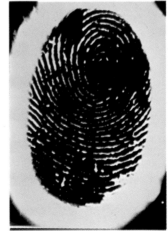

Figure 6

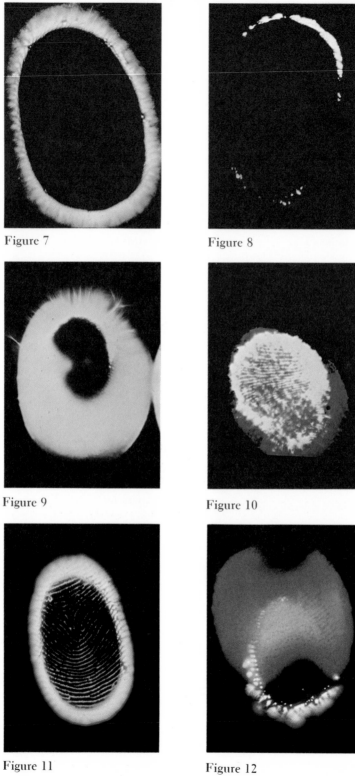

Figure 7

Figure 8

Figure 9

Figure 10

Figure 11

Figure 12

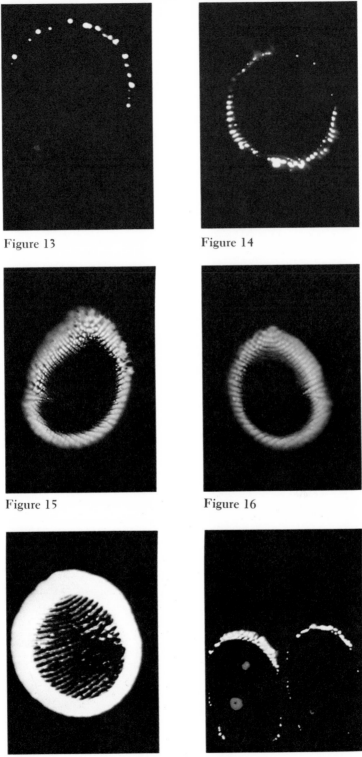

Figure 13

Figure 14

Figure 15

Figure 16

Figure 17

Figure 18

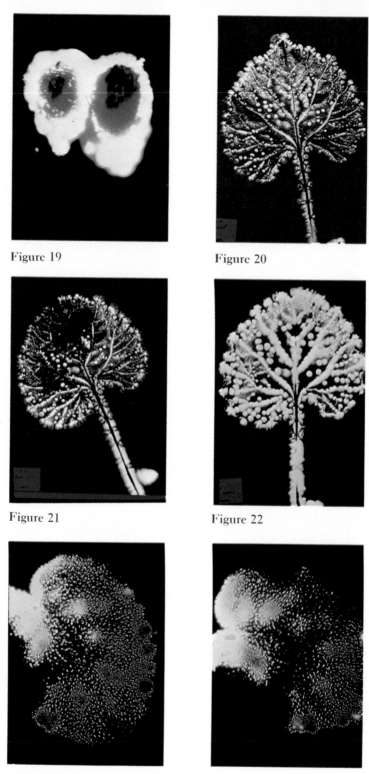

Figure 19

Figure 20

Figure 21

Figure 22

Figure 23

Figure 24

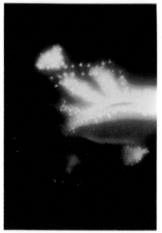

Figure 25

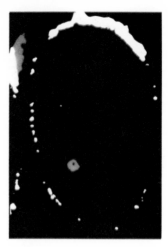

Figure 26

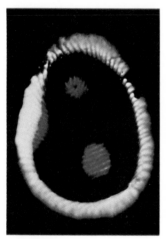

Figure 27

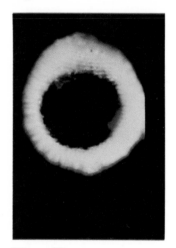

Figure 28

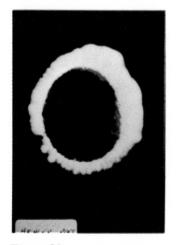

Figure 29

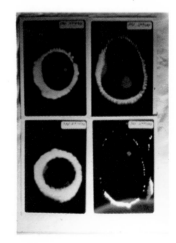

Figure 30

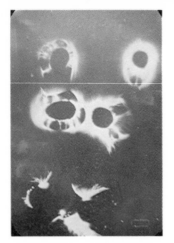

Figure 31

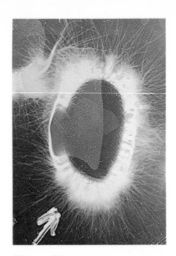

Figure 32

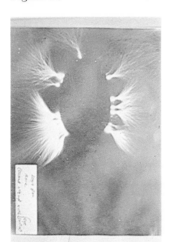

Figure 33

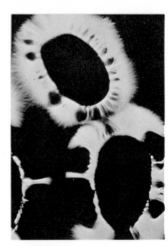

Figure 34

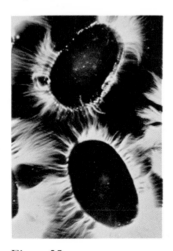

Figure 35

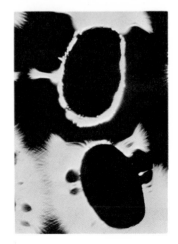

Figure 36

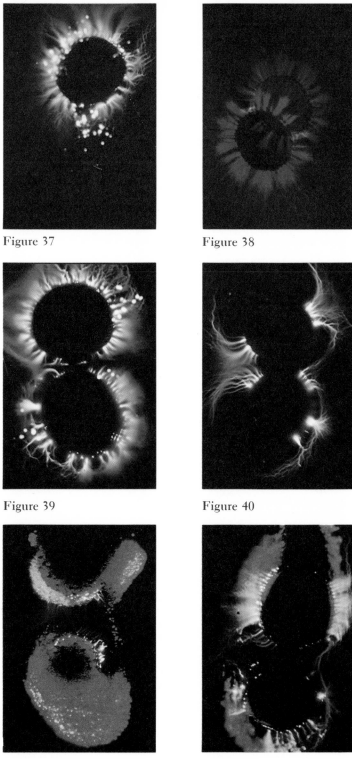

Figure 37

Figure 38

Figure 39

Figure 40

Figure 41

Figure 42

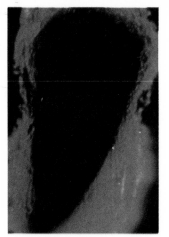

Figure 43

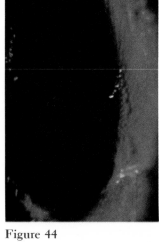

Figure 44

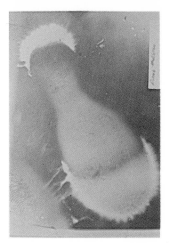

Figure 45

ties in being able to make comparisons with other laboratories doing research with this photography—a disadvantage. On the other hand, there is an advantage in exploratory work, comparing the results of one instrument with another. For example, one instrument developed by Dakin (1974) gave us much more pronounced, longer emanations—which made it easier to observe the effects of the next study in interactions. The following photographs were taken exclusively on the Dakin instrument; and you will observe that the pictures have a very different look than the previous ones, all of which were taken on Kendall Johnson's device (Moss & Kendall, 1972).

Now, to explore these energetic interactions (if that is what they were), we began to investigate *pairs* of presumably normal and healthy people under a specific psychological state. In a typical experiment, we would photograph, individually, the finger pad of each person, as can be seen in this contact print, on the top row (Figure 31). On the left is the finger pad of one member of the pair; on the right, the finger pad of the other member, each taken separately. Then we asked both persons to place their fingers close together, but not touching each other (approximately an eighth of an inch apart); and then we photographed both fingers simultaneously. This picture, on row two, shows how the two finger pads looked when neither member of the pair was engaged in a specific activity. This picture served as the baseline. Then we imposed a particular condition: that the subjects look into each other's eyes for as long as necessary to make strong eye contact (usually a period of between one and two minutes). When both persons indicated by a verbal sign that they had achieved good eye contact, the picture was taken. Here, on row three, is a typical—and surprising—result. The subject on the right is shown to have increased emanations, while the subject on the left has all but disappeared! We have, as yet, no explanation for this result, which has occurred frequently with different couples. We would change their positions, the subject on the right going on the left, and vice versa, but consistently it was found that *one* member of the pair would "blank out" the other member of the pair.

This situation was particularly obvious in the case of one of our veteran volunteers, a professional hypnotherapist. We found that he would repeatedly "blank out" any one of a number of partners. One possible (perhaps fanciful) outcome of further research in this area might be a method to screen good hypnotists from bad—a method which has thus far proved to be elusive. We know that certain people, like Milton Erickson, are masterful hypnotists, while other equally expert therapists—notoriously, Sigmund Freud—were so inept with hypnosis that they abandoned that treatment modality. But an **explana-**

tion for this phenomenon has not yet appeared. Could it be related to this strange "blanking-out" effect?

Another Instance of "Blanking-Out"

From time to time, persons have appeared in the lab who do not show any picture at all. In an effort better to understand this effect, certain members of the lab learned to "blank–out" deliberately by a process which they could not define verbally. On other occasions, a person who usually has a vivid corona will show a temporary "blanking-out," for no discernible reason. And on a few occasions, the reason seems to be psychological.

One of the most recent instances of this last occurred when a lady pediatrician spent a week in the lab, familiarizing herself with the technique of taking pictures, using herself as the subject in a variety of conditions. Generally, in a baseline picture, she revealed a bright corona, as in this picture (Figure 32). When she felt competent with the technique, she invited her skeptical psychiatrist husband to join her in an interaction study, hoping to persuade him to do a research project with Kirlian photography. Unfortunately, that entire morning, each time her picture was taken, she "blanked-out." Her husband, a kind man, kept urging her to relax, but to no avail. Here is one of their interaction pictures (Figure 33): we can see that the husband has a brilliant corona, but the wife's finger pad can hardly be seen. We might surmise that with this lady's keen desire to demonstrate the value of this research, she became, in the graphic language of slang, up tight, with the result that she "blanked–out" in the pictures.

The important question is, of course: by what process does this "blanking–out" occur, and what is its significance, physiologically, psychologically, and/or electrically?

Interaction Studies Involving Visualization

It gradually occurred to us that we were observing extreme changes *between* people in a variety of situations that had arisen spontaneously in the course of the lab work. Now it seemed a good idea to try deliberately to evoke specific reactions between people. Psychiatrists and psychologists speak frequently of "empathic" or "nonempathic" reactions, and of positive or negative transferences in psychotherapy. The question presented itself: could we obtain visual evidence of these attractive and repellent forces? We decided to explore that possibility by employing a role-playing or method-acting technique.

In that study a pair of subjects would first have a baseline picture taken of their two finger pads held close together, but with no particular thought or emotion in their conscious awareness. Here is an example (Figure 34) of such a baseline picture: the emanations of the two fingers billow out, but show no special kind of interaction. On the next photograph, the couple tried to feel strong attraction to each other (not sexual attraction, but rather a feeling of mutual appreciation and admiration). This is the picture obtained (Figure 35). It seems clear that the pattern of the emanations has changed radically, and there can be seen emanations which seem to be blending with each other, or attracting each other. Immediately after this picture was taken, the couple was asked to hold strong negative feelings about each other: intense dislike and repulsion. Here (Figure 36) is the result. Very obviously, the pattern of the emanations has changed. The emanations, instead of reaching out and connecting with each other, have cut off from each other, leaving a large gap between fingers. We describe this effect, which is quite repeatable with different subjects, "giving each other a haircut."

Our next project was to ask couples to visualize specific dramatic situations with each other. In one such study each person's finger pad was photographed separately. Here is one member of the pair (Figure 37), revealing in her baseline large emanations in a brilliant blue, with lots of tiny bubbles in a pinkish orange hue. The other subject, in her baseline picture, showed large sharp emanations, but no bubbles (Figure 38). Now the two people placed their finger pads in close proximity to each other, and a baseline photograph of the two ladies together was taken (Figure 39). We can clearly see that the bubbles which had belonged to only *one* of the subjects, when the pictures were taken separately, have now become the common property of both subjects. Some kind of nonvisual interaction had already taken place, without conscious awareness (for this was supposed to be the baseline picture). In the next photograph the two subjects were asked to hold strong negative feelings about each other, with this result (Figure 40). Please observe that the emanations, which on the previous picture—taken no more than a minute before—had bubbled around each other, now are retreating from each other, with no bubbles to be seen. The negative feelings had apparently caused a repulsion of emanations, and the disappearance of the bubbles.

On another occasion, two subjects volunteered to participate in a pretended act of aggression. One subject was asked to visualize that she was sticking a needle into her partner, who had confessed to a strong fear of needles. This next picture shows the result—so startling as to be almost unbelievable (Figure 41). Here one can see, from out of the brilliant red blotch of the aggressor, a red line darting out toward the person she is *imagining* to be sticking with a needle; and the lady who is afraid of needles is shown to have emanations retreating from the imaginary, inflicted pain.

Unfortunately, we have not yet been able to repeat this result, perhaps because it is difficult to find persons who can visualize strongly, who are also afflicted with a needle phobia. But in a similar study with a different pair of subjects, the same visualization technique was contrasted with the actual sticking of a needle into a brave volunteer. This is what the picture looked like when the subject on the left was stuck so hard with a needle that blood literally flowed (Figure 42). One can see the vivid red blotch of arousal, but without the darting line from the aggressor. On their next experiment, the young man who had been wounded with the needle was given an opportunity for revenge, in *fantasy*. He was asked to visualize sticking a needle into the lady partner who had drawn his blood. This is what emerged on film (Figure 43). Apparently this gentleman had been so aroused that his *imagined* assault caused an almost complete red blotchy ellipse around the two finger pads.

Shortly after that picture was taken (in the same experimental session), this couple was asked to fantasize sexual interaction, which, in spite of the earlier aggressive acts, seemed to be a pleasant task for both, at least according to the sounds that were emitted in the total darkness which is required for color photographs. Here is their rendition of fantasized sexual interaction (Figure 44). In an even more pronounced manner, we find that the emanations from the two individual subjects have merged into one complete red ellipse, obliterating the two individual finger pads in an apparent "blending" of fields.

Blending Interactions Caused by Another Variable

The question presented itself: would it be possible to show other types of blending, which are not considered to be related either to sex or aggression? A series of experiments was attempted with persons who had done a fair amount of meditation. In these studies, we asked that two subjects meditate together, each keeping his finger tip on film, in close proximity to the other. When both felt they had reached a good level of meditation, the picture was taken. Here, in a typical result, we can see on black-and-white film that a field has been formed, uniting the individual finger tips (Figure 45).

A Possible Area for Research

Our investigations into interactions between people have barely begun. Yet already we believe that the patterns of emanations revealed in this photography may be carrying specific information—information about what occurs between people on a nonverbal, sometimes unconscious level. At least the possibility exists that these photographic hieroglyphics may one day be deciphered. It is conceivable that these various corona patterns—the "haircut" of repulsion, the blending of attraction, the combined fields of aggression, or sex, or meditative rapport—may each have a characteristic, identifiable shape. If that proves to be the case, then electrical or Kirlian photography may provide a useful tool for both psychiatry and psychology, in defining more specifically the reactions that occur between people.

References

Adamenko, V. Electrodynamics of living systems. *Journal of Paraphysics,* 1970, **4,** 113–212.

Burr, H. S. *Blueprint for immortality.* London: Neville-Spearman, 1972.

Dakin, H. *High-voltage photography.* San Francisco: 1974.

Grad, B. Some biological effects of the "laying on of hands": a review of experiments with animals and plants. *Journal of the American Society for Psychical Research,* 1965, **59,** 95–127.

Inyushin, V. *Problems in bioenergetics,* Symposium, Kazakh State University, Alma-Ata, Kazakhstan, USSR, 1969.

Kirlian, S., & Kirlian, V. Photographic and visual observation by means of high-frequency currents. *Journal of Scientific and Applied Photography,* 1961, **6,** 397–403.

Krippner, S., & Rubin, D. (Eds.). *The kirlian aura.* New York: Doubleday, 1974.

Moss, T., & Johnson, K. Photographic evidence of healing energy in plants and people. *Dimensions of Healing Symposium, Proceedings.* Academy of Parapsychology and Medicine, Los Altos, California, 1972.

Smith, J. The influence on enzyme growth by the "laying on of hands." *Dimensions of Healing Symposium, Proceedings.* Academy of Parapsychology and Medicine, Los Altos, California, 1972, 121–131.

Paul L. Adams

Metapsychiatry and Quaker Meditation

ANY DEEP MEDITATION is a splendid way of getting high, so it is often advertised for its very personal hedonistic benefits irrespective of how the meditator loves and works with other human beings. Often meditators feel impelled either to "renounce the world" or to put all their energies to work against little personal sins, not major social evils. Quaker meditation is not merely an isolated way for an individual to achieve inner spiritual change; the meditation also drives the meditator into vigorous social action.

How is it of psychiatric relevance, that on a Sunday morning a small group of demonstrators lay down their placards beside the front door of a plain meetinghouse, and walk inside to sit for an hour as a circle of silent meditators? Once or twice their silence is broken by a spoken message of only a few phrases, and after an hour has elapsed, the assembled group arises with embraces and handshakes all around. Can a social psychiatry, pluralistic and eclectic, and Quaker group meditation coexist, share, and learn from each other?

Friends, Romans, Protestants

The Religious Society of Friends has only an estimated 200,000 members throughout the world (*Encyclopedia Americana,* 1972). These members range from 1) unaffiliated groups to 2) the Evangelical Friends, who are much like rural Methodists or Pentecostals in their fervid experiences to 3) those congregations with pastors who comprise the Friends United Meeting in North America (national office at Richmond, Indiana) and, finally, to 4) the group described by Richard M. Nixon as "radical humanists on the Eastern seaboard" (Friends General Conference, Philadelphia, Pennsylvania) who meditate in silent worship groups without any clergy. In the fourth group, meditation is their most characteristic way of worship. More accurately, there is for those "unpastorized Friends" no division into clergy and laity since *every* member of the Quaker gathering is constrained to carry out any and all clerical functions. Fired by the spirit of early Christians, and of those seventeenth-century Protestants who founded Quakerism, each woman and man is considered to be her or his own priest.[1] These Quakers do without intermediaries and intercessors, as they stress a religion of direct experiencing, as opposed to an intellectual, formulated creed or litany. As George Fox, the seventeenth-century Quaker founder, said, religion was "experimental" and not "notional."

Most Quakers are theists, however, and most count themselves as Christians, albeit, nondoctrinaire ones. Yet Quaker silent meetings throughout the world contain Buddhists, Jews, Moslems, Bahais, Christians, and some few people who have no theology and disbelieve the God which most Quakers do worship. Long before Roman Catholic ecumenism became popular, a few Roman Catholic priests regularly attended Quaker meetings for worship, feeling perhaps that at least Friends were as un-Protestant as they were un-Roman.

Seventeenth-century England was marked by a bitter and bloody three-way struggle among three factions of Christendom—Roman Catholics, Anglicans, and Puritans—reminding us, if we need to be, that people who meditate and strive for personal piety are not constrained from being fanatical killers. From the fringes of Puritanism there emerged the Quakers, "seekers" who found a viable voice and style in a religion of nonviolence that emphasized meditation and was—to use William James's terms—not religion as a dull habit but as an acute fever. Meditation, largely because of the Catholics' pervasive influence on spirituality, was more widely practiced by individual members of all parties in that era than appears to be true of twentieth–century Christians. However, it was the Quaker genius to elevate meditation to a paramount place in their group life of faith and practice, for, while some Anglicans, Catholics, and others might meditate, *all* Quakers did.

Catholics in seventeenth–century England were identified as a deposed

---

[1] In Quaker groups, females and males are equally free, equally weighty. This practice of female equality brought seventeenth-century Friends much persecution from their more sexist Christian contemporaries (Vann, 1969).

Ecclesia but constituted an underground group—with some aid and comfort from the royal Stuarts, Charles I and Charles II—who poured clandestinely into England dozens of priests who espoused meditation by propagating the translations of numerous continental treatises on meditation including manuals, guidebooks, poems, and lists of spiritual exercises to enhance private devotion, all of these prescribing a methodical approach to disciplined meditation (Martz, 1962).

Anglicans represented *Ecclesia* in ascendancy and circulated a plethora of theological, highly theoretical works on meditation. Anglican sentiment in the seventeenth century was sometimes anticlerical and Protestant, but assuredly reflected an establishment religion, a national church.

Puritans of that era were sectarian in rhetoric, advocating good thoughts, debunking outward forms, yet believing not in works but in faith and the individual's predestined relation to God's unmerited and unearned grace. Still, we, from a perspective safely outside of both Puritan and Catholic spirituality of the sixteenth and seventeenth centuries, can see little difference—but considerable commonality—in their respective self-examining and self-purifying exercises.

Quakers were a small group among the Christians who were forlorn and despairing of theology, church, and methodical exercises, but given to "expect only Enthusiastick Consolations" (Baxter, 1649), and to believe that no outward symbol but only one's own deepest nature gives spiritual promptings and directions. The Quakers developed into a fine art a simple religious belief system in which nondirective meditation occupied a central place (Jones, 1914).

Ingredients of Quaker Meditation

Quaker meditation has nothing unique, save perhaps the way that its ingredients are combined together. Like many other forms of meditation, the Quaker form brings special motoric, cognitive, affective, ecstatic, ethical, and utopical components into a complex interplay with each other and with a larger belief system that overarches and enfolds the meditative practices. The Quaker belief system is contained in "testimonies"—the Quaker alternative to a simple creed. The testimonies are taken as axiomatic as the Quakers go about the meditation of worship meetings and the dialogue of business meetings. Their basic testimony is to "that of God in every person," often called the Testimony to the Inner Light, or to Community and Equality. Closely related are the corollary testimonies to Peace and Simplicity, the former leading Quakers to oppose war and the latter prompting them to be direct and open in all their dealings—by refusing to take oaths, by adopting quite plain speech and dress. The Testimonies are also reflected in the set of "queries" which lead Quakers in their business meetings to approach the practical matters affecting the group in a spirit of quiet reverence and simplicity. The query for April, for example, is, "Are love and unity maintained among you? Do you manifest a forgiving spirit and a care for the reputation of others? When differences arise are endeavors made to settle them speedily and in a spirit of meekness and love?" Quaker business meetings often begin and end with silent meditation and may resort to silent meditation during the meeting's deliberations if full unanimity of the members is not obtained on some thorny question.

The Quaker belief system is neither antiscientific nor antiintellectual. Indeed, Quaker natural scientists have been more numerous than the proportion of Quakers in the world's population would dictate. Likewise, Quaker beliefs emphasize everyday hard work (especially working at humanitarian service), common sense empiricism, and the spiritual value of material things. Quaker practicality and efficiency have cut down their overhead expenses to such a degree that their know-how has been sought out by nonprofit organizations carrying out fund-raising projects. A joke among Quakers holds that Quakers aimed to do good for their fellowman, and in the process did very well for themselves.

In the context of their history and of their overall belief system, as I have sketched them in the foregoing, we can see how Quaker meditation falls into place as we now briefly characterize the various components of Quaker meditation.

Motoric. The bodily posture is one of just sitting comfortably with the eyes often closed. Many Quakers describe this as a pose of "watchful waiting" and of "alert relaxation." Silent and nonverbal, the meditator may become fearful and anxious if "the Spirit moves him" to make an utterance. He literally quakes at such a moment. The messages delivered during Quaker meetings are rarely the "strange utterances" of the Pentecostals, but are sometimes terse and crisp, usually brief, fumbling, yet sensible.

Cognitive. Some of the Quaker meditators' thinking is conceptual, and substantively centered, but in the main it is not focused on any particular topic and involves a dismantling of common logic and cognitive schemata. Memory and attention are often regarded as annihilated during meditation, but the meditator attests to feeling as if his mind were quickened, opened up, illuminated—so that he is attuned to his innermost depths of understanding. Intuitive insight is valued very highly by the Quaker in meditation.

Therapeutic. A sense of relief or release is an almost universal attendant of Quaker meditation. One feels divested of his habits, conventions, defenses, and personal traits. He senses an enhancement of his autonomy, or wholeness, as, in meditation, he drops off his customary ways of experiencing the world, as he "derepresses," we might say, although less in agitated frenzy than in a "quiet leading." George Fox, the Quaker founder, experienced this therapeutic release in the form of a keener sense of smell (Jones, 1914), a heightening of a proximate sensory mode that was often tabooed in Fox's day, as it is in ours (Schachtel, 1959). The extent of the therapeutic release derived in meditation can go to the extreme of ecstatic (out of one's body) or enthusiastic (in God) experience. The meditator is transported into the farthest stage of meditation, namely, *contemplation,* wherein he is capable of truly mystical experiences. As St. François de Sales (1630) wrote:

> Meditation considereth by peecemeale the objectes proper to move us; but contemplation beholds the object it loves, in one simple and recollected looke. . . .

Ethical. The Quaker meditator often is absorbed in self-scrutiny or self-analysis, in the work of know thyself. Personal change toward self-improvement is the ethical goal of meditation, quite as it is the ethical goal of psychoanalysis. Some personal problem-solving occurs in Quaker meditation.

Utopical. Almost singly distinctive of the several ingredients of Quaker meditation is the strong utopical imperative that overcomes the Quaker meditator. Many forms of meditation augment the meditator's compassion for his fellow beings, his sociability, or sensitivity to affiliation (Naranjo, 1971). Assuredly, the Quaker meditator does not value "inner space" (Kelly, 1944) as an escape from the world of citizenship and the engagement of changing the world. He does not believe his own navel is the center of any important universe, and he asserts that the goal of the human condition is not to strive for personal salvation or merely "doing one's own thing." The Quaker gospel is one of high social relevance, bringing the meditator to fight against major institutionalized evils such as economic injustice and exploitation, racism, childism, sexism, imperialism, war. Thomas Kelly (1941) wrote:

> Social concern is the dynamic Life of God at work in the world, made special and emphatic and unique, particularized in each

individual or group who is sensitive and tender in the leading strings of love [p. 111].

We fear a life of wallowing in ecstasies of spiritual sensuality while cries of a needy world go unheeded. And some pages of history seem to fortify our fears [p. 48].

Five Stages in Quaker Group Meditation

The aforementioned components of Quaker meditation may be given clearer exposition if we examine in temporal sequence some stages in Quaker group meditation:

Stage 1: Listening. The meditator enters the meetinghouse, sits on a chair, or bench, or on the floor. He makes his body a part of his surroundings and has some awareness that others, too, are searching, striving to become a "gathered meeting." The meditator listens, much as the student of the Stanislavsky method of acting is trained to listen—to his own breathing, to all sounds in his environment, to all the utterances of nature and human culture. While listening, he aims for a transcendence of the sounds around him, for listening to the silence—for a "naked intent unto God." Common logic is suspended and although his thoughts may be said to ramble, it would hit the mark more nearly if we said the meditator relaxes and enters "a time of letting go and shutting out, letting go of internal problems and shutting out of external distractions (Chase, 1951)."

Stage 2: Substantive. From out of nowhere in particular, one's thoughts emerge, dwelling upon a topic such as a saying of Gandhi, Jesus, James Nayler, Martin Luther King, Jr., a Hassidic master, or a Zen koan. Or in a less verbal mode, one may dwell upon the star of David, the cross of Jesus, the peace symbol. The conscious cooperation of the surface level of attending and concentrating may be needed at first. Meditation progresses.

Stage 3: Nondirective. A period of greater patience occurs, as one waits without even giving a thought to waiting. Some have referred to this stage as a topicless wandering of an empty-headed mind—for awareness flits from money shortages to love life to daydreams, all transient half-articulated thoughts of self and of interpersonal relations.

Stage 4: Radiant. The feelings of struggle subside further in the meditator and he feels an inward glow which is greatly reinforced by the radiance he perceives in his fellow meditators. Good vibrations abound. This phase of worship is the time of the deepest corporate feeling among the gathered meditators, for in other stages there is awareness of a group but the group's presence is not the heart of the experience as it is in the radiant phase. During this phase, verbal messages may be given and since the group's attention is so centered and so steeped in mutuality, every message spoken "speaks to the condition" of many of the assembled meditators. What is said seems just right, loving, and radiant. It is as if the group were being readied for the succeeding stage, in which the group persists but is not so keenly the focus of warmth and attention.

Stage 5: Ecstatic. This is the peak experience according to Quakers. It is the mystical Divine Encounter, made only by an individual, but after all it can be shared with others, as it is reputed to have been shared at Pentecost. This is the stage of pure contemplation, in which George Fox and many other Quakers felt "a great opening" and suffusion with the conviction that God is Within. An unbridgeable gap has been transcended. No alienation remains. Glatthorn (1961) wrote:

> None of us can say for sure how this happens; we know no magic formulas, and we can teach no easy method. All we know is that out of the endless searching and seeking there will come surely a divine revelation when we will feel deep in our being that God is speaking to us, is showing us a new way, is opening up a new truth [pp. 484–485].

Like almost all other mystics, Quakers are reluctant to describe verbally what the mystical encounter is like, claiming that it cannot be described and that no words are adequate, and so on. Some Quakers would insist that their deficit in accounting for what happened during the ecstatic experience is due to the fact that they were "seized in divinity" for a time but, immediately after, experienced a postlude of such calm that upon "reentry" the describable details of the whole event became lost in amnesia.

Quaker Meditation and Psychiatry

Although the Quakers have not been very informative to psychiatrists concerning the quintessential mysticism of their meditation, there are many other areas relative to psychiatry in which Friends have been considerably more explicit and articulate. Some of the major interfaces between Quakers and psychiatry can be pointed to in the following brief comments.

Quakers long have contributed to the humane care of mentally ill persons because they believed that the mentally ill were treated unwisely and unjustly. Quaker involvement in bettering the conditions of the mentally ill has ranged from the founding of the York Retreat in 1796, the founding of Friends Asylum in Frankford, Pennsylvania, in 1817, to political work to help improve the lot of such victims, to recent work to guarantee their civil rights and civil liberties, including their right to treatment. During various wars, Quakers have set up programs for service by conscientious objectors attending to mentally ill people, in World War II notably, and played a pace setting role in establishing the new career of psychiatric aide.

A second contribution to human relations has been derived from the non-manipulative manner of conducting the Quaker meeting for business. Most theories of group dynamics rely upon the Quaker business meeting for their fund of certain principles—unanimous decisions, silent periods, a moratorium or cooling-off, full participation, encouragement to dissent and to uncover contradictory facts, learning to listen, absence of energetic leader, nobody outranks anybody, and meetings kept personal and small (Chase, 1951).

A third contribution may be seen in the Quaker view that prophetic religion is an "adjustive" or balancing force at the same time it is socially revolutionary. Quaker religious values run counter to religious values that alienate and trouble people; and the Quakers, while refraining from judging their religious neighbors, have often exhorted their own members to shun religious attitudes that promote fear, anxiety, intolerance, dogmatism, guilt, self-mortification, hatred, sadism, cruelty, and resistance to inquiry. Also they have railed against religion which encourages trickery (as in praying for rain and wealth), which promotes frenzy, and depreciates human life. Established, churchly religion has a very dark side from a moral or psychiatric standpoint; Quakers know this and try to keep level-headed as well as God-possessed. They acknowledge that imagination, deserted by reason, creates monstrosities. Quakerism joins psychiatry most notably perhaps in the quest for reasonableness in human affairs, for both psychiatrists and Quakers value the life of the intellect.

A fourth area of interfacing between psychiatry and Quaker meditation lies in their shared, augmented view of the whole man. For both of them, the altered and expanded consciousness as well as everyday, commonsense reasoning is acceptable. The Quaker meditator joins with the social psychiatrist in pursuit of an inward-looking ethical pursuit, fused as part and parcel of a utopical imperative to change the world. The inner man is indeed a man of sensible social action, holding to the logic of scientific propositions as well as to the logic of heartfelt commitments.

References

Baxter, R. *The saints everlasting rest.* London: Underhill and Lyton, 1649.

Chase, S. *Roads to agreement.* New York: Harper Brothers, 1951.

De Sales, St. F. A treatise of the loved of God. In Martz, L. L., *The poetry of meditation.* New Haven, Conn.: Yale University Press, 1962.

Glatthorn, A. The stages of worship. *Friends Journal,* 1961, 484–485. (Reprints available from Friends General Conference, 1520 Race Street, Philadelphia, 19102.)

Jones, R. M. *Spiritual reformers in the sixteenth and seventeenth centuries.* New York: Macmillan, 1914.

Kelly, T. R. *A testament of devotion.* New York: Harper Brothers, 1941.

Martz, L. L. *The poetry of meditation.* New Haven, Conn.: Yale University Press, 1962.

Naranjo, C. & Ornstein, R. E. *On the psychology of meditation.* New York: Viking, 1971.

Schachtel, E. On memory and childhood. In *Metamorphosis: on the development of affect, perception, attention, and memory.* New York: Basic Books, 1959.

Vann, R. T. *The social development of English Quakerism.* Cambridge, Mass.: Harvard University Press, 1969.

Gary E. Schwartz

Positive and Negative Aspects of Meditation

STIMULATED BY THE efforts of the Maharishi Mahesh Yogi and his organization, transcendental meditation is booming in America, and the scientific research on TM seems to be growing just as fast. TM is an easily learned meditational technique. A person sits down with his eyes closed for two 20-minute periods a day, once in the morning and again before dinner, and directs his attention to the imagined sound of a Sanskrit *mantra* ("tool for thinking") chosen for him by his teacher. It's as simple as that. The results, moreover, are said to be astonishing. Recent advertisements claim that TM reduces tension, improves personal relationships, and make meditators more energetic and efficient. Thousands of Americans who practice TM insist that it has changed their lives.

A considerable amount of psychological and physiological research, much of which is still unpublished, backs up some of these extraordinary claims. Certain other research suggests that the proponents of TM have promised more than they can deliver. In either case, the movement stays abreast of scientific findings on meditation and uses them extensively to explain and advertise TM to the American public. The research is therefore worth reviewing.

TM is, first of all, a method of altering consciousness, about which Western science has learned a few things in the past decade; and second, TM is one of many meditational techniques.

Changing Consciousness

There are several different "states of consciousness." We experience sleep differently from wakefulness, and physiologically they are distinct. Moreover, we all know how to change our state of consciousness, as when we lie down and close our eyes at night, confident that we shall fall asleep. The most skeptical Western observers should keep these facts in mind, since a large part of TM is simply the recognition that various states of consciousness exist and that a person can regulate them in order to feel better.

Man's consciousness is forever changing. Normally, 24-hour rhythms modulate waking, sleeping, and dreaming—the three major states, according to most Western scientists. Within the waking and dreaming states, certain internal fluctuations, such as the desires to eat and drink, exert their influence. At the same time, prior learning and the environment affect our consciousness at any given time. I may want to eat, for example, because I haven't eaten all day and am therefore very hungry—or because I've just watched a commercial for a chocolate layer cake.

Special environments influence our consciousness in ways that have only recently been scrutinized by scientists. When looking at mountains, for instance, we tend to feel relaxed; it's the same with clouds and seascapes and the interiors of great churches. Part of the reason for this sense of relaxation is that we don't *focus* on such vast scenes. Focusing the eyes on limited objects blocks the alpha and theta waves of the brain, and these brain rhythms relate closely to relaxation and drowsiness. Unfocusing the eyes, on the other hand, results in more sustained alpha waves.

We can, if we wish, regulate our consciousness more than we do normally. We can discipline our bodies to breathe in certain ways, or we can suggest to ourselves that we are "floating above the clouds" and begin to feel calm and buoyant. Recent research in biofeedback has presented evidence that we can even modify the autonomic nervous system, which means that the autonomic system isn't so autonomic as once supposed. We should view meditation as the deliberate attempt to influence the ebb and flow of normal consciousness, even though the attempt may be "passive" in nature.

All meditation is not alike. There are dozens of meditative disciplines. The proponents of TM have tended to present research data as if TM were the only good way of producing beneficial and systematic changes in consciousness. This is hardly the case. Admittedly, TM is simple to perform and requires little training. Nevertheless, there are other ways of achieving deep relaxation.

These include Zen, Sufi, and Christian meditation, as well as autogenic training and progressive relaxation. Each of these techniques directs a person's attention somewhat differently. Zen meditation usually involves respiration. Although some Sufi techniques require active dancing and produce high arousal, Sufis also practice a form of meditation called *zikr* which involves attention to a mantra as in TM. Autogenic training uses images of warmth and heaviness in one's hands and arms. And progressive relaxation does pretty much what it says, relaxing the muscle groups in sequence. All these techniques may lead to deep and beneficial rest. So may prayer, or even a day at the beach.

Western psychology and other sciences have advanced to the point where we are now able to look into how Eastern meditative procedures work. But we should always be cautious in separating fact from fiction. In 1935, Thérèse Brosse (1950) went to India with a portable electrocardiograph and claimed that a yogi could stop his heart. A follow-up study by Marion Wenger and Basu Bagchi (1961) in 1957 decided that Brosse's observation was probably an artifact of her recording procedure. This is not to say that yogis can't do remarkable things. Wenger and Bagchi also observed that the valsalva maneuver (in which a yogi raises the pressure within his chest by holding his breath and straining downward) did indeed change heart rate and rhythm as physiological theory would predict.

Disillusionment, however, lies in store for those who believe every astounding yogic feat they hear about. T. X. Barber proposed recently that certain yogis can walk barefooted across hot coals by a) developing hard calluses on their feet, b) taking powerful drugs, such as heroin, and c) walking very fast.

The Physiology of TM

Transcendental meditation came to the foreground of the scientific view in 1970, when Robert Keith Wallace (1970), now president of the Maharishi International University, published his UCLA doctoral thesis on the physiology of TM in *Science*. Wallace, a meditator himself, had measured various physiological responses to meditation, including changes in oxygen consumption, brain waves, and skin resistance. He observed increases in alpha and theta waves during meditation, particularly in the frontal areas of the brain; and yet the meditators' brain waves kept responding to auditory and light stimuli. The alpha waves were more intense during TM than when his subjects merely closed their eyes; the occasional theta waves resembled those of drowsiness or the early stages of sleep. The meditators were deeply relaxed, in other words; they were also awake, as their reactions to light and sound demonstrated.

Wallace's meditators consumed 20 percent less oxygen while they were meditating, and their skin resistance seemed to rise by more than 100 percent. A 20 percent drop in oxygen consumption indicates a greatly lowered metabolism. The rise in skin resistance seemed just as remarkable. Generally speaking, the resistance of the skin to the passage of an electric current across it is a measure of arousal; the more aroused or alert a person is, the more freely a current flows, perhaps because of sweating. In any case, Wallace suggested that meditators had the skin of relaxed and confident people.

Overall, Wallace distinguished the state of transcendental meditation from both sleep and hypnosis. He decided that TM represented a fourth major state of consciousness, in addition to waking, sleeping, and dreaming.

Working later with Herbert Benson (1971) a cardiologist at the Harvard Medical School, Wallace tested additional meditators, repeating some of his earlier measurements and adding a few new ones. During meditation, they reported, oxygen consumption certainly decreased, elimination of CO_2 decreased, and the rate of respiration fell; skin resistance increased (this finding was a re-presentation of the old data) and blood lactate declined. Lactate is a body chemical which may be associated with anxiety. The authors concluded that, by traditional scientific standards, TM represented an anomaly: "a wakeful hypometabolic state." They left open the question of whether other forms of meditation might yield comparable results.

One of Wallace's colleagues at the Maharishi International University, David Orme-Johnson, published another major report on the hysiology of TM in 1973. Using skin-resistance response as a measure of stress, he found that meditators adjusted to loud, unpleasant noises more quickly than control subjects. Moreover, the skin resistance response of meditators appeared generally more stable than that of nonmeditators. He interpreted these findings to mean that TM, besides enhancing relaxation and reducing stress, made people able to live more easily with unpleasant aspects of the environment.

Orme-Johnson failed to report, however, the precise magnitude of skin-resistance changes. Perhaps he was unable to reproduce the strikingly large differences that Wallace had observed. In a series of studies at Harvard, Daniel Goleman, Lynn Levin, and I have never observed large increases in skin resistance during meditation. It is possible that Wallace's original measurements were in error, or that one's depth of meditation varies depending upon the conditions under which one meditates.

The significance of changes in skin resistance remains somewhat obscure in either case. The obscurity is compounded by the imprecision of words like "relaxed," "alert," and "aroused." Goleman and I believe that the practice of TM can make a person more alert mentally, or cortically, while at the same time less aroused emotionally, or subcortically. This view corresponds fairly closely with the way meditators themselves describe their experience.

TM: Antidote for Drugs?

In 1969, while using meditators in a study of blood pressure, Herbert Benson (1972) noticed that 19 of his 20 volunteers had given up the use of drugs. According to their own testimony, changes in consciousness due to marijuana, LSD, and heroin had become distasteful since their discovery of TM.

Benson and Wallace followed up this finding by questioning 1,862 experienced meditators. The results confirmed Benson's earlier observation that many practicing meditators had abandoned drugs. Moreover, the longer a person had meditated, the greater the change in his drug habits.

These and similar studies have encouraged the U.S. Army and several state governments to investigate TM as a possible alternative to drug abuse. And yet the findings are hard to interpret without more information. It is tempting to accept Benson's and the meditators' own interpretation—that meditation changed their consciousness more pleasantly than the drugs had. This view is consistent with Andrew Weil's (1972) concept that human beings have a *need* to alter consciousness. On the other hand, we should look into several other possibilities, as suggested in our own studies at Harvard. For instance, in order to learn TM a person must voluntarily abstain from drugs for two weeks. Some people are ready to commit themselves; in other words, they give up drugs provisionally even *before* meditation.

There is a process of self-selection involved here. There are also strong group pressures to conform to the model of the successful meditator, who presumably has transcended drugs. Group dynamics like these are used by Alcoholics Anonymous and Weight Watchers very effectively. Placebo factors may also be operating. Finally, the lifestyle of youthful meditators becomes more ordered and relaxed than the lifestyle of most drug users. This regularity alone could reduce a tremendous amount of stress, and hence a need for drugs. The assertion, in short, that TM cures drug abuse may be true but remains unproven.

Practitioners of TM have recounted thousands of stories about how their personalities have improved since taking up TM. They feel happier, stronger, more tolerant—healthier in body and mind. These stories are interesting in themselves. But to determine strictly whether the changes took place as a result of TM, it is necessary to measure personalities before and after people begin meditating, and to compare these changes with appropriate control groups. Leon Otis (1974) at the Stanford Research Institute has been examining this tricky problem for over two years. Another study, by William Seeman, Sanford Nidich, and Thomas Banta (1972) of the University of Cincinnati, assessed the influences of TM on "self-actualization" using the Personal Orientation Inventory. The results of that experiment speak favorably for meditation. In comparison to control subjects, the group that took up TM improved in several ways: in their capacity for intimate contact, in self-regard and spontaneity. Similar data from our laboratory (1973) indicate that personality changes, rather than the experience of altered consciousness itself, may account for the fact that many people who take up meditation give up drugs.

Intelligence and Creativity

Probably the most controversial claim made for transcendental meditation is that it increases "creative intelligence." By creative intelligence, the Maharishi doesn't simply mean an enhanced ability to produce creative products or raise IQ, but rather a more global change in one's perceptions of the world and other people, as well as better choices of activity.

Creativity and intelligence are both hard to measure. But there is some evidence that meditation can improve a person's performance in some intellectual subjects. A recent experiment by William Linden (1973) indicated that third-graders trained in meditation were less anxious when taking tests. Certainly there is a good deal of evidence from other studies that the less anxious a person is, within limits, the more effectively he or she can think and act.

It is worth asking, though, if relaxation is the right state for *all* kinds of activities. Basic research indicates that too much or too little arousal can lead to inferior performance. Moreover, there appears to be an optimal level of arousal for a given person doing a given task.

I recently (Schwartz, 1974) tested 16 teachers of meditation and a group of 16 controls using two standardized measures of creativity, the Barron-Welsh Art Scale and a battery of tests devised by M. A. Wallace and Nathan Kogan. Surprisingly, the meditators scored no better than the nonmeditators. On some scales, in fact, the meditators did consistently worse. The result was especially interesting because the meditators were trying hard to succeed. On other tests, however, including a story-telling task used as a philosophical or projective measure of creativity, the meditators scored consistently higher than the controls.

Perhaps the explanation lies in Robert Ornstein's (1971) distinction between the left and right sides of the brain. To the extent that meditation leads to the kind of low arousal and self-reflective behavior typical of right-hemispheric processes, meditation enhances spontaneity and creativity, especially in free-associational tasks like story-telling. On the other hand, too much meditation may interfere with a person's logical, left-hemispheric processes, or the sort of problem-solving creativity required by the Wallace-Kogan Test.

Thus, TM may enhance the germinal stages of creativity, but if practiced to excess, it may reduce the chance of the meditator's producing a recognizably creative product. The distinction is important. The creative process allows for novel integrations, or gestalts, and creative ideas often emerge in drowsy or twilight states of consciousness. But the *expression* of these ideas often requires activity, excitement, and a good deal of rational and sequential thought. Creativity in the fullest sense involves both sides of the brain. It remains to be seen whether or not meditators typically respond well to what we might call the "necessities" of creation.

Cosmic Language

Many people are curious to know how transcendental meditation "works." The Maharishi has supplied one kind of explanation, but Westerners sometimes find his language too cosmic to follow. The TM movement in America has gone to great lengths to make TM understandable to nonmeditating non-Indians, perhaps especially by publicizing the scientific research on TM. I believe we can go even further along the road of demystification, and I don't think TM will wither under the light.

For one thing, there's the matter of the *mantra*. Westerners like to think that repeating a meaningless sound is an absurd thing to do; and yet the mantra is an integral part of TM. One of the keys to the mantra is that it has "signal value." The teacher chooses a mantra for each student, who must never disclose it. It becomes special for the student and therefore more likely to hold his attention and be used. It signals to the meditator that he is about to feel deeply relaxed. Perhaps the choice of the mantra is less important than the teacher's and student's belief that it is the correct one.

The euphonics of the mantra are probably important too. Psychophysiological research indicates that sounds which rise slowly and are resonant can decrease the heart rate, inducing relaxation. Thus the mantra can help a person relax for physical reasons, as well as for reasons of expectation and suggestibility.

The pleasant-sounding mantra also diverts a meditator's attention from unpleasant sensations and thoughts. The process is somewhat like counting sheep. Whenever problems or images threaten to attract the meditator's attention, he quietly focuses again on the mantra, which blocks them out. Then nothing but the mild word remains in consciousness.

Another difficulty many Westerners run into is the Maharishi's concept of "transcending" thought. The Maharishi has described the fourth, or transcendent, state of consciousness as the state in which one goes beyond specific and transient thoughts and arrives at what he calls the *source* of thought. Robert Ornstein (1971) has provided a simple and convincing explanation for this experience. When a person concentrates on a single stimulus, it seems eventually to disappear, leaving pure attention without any specific content. Scientists have studied this process of habituation behaviorally and physiologically; it reflects a basic process of neural function. In TM, the single object of attention, the mantra, first reduces a person's attention to other stimuli, and then, with repetition, vanishes itself, leaving awareness of *nothing* in particular—or "pure consciousness." People react in similar ways to any repetitive stimulus that isn't objectionable.

The Maharishi has suggested that a process of "unstressing" goes on during meditation. The therapeutic aspect of TM suggests that this meditative state may not be without content after all, but may (like sleep) combine effortless relaxation with spontaneous imagery and emotion. Researchers have known for a long time that under conditions of low arousal and low sensory input, images and feelings arise naturally. Sometimes they're disturbing images. Teachers of meditation tell their students not to be alarmed by any thought that comes to mind, but to notice it as they would any passing thought and then attend once again to the mantra. It is quite possible that "unstressing" takes place as a result of this soothing yet instructive dialectic. In a way, it resembles Freud's notion of catharsis during free association.

And yet TM is quite effortless, and like any task, it becomes easier with practice. The ease of the technique is probably essential for lowering the metabolism. The lowered metabolism, in turn, relaxes a person generally, so that during meditation he moves, feels, and thinks less.

Genuine relaxation helps explain why meditators seem to feel so alive and sensitive to sights and sounds after coming out of meditation. It's a matter of contrast. A person's perceptual response to a change in stimulation depends on his prior stimulation. Harry Helson's research (1964) on adaptation level illustrates the phenomenon perfectly. If you put one hand in hot water and the other in cold water, and then after a few minutes put both hands in lukewarm water, the hand that was in the cold water will feel the warm water as hot, while the hand that was in the hot water will feel the warm water as cold. Meditators undoubtedly are subject to the same contrasting perceptions —accentuated perhaps by the unusual nature of the meditative process.

Glowing Belief

Meditators seem to value TM very highly. The most obvious reason for their attachment is that TM feels good. But psychologically the situation is more complicated than that. The sheer novelty of meditation for most Americans probably affects their view of it quite strongly, intensifying either their enthusiasm or hostility. The experience of meditation also puts people into a receptive frame of mind, since it relaxes them thoroughly. They are more likely to say yes to the first available explanation for their experience, and teachers of meditation, whether dedicated to TM or to other schools, explain things in glowing terms.

A person's beliefs can be crucial to the way he experiences something. The difference between "relaxation," for instance, and "depression" may depend in part on one's expectations. Meditators hope, believe, and expect that TM will be a good thing. It's *supposed* to be a good thing, and the supposition helps define the eventual experience.

We have to remember that the meditative state is self-induced, that people are seeking changes in consciousness and can predict more or less what the changes will be. The fact that meditators control the experience almost insures that it will seem worthwhile. Someone who knowingly takes LSD stands a better chance of enjoying the trip than someone who has been fed the drug on the sly. Similarly, the extreme meditator who, after 14 solid days of meditation, starts seeing halos around the heads of his fellow meditators differs importantly from the unhappy mental patient who enters the hospital with "hallucinations —claims to see halos" on his history.

Not long ago, researchers would isolate experimental subjects from all sensory experience. The result would be hallucinations and other symptoms of psychosis. Sensory deprivation became, for many psychologists, a model for insanity. Today some people *choose* to enter a condition of sensory deprivation. Their goal is not to go crazy but to experience "altered states of consciousness." Accordingly, whatever else we may think of their taste or wisdom, we wouldn't necessarily call them psychotic.

Meanwhile, Brendan Maher (1972) at Harvard has suggested that one of the reasons "schizophrenic" patients are so anxious and upset is that they label themselves "crazy." Their perceptions and thinking begin to change, and they can think of only one way to characterize their new state. But since part of the syndrome of schizophrenia can be caused by physiological deficits, it might help the patient considerably if he could relabel his problem.

Differences in *who controls* our experiences, and differences in how we classify and interpret them, separate the meanings of those experiences profoundly.

Evolutionary Precedent

Meditative practices have existed for thousands of years. Very broadly, we may think of meditation as an act of sustained self-reflection: in this sense it is a natural act. I suspect that there is an evolutionary precedent for meditation. Primitive human societies and even certain apes typically spend part of each day sitting quietly, in what appears to be self-reflection. Who is to say they're not meditating? There may be a basic human need for something like TM.

If so, there is probably more need for it today than ever before. Modern technology showers us with new images, sounds, tastes, and chemicals. We pay a price for this flood of stimulation. Television and TV dinners don't require us to *act* in varied ways, and in our passiveness we lose contact with our natural modes of experience and their related skills.

Meditation, however, is not the "solution to all problems," as one of TM's brochures has stated in large type. If practiced to excess, it is conceivable that TM can itself become a problem. For just as too much activity and stress can interfere with the proper functioning of the human animal, I would predict that too much meditation can also harm the organism. The nervous system needs reasonably intense and varied external stimulation, and there is no evolutionary, ethological, or biological precedent for massive and prolonged meditation. A few people, with a tendency toward mental illness, may even aggravate their condition by meditating for long periods—just as some people react adversely to specific drugs. At worst, it is remotely possible that too much meditation can starve the brain of needed oxygen.

There are still a good many mysteries about meditation, and there are several versions of how it works. For this reason, I think we should remain wary of the claims and selective use of scientific data by well-meaning but scientifically unsophisticated practitioners. We should pay attention to the simple claim that meditation relaxes some people and makes them feel better. A skill that can do such things—that can lead us to be more self-sufficient and more aware of ourselves and others—is clearly a good thing. There are many routes to these important human goals, including traditional psychotherapy. Meditation is another route, and perhaps a more direct one.

References

Benson, H. and Wallace, R. K. Decreased drug abuse with transcendental meditation—a study of 1,862 subjects. In C. J. Zarafonetis (Ed.), *Drug Abuse: Proceedings of the International Conference.* Philadelphia: Lea & Febiger, 1972.

Brosse, T. Altruism and creativity as biological factors of human evolution. In P. A. Sorokin (Ed.), *Exploration in altruistic love and behavior.* Boston: Beacon Press, 1950.

Dalal, A. S. and Barber, T. X. Yoga, "yogic feats" and hypnosis in the light of empirical research. *American Journal of Clinical Hypnosis,* 1969, 11, 155–166.

Helson, H. *Adaptation level theory; An experimental and systematic approach to behavior.* New York: Harper and Row, 1964.

Linden, W. Practicing of meditation by school children and their levels of field independence-dependence, test anxiety and reading achievement. *Journal of Counselling and Clinical Psychology,* 1973, 41, 139–143.

Maher, B. The language of schizophrenia; A review and interpretation. *British Journal of Psychiatry,* 1972, 120, 3–17.

Orme-Johnson, D. W. Autonomic stability and transcendental meditation. *Psychosomatic Medicine,* 1973, 35, 341–349.

Ornstein, R. E. The techniques of meditation and their implications for modern psychology. In C. Naranjo and R. E. Ornstein, *On The Psychology of Meditation.* New York: Viking Press, 1971.

————. *The psychology of consciousness.* San Francisco: Freeman, 1973.

Otis, L. S. If well-integrated but anxious, try T. M. *Psychology Today,* 1974, 7, 45–46.

Schwartz, G. E. Pros and cons of meditation: current findings on physiology and anxiety, self-control, drug abuse and creativity. Paper presented at the 81st Annual Meeting of the American Psychological Association, Montreal, 1973.

_____. Meditation as an altered trait of consciousness: Current findings on stress reactivity and creativity. Paper presented at the 82nd annual meeting of the American Psychological Association, New Orleans, 1974.

Seeman, W., Nadich, S., and Banta, T. Influence of transcendental meditation on a measure of self-actualization. *Journal of Counseling Psychology,* 1972, **19**, 184–187.

Wallace, R. K. Physiological effects of transcendental meditation. *Science,* 1970, **167**, 1751–1754.

Wallace, R. K., Benson, H., and Wilson, A. F. A wakeful hypometabolic physiologic state. *American Journal of Physiology,* 1971, **221**, 795–799.

Wenger, M., Bagchi, B., and Anand, B. Experiments in India on "voluntary" control of the heart and pulse. *Circulation,* 1961, **24**, 1319–1325.

Weil, W. *The Natural Mind.* New York: Houghton-Mifflin, 1972.

Herbert Benson, John F. Beary, Mark P. Carol

Meditation and the Relaxation Response

In the Western world today, there is a growing interest in nonpharmacological, self-induced, altered states of consciousness because of their alleged benefits of better mental and physical health and improved ability to deal with tension and stress. During the experience of one of these states, individuals claim to have feelings of increased creativity, of infinity, and of immortality; they have an evangelistic sense of mission, and report that mental and physical suffering vanish (Dean). Subjective and objective data exist which support the hypothesis that an integrated central nervous system reaction, the *"relaxation response,"* underlies this altered state of consciousness. Physicians should be knowledgeable of the physiological changes and possible health benefits of the relaxation response.

The Physiology of the Relaxation Response

The relaxation response appears to be an integrated hypothalamic response which results in generalized decreased sympathetic nervous system activity, and perhaps also increased parasympathetic activity. This response, termed the "trophotropic response," was first described by Hess in the cat (Hess, 1957). The trophotropic *zone* is located in the area of the anterior hypothalamus. It extends into the supra- and pre-optic areas, septum, and inferior lateral thalamus. The response is mediated by the parasympathetic nervous system, and electrical stimulation of this zone results in hypo- or adynamia of skeletal musculature, decreased blood pressure, decreased respiratory rate, and pupil constriction. Hess stated, "Let us repeat at this point that we are actually dealing with a protective mechanism against overstress belonging to the tro-photropic-endophylactic system and promoting restorative processes. We emphasize that these adynamic effects are opposed to ergotropic reactions which are oriented toward increased oxidative metabolism and utilization of energy" (1957, p. 40). The "ergotropic" reactions of Hess correspond to the "emergency reaction" first described by Cannon, popularly referred to as the fight or flight response and also called the "defense reaction" by others (Hess and Brugger; Abrahams et al.).

To better understand the relaxation response (the trophotropic response), a discussion of its counterpart, the fight or flight response (the ergotropic response) is appropriate. The ergotropic *zone* extends from the anterior midbrain toward the hypothalamus. The response is mediated by the sympathetic nervous system. When the zone is electrically stimulated, it consistently produces dilation of the pupils, increased blood pressure, increased respiratory rate, and heightened motor excitability. Although at times one of these responses may be emphasized, Hess stresses that there are no foci that correspond to individual isolated responses such as in the cortical motor zone. Rather, "In the diencephalon, we are dealing with a *collective* representation of a group of responses which includes responses of the autonomic system as they make their appearance in the form of synergically associated mechanisms" (1957, p. 35). Cannon reasoned that this integrated response prepared the animal for "fight or flight" when faced with a threatening environmental situation. Man also responds to threatening environmental conditions or to environmental situations which require behavioral adjustment by a coordinated physiological response which mimics that of the increased sympathetic nervous system activity of the fight or flight response (Gutmann and Benson).

The relaxation response in man consists of changes opposite to those of the fight or flight response.[1] During the practice of one well-investigated technique called Transcendental Meditation, the major elements of the relaxation response occur: decreases in oxygen consumption, carbon dioxide elimination, heart rate, respiratory rate, minute ventilation, and arterial blood lactate. Systolic, diastolic, and mean blood pressures remain unchanged compared to control levels. Rectal temperature also remains unchanged while skin resistance markedly increases and skeletal muscle blood flow slightly increases. The electroencephalogram demonstrates an increase in the intensity of slow alpha waves and occasional theta wave activity. Muscle tonus, not yet measured in Transcendental Meditation, decreases in other relaxation

---

[1]See Wallace and Benson; Wallace, Benson and Wilson; Levander et al.

techniques (Jacobson; Luthe, 1969). These changes are consistent with generalized decreased sympathetic nervous system activity and are distinctly different from the physiological changes noted during quiet sitting or sleep. The changes occur simultaneously and are consistent with those noted by Hess.

The Technique of Eliciting the Relaxation Response

Four basic elements are usually necessary to elicit the relaxation response in man:
1. *Mental Device*—There should be a constant stimulus—e.g., a sound, word, or phrase repeated silently or audibly, or fixed gazing at an object. The purpose of these procedures is to shift from logical, externally-oriented thought.
2. *Passive Attitude*—If distracting thoughts do occur during the repetition or gazing, they should be disregarded and one's attention should be redirected to the technique. One should not worry about how well he is performing the technique.
3. *Decreased Muscle Tonus*—The subject should be in a comfortable posture so that minimal muscular work is required.
4. *Quiet Environment*—A quiet environment with decreased environmental stimuli should be chosen. Most techniques instruct the practitioner to close his eyes. A place of worship is often suitable, as is a quiet room.
The efficiency of learning the various relaxation techniques appears enhanced when taught by trained instructors.

Historical Subjective Writings Supporting Existence of the Relaxation Response

Techniques have existed for centuries, usually within a religious context, which allowed an individual to experience the relaxation response. For example, in the West a fourteenth-century Christian treatise entitled *The Cloud of Unknowing* discussed how to attain an altered state of consciousness which was required to attain alleged union with God (Progoff). The anonymous author stated that this goal could not be reached in the ordinary levels of human consciousness, but rather by use of "lower" levels. These levels were reached by eliminating all distractions and physical activity, all worldly things including all thoughts. As a means of ". . . beating down thought," the use of a single-syllable word, such as "god" or "love," should be repeated.

> Choose whichever one you prefer, or, if you like, choose another that suits your taste, provided that it is of one syllable. And clasp this word tightly in your heart so that it never leaves it no matter what may happen. This word shall be your shield and your spear. . . . With this word you shall strike down thoughts of every kind and drive them beneath the cloud of forgetting. After that, if any thoughts should press upon you . . . answer him with this word only and with no other words [Progoff, pp. 76–77].

There will be moments when ". . . every created thing may suddenly and completely be forgotten. But immediately after each stirring, because of the corruption of the flesh, it [the soul] drops down again to some thought or some deed" (Progoff, p. 68). An important instruction for success is ". . . do not by another means work in it with your mind or with your imagination" (Progoff, p. 69).

Another Christian work, *The Third Spiritual Alphabet,* written in the tenth century by Fray Francisco de Osuna, dealt with an altered state of consciousness. He wrote that "Contemplation requires us to blind ourselves to all that is not God" (p. viii), and that one should be deaf and dumb to all else (p. 50) and must ". . . quit all obstacles, keeping your eyes bent on the ground . . ." (pp. 293–294). The method can be either a short, self-composed prayer, repeated over and over, or simply saying "no" to thoughts when they occur. This exercise should be performed for one hour in the morning and evening and should be taught by a qualified teacher. Fray Francisco wrote that such an exercise would help in all endeavors, making us more efficient in our tasks and the tasks more enjoyable. All men, especially the busy, secular as well as religious, should be taught this meditation, for it is a refuge to which one can retreat when faced with stressful situations (Osuna).

The famous fifteenth-century Christian mystics Saints John and Terese described the major steps required to achieve the mystical state (Anon.; Saint Terese), which included ignoring distractions, usually by repetitive prayer.

Christian meditation and mysticism were well-developed within the Byzantine church and known as Hesychasm (Norwich and Sitwell, pp. 56–57). This method of repetitive prayer was described in the fourteenth century at Mount Athos in Greece by Gregory of Sinai and is called "The Prayer of the Heart" or "The Prayer of Jesus." It dates back to the beginnings of the Christian era. The prayer itself was called secret meditation and was transmitted from older to younger monks through an initiation rite. Emphasis was placed on having a skilled instructor. The method of prayer recommended by these monks was:

> Sit down alone and in silence. Lower your head, shut your eyes, breathe out gently, and imagine yourself looking into your own heart. Carry your mind, i.e., your thoughts, from your head to your heart. As you breathe out, say 'Lord Jesus Christ,' have mercy on me.' Say it moving your lips gently, or simply say it in your mind. Try to put all other thoughts aside. Be calm, be patient and repeat the process very frequently [French, p. 10].

To reach such a state, a tranquil environment is necessary. "It may happen that a man who has been busy all day gives himself to prayer for an hour . . . so that during that time the thoughts of his earthly preoccupations are forgotten" (Ross, p. 87).

In Judaism, similar practices leading to this altered state of consciousness date back to the time of the second temple in the second century B.C. and are found in one of the earliest forms of Jewish mysticism, Merkabalism (Scholem). In this practice of meditation, the subject sat with his head between his knees, whispered hymns and songs, and repeated a name of a magic seal. In the thirteenth century A.D., the works of Rabbi Abulafia were published and his ideas became a major part of Jewish Kabbalistic mysticism (Scholem). Rabbi Abulafia felt that the normal life of the soul is kept within limits by our sensory perceptions and emotions, and since these perceptions and emotions are concerned with the finite, the soul's life is finite. Man therefore needs a higher form of perception, which instead of blocking the soul's deeper regions, opens them up. An "absolute" object upon which to meditate is required. Rabbi Abulafia found this in the Hebrew alphabet. He developed a mystical system of contemplating the letters of God's name. Bokser describes Rabbi Abulafia's prayer:

> . . . immersed in prayer and meditation, uttering the divine name with special modulations of the voice and with special gestures, he induced in himself a state of ecstasy in which he believed the soul had shed its material bonds, and, unimpeded, returned to its divine source. [p. 9]

The purpose of this prayer and methodical meditation is to experience a new state of consciousness, described as harmonious movement of pure thought, which has severed all relation to the senses. This is compared by Scholem to music and yoga (pp. 733–734). Scholem felt that Rabbi Abulafia's

... teachings represent but a Judaized version of that ancient spiritual technique which has found its classical expression in the practices of the Indian mystics who follow the system known as *Yoga.* To cite only one instance out of many, an important part in Abulafia's system is played by the technique of breathing; now this technique has found its highest development in the Indian *Yoga,* where it is commonly regarded as the most important instrument of mental discipline. Again, Abulafia lays down certain rules of body posture, certain corresponding combinations of consonants and vowels, and certain forms of recitation, and in particular some passages of his book "The Light of the Intellect" give the impression of a Judaized treatise on *Yoga.* The similarity even extends to some aspects of the doctrine of ecstatic vision, as preceded and brought about by these practices. [p. 139]

The basic elements which elicit the relaxation response in certain practices of Christianity and Judaism are also found in Islamic mysticism or Sufism (Trimingham). Sufism developed as a reaction against the external rationalization of Islam and made use of intuitive and emotional faculties which were claimed to be dormant until they were utilized through training under the guidance of a teacher. The method of employing these faculties is known as Dhikr. It is a means of excluding distractions and of drawing nearer to God by the constant repetition of His name, either silently or aloud, and by rhythmic breathing. Music, musical poems, and dance are also employed in the ritual of Dhikr, for it was noticed that they could help induce states of ecstasy. Originally, Dhikr was only practiced by the members of the society who made a deliberate choice to redirect their lives to God as the preliminary step in the surrender of the will. Upon initiation to his order, the initiate received the *wird,* a secret, holy sound. The old Masters felt that the true encounter with God could not be attained by all, for most men are born deaf to mystical sensitivity. However, by the twelfth century, this attitude had changed. It was realized that this ecstasy could be induced in the ordinary man in a relatively short time by rhythmic exercises involving posture, control of breath, coordinated movements, and oral repetitions (Trimingham, p. 199).

In the Western world, the relaxation response elicited by religious practices was not part of the routine practice of religions, but rather was within the mystical tradition. In the East, however, meditation which elicited the relaxation response was developed much earlier and became a major element in religion and in everyday life. Writings from Indian scriptures, the Upanishads, dated sixth century B.C., note that individuals might attain "... a unified state with the Brahman [the Deity] by means of restraint of breath, withdrawal of senses, meditation, concentration, contemplation and absorption" (Organ, p. 303).

There are a multitude of Eastern religions and ways of life, including Zen and Yoga with their many variants, which can elicit the relaxation response. They employ mental and physical methods including the repetition of a word or sound, the exclusion of meaningful thoughts, a quiet environment, and a comfortable position, and they stress the importance of a trained teacher. One of the meditative practices of Zen Buddhism, Zazen, employs a yoga-like technique of the coupling of respiration and counting to ten—i.e., one on inhaling, two on exhaling, and so on, to ten. With time, one stops counting and simply "follows the breath" (Johnston, p. 78) in order to achieve a state of no thought, no feeling, to be completely in "nothing" (Ishiguro).

Shintoism and Taoism are important religions of Japan and China respectively. In Shintoism, one method of prayer consists of sitting quietly, inspiring through the nose, holding inspiration for a short time, and expiring through the mouth, with eyes directed toward a mirror at their level. Throughout the exercise, the priest repeats ten numbers, or sacred words, pronounced according to the traditional religious teachings (Herbert, p. 83). Fujisawa noted, "It is interesting that this grand ritual characteristic of Shintoism is doubtlessly the same process as *Yoga* . . ." (p. 23). Taoism, one of the traditional religions of China, employs, in addition to methods similar to Shinto, concentration on nothingness to achieve absolute tranquility (Chang, p. 167).

Similar meditational practices are found in practically every culture of man. Shamanism is a form of mysticism associated with feelings of ecstasy and is practiced in conjunction with tribal religions in North and South America, Indonesia, Oceania, Africa, Siberia, and Japan. Each shaman has a song or chant to bring on trances, usually entering into solitude to do so. Music, especially the drum, plays an important part in Shamanistic trances (Johnson; Segal, p. 29).

Many less traditional religious practices are flourishing in the United States. One aim of the practices is achievement of an altered state of consciousness which is induced by techniques similar to those that elicit the relaxation response. Subub, Nichiren Sho Shu, Hare Krishna, Scientology, Black Muslimism, Meher Baba, and the Association for Research and Enlightenment are but a few of these (Needleman).

In addition to techniques which elicit the relaxation response within a religious context, secular techniques also exist. One method often used is gazing upon an object and keeping attention focused upon that object to the exclusion of all else (Lowell, p. 303, p. 343; Underhill, pp. 301–302). Others, the so-called nature mystics, have been able to elicit the relaxation response by immersing themselves in quiet, often in the quiet of nature. Wordsworth believed ". . . that when his mind was freed from preoccupation with disturbing objects, petty cares, 'little enmities and low desires,' that he could then reach a condition of equilibrium, which he describes as a 'wise passiveness' or 'a happy stillness of the mind' . . ." (Spurgeon, p. 61). Wordsworth believed that anyone could deliberately induce this condition in himself by a kind of relaxation of the will. Thoreau made many references to such feelings attained by sitting for hours alone with nature. Indeed, Thoreau compares himself to a Yogi (Sanborn, pp. 210–211). William James describes similar experiences (pp. 76–77). A treatise on other such experiences may be found in Johnson's *Watcher on the Hills.*

Objective Data Supporting the Widespread Existence of the Relaxation Response

Physiologic changes occurring during the practice of various techniques which elicit the relaxation response are summarized and referenced in the table. These consist, in part, of decreased oxygen consumption, respiratory rate, heart rate, and muscle tension. Increases are noted in skin resistance and EEG alpha wave activity. These changes are hypothesized to result from an integrated, hypothalamic response leading to decreased sympathetic nervous system activity. The neurophysiologic and neuroanatomic pathways from the cortex to the diencephalon remain to be definitely established (Gellhorn).

Autogenic training is a technique of medical therapy which is said to elicit the trophotropic response of Hess or the relaxation response. Autogenic therapy is defined as ". . . a self-induced modification of corticodiencephalic interrelationships" which enables the lower brain centers to activate "trophotropic activity" (Luthe, 1969). The method of autogenic training is based on six psychophysiologic exercises devised by a German neurologist, H. H. Shultz, which are practiced several times a day until the subject is able to voluntarily shift to a wakeful *low-arousal* (trophotropic) state. The "Standard Exercises" are practiced in a quiet environment, in a horizontal position, and with closed eyes (Luthe, 1969). Exercise 1 focuses on the feeling of heaviness in the limbs, and Exercise 2 on the cultivation of the sensation of warmth in the limbs. Exercise 3 deals with cardiac regulation, while Exercise 4 consists of passive concentration on breathing. In Exercise 5, the subject cultivates the sensation of warmth in his upper abdomen, and Exercise 6 is the cultivation of feelings of coolness in the forehead. Exercises 1 through 4 most effectively elicit the trophotropic response, while Exercises 5 and 6 are reported to have different effects (Luthe, 1969). The subject's attitude toward the exercise must not be intense and compulsive, but rather of a quiet, "let it happen," nature. This is referred to as *passive concentration* and is deemed absolutely essential (Luthe, 1972).

Progressive relaxation is a technique which seeks to achieve increased discriminative control over skeletal muscle until a subject is able to induce very low levels of tonus in the major muscle groups. Jacobson, who devised the technique, states that anxiety and muscular relaxation produce opposite physiologic states, and therefore cannot exist together. Progressive relaxation is practiced in a supine position in a quiet room; a passive attitude is essential because mental images induce slight, measurable tensions in muscles, especially those of the eyes and face. The subject is taught to recognize even slight contractions of his muscles so that he can avoid them and achieve the deepest degree of relaxation possible.

Hypnosis is an artificially induced state characterized by increased suggestibility (Gorton). A subject is judged to be in the hypnotic state if he manifests a high level of response to test suggestions such as muscle rigidity, amnesia, hallucination, anesthesia, and post-hypnotic suggestion, which are used in standard scales such as that of Weitzenhoffer and Hilgard. The hypnotic induction procedure usually includes suggestion (autosuggestion for self-hypnosis) of relaxation and drowsiness, closed eyes, and a recumbent or semisupine position (Barber, 1971). Following the induction procedure, an appropriate suggestion for the desired mental or physical behavior is given.

So far it has not been possible to find a unique physiologic index which defines the hypnotic state (Barber, 1971). Physiologic states vary the same way during hypnosis as they do during waking behavior. Suggested states of arousal or relaxation are accompanied by *either* increased or decreased metabolic rate, heart rate, blood pressure, skin conductance, and respiratory rate, corresponding to the changes seen when these states are induced by nonhypnotic means (Barber, 1971). If the control state is the same as the suggested state, then, of course, no change in physiologic parameters will be seen (Barber, 1961). For example, the study by Whitehorn et al. reported that the control oxygen consumption value of 217 ml/min was not significantly changed by hypnosis. However, subjects in this experiment were trained to relax before control readings were taken. Therefore, hypnotic suggestion to relax produced no further change.

Sentic cycles is another psychophysiologic technique, devised by Manfred

PHYSIOLOGIC PARAMETERS SUPPORTING THE EXISTENCE OF THE RELAXATION RESPONSE DURING THE PRACTICE OF VARIOUS MENTAL TECHNIQUES

Technique

(General references indicated under each technique heading; specific references with each parameter; key below)

Parameter	Transcendental Meditation (22)	Autogenic Training (16)	Hypnosis* (5, 12, 4, 8)	Zen and Yoga (13, 17)	Cotention (6)	Sentic Cycles (7)	Progressive Relaxation (14)
Oxygen consumption	↓ (22, 21)	N.M.**	↓ (10)	↓ (2, 20)	N.M.	↓ (7)	N.M.
Respiratory rate	↓ (1, 22)	↓ (16)	↓ (5)	↓ (3, 17, 20)	↓ (19)	↓ (7)	N.M.
Heart rate	↓ (22, 21)	↓ (16)	↓ (5)	↓ (3, 20)	N.M.	↓ (7)	N.M.
Alpha waves	↑ (22, 21)	↑ (16)	N.M.	↑ (13, 20)	Present (18)	N.M.	N.M.
Skin resistance	↑ (22, 21)	↑ (16)	↑ (9, 11)	↑ (3)	N.M.	N.M.	N.M.
Blood pressure	No change (22)	?*** (16)	? (8)	No change (15, 20)	N.M.	N.M.	N.M.
Muscle tension	N.M.	↓ (16)	N.M.	N.M.	N.M.	N.M.	↓ (14)

*Suggested deep relaxation
**N.M. = Not measured.
***? = Inconclusive results.

1. Allison.
2. Anand et al.
3. Bagchi and Wenger.
4. Barber, 1961.
5. Barber, 1971.
6. Burrow.
7. Clynes.
8. Crasilneck and Hall.
9. Davis and Kantor.
10. Dudley et al.
11. Estabrooks.
12. Gorton.
13. Hoenig.
14. Jacobson.
15. Karambelkar et al.

16. Luthe, 1969.
17. Onda.
18. Segal.
19. Shiomi.
20. Sugi and Akutsu.
21. Wallace, 1970.
22. Wallace, Benson, and Wilson.

Clynes. A sentic "cycle" is composed of eight sentic states. A sentic "state" is a self-induced emotional experience, and the sequence of states used by Clynes is: no emotion, anger, hate, grief, love, sex, joy, reverence. A subject practices a cycle by thinking the state—e.g., anger—and responding with finger pressure on a key (which transduces the pressure for recording) as he sits and listens to a tape recording. The recording states which sentic state is present and when the subject should press the key.

Burrow described two kinds of attention: *cotention* and *ditention* (Burrow; Shiomi). Cotention is the subject's ". . . focus on the object of its environment." It is concentration on one thing exclusively. Ditention is described as "ordinary" wakefulness, in which state the subject's interest shifts from object to object. The state of cotention is induced by relaxing the muscles, closing the eyes, and resting them on a point imagined to be the center of a curtain of darkness in front of the subject.

Yoga has been an important part of Indian culture for thousands of years. It is claimed to be the culmination of the efforts of ancient Hindu thinkers to "give man the fullest possible control over his mind" (Hoenig). Yoga consists of meditation practices and physical techniques usually performed in a quiet environment, and it has many variant forms. Yoga began as Raja Yoga, which sought "union with the absolute" by meditation. Later, there was an emphasis on physical methods in attempts to achieve an altered state of consciousness. This form is termed Hatha Yoga. It has developed into a physical culture and is claimed to prevent and cure certain diseases. Essential to the practice of Hatha Yoga are appropriate posture and control of respiration (Ramamurthi). The most common posture is called Lotus (seated on the ground with legs crossed). This posture helps the spine stay erect without strain and is claimed to enhance concentration. The respiratory training promotes control of duration of inspiration and expiration, and the pause between breaths, so that one eventually achieves voluntary control of respiration. Bagchi and Wenger, in studies of Yoga practitioners, reported that Yoga could produce a 70% increase in skin resistance, decreased heart rate, and EEG alpha wave activity. These observations led them to suggest that Yoga is "deep relaxation of a certain aspect of the autonomic nervous system without drowsiness or sleep."

Transcendental Meditation is currently a widely practiced form of Yoga. The technique, as taught by Maharishi Mahesh Yogi, comes from the Vedic tradition of India. Instruction is given individually, and the technique is allegedly easily learned at the first instruction session. It is said to require no physical or mental control. The individual is taught a systematic method of repeating a word or sound, the mantra, without attempting to concentrate specifically on it. It involves little change in lifestyle, other than the meditation period of 15 to 20 minutes twice a day when the practitioner sits in a comfortable position with closed eyes.

Zen is very like Yoga, from which it developed, and is associated with the Buddhist religion (Onda). In Zen meditation, the subject is said to achieve a "controlled psychophysiologic decrease of the cerebral excitatory state" by a crossed-leg posture, closed eyes, regulation of respiration, and concentration on the Koan (an alogical problem—e.g., What is the sound of one hand clapping?), or by prayer and chanting. Respiration is adjusted by taking several slow deep breaths, then inspiring briefly and forcelessly, and expiring long and forcefully, with subsequent natural breathing. Any sensory perceptions or mental images are allowed to appear and leave passively. A quiet, comfortable environment is essential. Experienced Zen meditators elicit the relaxation response more efficiently than novices (Sugi and Akutsu).

Possible Therapeutic Benefits and Side Effects of the Relaxation Response

Although advocates of many of the techniques which elicit the relaxation response offer anecdotal evidence to support claims of healthful and therapeutic benefits, only preliminary objective data exist at the present time which establish the place of the relaxation response in medicine. The regular practice of Transcendental Meditation leads to decreased systolic blood pressure in hypertensive subjects (Benson, Rosner, and Marzetta) and, in an uncontrolled retrospective study, was associated with decreased drug abuse (Benson and Wallace). The daily elicitation of the relaxation response predictably may be of value in situations where excessive sympathetic activity is present, situations which chronically evoke the fight or flight response and which may lead to prevalent, serious diseases such as hypertension (Gutmann and Benson).

The side effects of the chronic practice of the relaxation response have not been well documented. When the response is elicited for two limited daily periods of 20 to 30 minutes, no adverse side effects have been observed (personal observations, H. B.). When elicited more frequently, some subjects experience a withdrawal from life and symptoms which range in severity from insomnia to psychotic manifestations, often with hallucinatory behavior (personal observations, H. B.; Ornstein). These side effects are difficult to evaluate on a retrospective basis since many people with preexisting psychiatric problems would be drawn to any technique which evangelistically promises relief from tension and stress. Extensive prospective investigations of the relaxation response are underway in subjects suffering from hypertension, headache, drug abuse, psychoses, and anxiety neuroses, and results soon should be available.

If the relaxation response proves to be of value in medicine, there exist many religious, secular, or "therapeutic" techniques which elicit it. This should not be construed so as to interpret religion in mechanistic terms. *Belief* in the technique in question may well be a very important factor in the elicitation of the relaxation response. Future studies should establish the most efficient method for a given individual.

References

Abrahams, V. C., et al. "Active Muscle Vasodilatation Produced by Stimulation of the Brain Stem: Its Significance in the Defense Reaction," *J. Physiology* (1960) 154:491.

Allison, John. "Respiration Changes during Transcendental Meditation," *Lancet* (1970) 1:833–834.

Anand, B. K., et al. "Studies on Shri Ramananda Yogi during His Stay in an Air-tight Box," *Indian J. Med. Res.* (1961) 49:82–89.

Anonymous: A Benedictine of Stanbrook Abbey. *Mediaeval Mystical Tradition and Saint John of the Cross;* London, Burns and Oates, 1954.

Bagchi, B. K., and Wenger, M. A. "Electrophysiological Correlations of Some Yoga Exercises," *Electroencephalog. Clin. Neurophysiology Suppl.* (1957) 7:132–149.

Barber, Theodore X. "Physiological Effects of Hypnosis," *Psychol. Bull.* (1961) 58:390–419.

―――. "Physiological Effects of Hypnosis and Suggestion," in *Biofeedback and Self-Control 1970;* Aldine-Atherton, 1971.

Benson, Herbert, and Wallace, Robert K. "Decreased Drug Abuse with Transcendental Meditation—A Study of 1,862 Subjects," in C. J. D. Zarafonetis (Ed.), *Drug Abuse—Proceedings of the International Conference;* Lea and Febiger, 1972.

Benson, Herbert, Rosner, Bernard A., and Marzetta, Barbara R. "Decreased Systolic Blood Pressure in Hypertensive Subjects Who Practiced Meditation," *J. Clin. Invest.* (1973) 52:8a.

Bokser, Rabbi Ben Zion. *From the World of the Cabbalah;* Philosophical Library, 1954.

Burrow, Trigant. "Kymograph Studies of Physiological (Respiratory) Concomitants in Two Types of Attentional Adaptation," *Nature* (1938) 142:156.

Cannon, Walter B. "The Emergency Function of the Adrenal Medulla in Pain and the Major Emotions," *Amer. J. Physiology* (1941) 33:356.

Chang, Chung-Yuan. *Creativity and Taoism;* Julian Press, 1963.

Clynes, Manfred. "Toward a View of Man," in M. Clynes and J. Milsum (Eds.), *Biomedical Engineering Systems;* McGraw-Hill, 1970.

Crasilneck, Harold B., and Hall, James A. "Physiological Changes Associated with Hypnosis: A Review of the Literature Since 1948," *Internat. J. Clin. and Exp. Hypnosis* (1959) 7:9–50.

Davis, R. C., and Kantor, J. R. "Skin Resistance During Hypnotic States," *J. General Psychology* (1935) 13:62–81.

Dean, Stanley R. "Is There an Ultraconscious Beyond the Unconscious?," *Canadian Psychiatric Assn. J.* (1970) 15:57–61.

Dudley, Donald L., et al. "Changes in Respiration Associated with Hypnotically Induced Emotion, Pain, and Exercise," *Psychosomatic Medicine* (1963) 26:46–57.

Estabrooks, G. H. "The Psychogalvanic Reflex in Hypnosis," *J. General Psychology* (1930) 3:150–157.

French, Reginald Michael, (Trans.). *The Way of a Pilgrim;* Seabury Press, 1968.

Fujisawa, Chikao. *Zen and Shinto;* Philosophical Library, 1959.

Gellhorn, Ernst. *Principles of Autonomic-Somatic Interactions;* Univ. of Minn. Press, 1967.

Gorton, Bernard E. "Physiology of Hypnosis," *Psychiatric Quart.* (1949) 23:317–343 and 457–485.

Gutmann, Mary C., and Benson, Herbert. "Interaction of Environmental Factors and Systemic Arterial Blood Pressure: A Review," *Medicine* (1971) 50:543–553.

Herbert, Jean. *Shinto: At the Fountain-head of Japan;* London, Allen and Unwin, 1967.

Hess, Walter R. *Functional Organization of the Diencephalon;* Grune & Stratton, 1957.

Hess, Walter R., and Brugger, M. "Das subkortikale Zentrum der affektiven Abwehrreaktion," *Helv. Physiol. Acta* (1943) 1:33–52.

Hoenig, J. "Medical Research on Yoga," *Confin. Psychiatr.* (1968) 11:69–89.

Ishiguro, H. *The Scientific Truth of Zen;* Tokyo, Zenrigaku Soc., 1964

Jacobson, Edmund, *Progressive Relaxation;* Univ. of Chicago Press, 1938.

James, William. *Letters;* Atlantic Monthly Press, 1920.

Johnson, Raynor Carey. *Watcher on the Hills;* Harper, 1959.

Johnston, William. *Christian Zen;* Harper & Row, 1971.

Karambelkar, P. V., et al. "Studies on Human Subjects Staying in an Air-tight Pit," *Indian J. Med. Res.* (1968) 56:1282–1288.

Levander, Victoria L., et al. "Increased Forearm Blood Flow during a Wakeful Hypometabolic State," *Fed. Proc.* (1972) 31:405.

Lowell, Percival. *The Soul of the Far East;* Houghton, Mifflin, 1892.

Luthe, Wolfgang. (Ed.) *Autogenic Therapy,* Vols. 1–5; Grune & Stratton, 1969.

Luthe, Wolfgang. "Autogenic Therapy: Excerpts on Applications to Cardiovascular Disorders and Hypercholesterolemia," in *Biofeedback and Self-Control 1971;* Aldine-Atherton, 1972.

Maharishi Mahesh Yogi. *The Science of Being and Art of Living;* London, Internat. SRM Pubs. 1966.

Needleman, Jacob. *The New Religions;* Doubleday, 1970.

Norwich, John Julius, and Sitwell, Reresby. *Mount Athos;* Harper & Row, 1966.

Onda, A. "Autogenic Training and Zen," in W. Luthe (Ed.), *Autogenic Training* (Internat. Ed.); Grune & Stratton, 1965.

Organ, Troy Wilson. *The Hindu Quest for the Perfection of Man;* Ohio Univ. Press, 1970.

Ornstein, Robert E. *The Psychology of Consciousness;* W. H. Freeman, 1972.

Osuna, Fray Francisco de. *The Third Spiritual Alphabet;* London, Benziger, 1931.

Progoff, Ira. (Ed. and Trans.) *The Cloud of Unknowing;* Julian Press, 1969.

Ramamurthi, B. "Yoga: An Explanation and Probable Neurophysiology," *J. Indian Med. Assn.* (1967) 48:167–170.

Ross, Floyd Hiatt. *Shinto, The Way of Japan;* Beacon Press, 1965.

Saint Terese of Avila. *The Way of Perfection,* A. R. Waller (Ed.); London, J. M. Dent, 1901.

Sanborn, Frank B. *Familiar Letters of Henry David Thoreau;* Houghton, Mifflin, 1894.

Scholem, Gershom Gerhard. *Jewish Mysticism;* Schocken Books, 1967.

Segal, Julius (Ed.). *Mental Health Program Reports—5;* Washington, D.C., Natl. Inst. of Mental Health, 1971.

Shiomi, K. "Respiratory and EEG Changes by Cotention of Trigant Burrow," *Psychologia* (1969) 12:24–28.

Spurgeon, Caroline Francis Eleanor. *Mysticism in English Literature;* Kennikat Press, 1970.

Sugi, Yasusaburo, and Akutsu, Kunio. "Studies on Respiration and Energy-Metabolism during Sitting in Zazen," *Research J. Physical Education* (1968) 12:190–206.

Thoreau, Henry David. *Walden;* Princeton Univ. Press, 1971.

Trimingham, John Spencer. *Sufi Orders in Islam;* Oxford, Clarendon Press, 1971.

Underhill, Evelyn. *Mysticism;* London, Methuen, 1957.

Wallace, Robert K. "Physiological Effects of Transcendental Meditation," *Science* (1970) 167:1751–1754.

Wallace, Robert K., and Benson, Herbert. "The Physiology of Meditation," *Sci. Amer.* (1972) 226:85–90.

Wallace, Robert K., Benson, Herbert, and Wilson, Archie F. "A Wakeful Hypometabolic State," *Amer. J. Physiology* (1971) 221:795–799.

Weitzenhoffer, Andre M., and Hilgard, E. *Stanford Hypnotic Suggestibility Scale;* Consulting Psychol. Press, 1959.

Whitehorn, J. C., et al. "The Metabolic Rate in Hypnotic Sleep," *New England J. Medicine* (1932) 206:777–781.

Arthur E. Gladman and Norma Estrada

Biofeedback in Clinical Practice

IN 1962, Gardner Murphy (1970) suggested the possibility of using electro-physiological instrumentation for measuring and presenting to a person some of his own normally unconscious physiological processes, that is, processes of which a person is normally unaware. To describe this process, the term "biofeedback" was coined at the founding meeting of the Biofeedback Research Society in 1969.

Through the use of biofeedback instruments it is becoming apparent that if a person can be aware of his (unconscious) physiological functioning, he or she can learn to modify it. Research has been conducted in many laboratories in an intensive exploration of this concept. Many pieces of intriguing information have evolved (Murphy, 1970). However, much of this information has yet to be communicated to the medical profession and, thus, it has yet to be applied in the clinical practice of medicine (treatment of psychosomatic disorders). Before discussing our preliminary observations it seems important to differentiate what we do from that which must be done in the research setting.

Research requires a discipline that eliminates as many variables as possible so that the effect of the subject's interaction with the biofeedback instrument can be clearly defined. In our clinical application the aim of using biofeedback instruments, however, is quite different. We treat the patient to help him do away with his symptoms and improve the quality of his life. To this end we help the patient train himself to control his internal states, using the biofeedback instruments as a starting point. We use the personal interaction between patient and therapists to encourage and support his efforts, to learn to control his internal states as quickly and effectively as possible, while modifying his way of dealing with problems.

In a personal communication (1973), Elmer and Alyce Green point out that we are using the "placebo effect," and we freely admit to this, (i.e., to alter the patient's emotional state so that whatever is offered will be assumed by the patient to have a favorable influence and thereby effect a favorable change in his physical state). Contrary to the research approach of trying to eliminate these factors, we seek to utilize them. We also feel free to make other individualistic therapeutic interventions helpful to a particular patient. Intervention may include interpretation of behavior patterns that produce a negative response in the patient and his environment, helping him to modify rigid value judgements and to achieve a more relaxed approach to his problems, and helping him to put into perspective those elements of his lifestyle which seem to be overemphasized (stressful).

In the past few years numerous papers have appeared in literature describing the use of biofeedback instruments in training individuals to control their internal states. Some observations make reference to the possibility that increased personal contact (interaction), not encompassed in research feedback training, can affect voluntary control substantially. The importance of this point has been grossly underestimated. With few exceptions, research projects have used healthy subjects, often of college age, whereas in the clinical setting we are treating patients who present themselves with complaints, usually chronic, for which they have sought help over a number of years. In those research projects where patients with specific complaints are treated with biofeedback, the research design, in order to be scientific, attempts to eliminate parameters, especially the interaction between subject and experimenter. We feel that the subject's relationship to the experimenter(s) and to his whole environment plays a vital role in the success or failure of the work. In a personal communication, Jack Schwartz[1], while working as a research subject, with Kenneth Pelletier, in Joe Kamiya's laboratory, points out that he was better able to control his internal states when the people around him had created a warm and friendly atmosphere. Our primary concern is to provide just such an atmosphere for the patient, not only by our attitude but also through the way in which we furnish the immediate environment. The treatment rooms contain a large, comfortable, reclining chair and footstool for the patient and comfortable chairs for the therapists. The nonverbal communication, or positive environment, in our treating is as important as the

---

[1]Jack Schwarz has considerable control over his internal states, including the ability to control bleeding, pain, and infection. He has been studied extensively, especially by Green and Green (1973) at the Menninger Foundation and Kenneth Pelletier at Langley Porter Clinic (1973).

treatment choice itself. If we are to treat the whole individual, we must include the world around him, the people who are important to him and to whom he is important, and the ways in which they interact, verbally and nonverbally.

Green, Green, and Walters state: "The psychophysiological principle, as we hypothesize it, affirms that every change in the physiological state is accompanied by an appropriate change in the mental/emotional state, conscious or unconscious, and conversely, every change in the mental/emotional state, conscious or unconscious, is accompanied by an appropriate change in the physiological state." If this is true, we have then an opportunity of making significant changes in the individual's way of functioning, not only physiologically, but also emotionally. It follows that control in the internal state would also modify the way the individual relates to his environment. If the individual can be taught to control his internal state, this provides us with an opportunity to teach him, with the use of biofeedback, to modify those illnesses which are termed "psychosomatic."

Armed with this information having to do with what has been observed in research, we decided to undertake the treatment of some "difficult psychosomatic problems" using biofeedback training and conjoint therapy. Consequently, we treated the patient as a team and approached the problem in a very direct fashion. We feel that biofeedback training, in conjunction with our team approach has been a significant factor in speeding symptom removal. We use conjoint therapy, primarily, in three ways: 1) the fact that there is a male and female therapist increases the possibility of the patient making a successful working relationship with one or both of us; 2) two heads are better than one; we can view the problems (usually complex) from two points of view; and 3) we are able to add considerable positive reinforcement by conversing with each other, in the patient's presence, on how he has improved his skill with the instrument. The fact that the patient (quickly) demonstrates to himself that he can modify an internal state seems to give many patients a sense of mastery, which spreads to everyday life. The fact that he can influence his own functioning seems to allow him to see his external world in a new way, no longer dictating how he must function (what he must do), but rather something over which he can influence some control.

It is useless to try to categorize the types of psychotherapy that can be used in conjunction with biofeedback. Each individual therapist must adapt his own style, using his own personality to achieve results. We are quite aware, in our situation, that we encourage our patients to identify with us, since we have worked with the instruments and we are capable of controlling the internal states that we monitor in others. This fact is conveyed to the patient.

The treatment atmosphere is relaxed and friendly, which nonverbally communicates a basic way of functioning that "feels good." The compulsive patient with intractable neck pain who has tried meditation, yoga, etc., who discusses her drive to get things done, is told that our compulsive needs have not disappeared, but we get things done in a much more relaxed way. It makes sense to go to the store early to avoid the crowd, but this can be done without the usual stress and push. Very soon, the patient is encouraged to carry the quiet state of mind, indicated by the production of high amplitude alpha waves in our treatment room, to the business of her everyday life.

Many instruments which convert autonomic nervous system and muscle activity into sounds and visual displays have been, and are being, developed. We chose three of those most commonly used: 1) A sensitive, large dial thermometer (temperature trainer) with a thermister which can be attached anywhere on the body, that we use for monitoring vasodilation and constriction; 2) an electromyograph, which picks up electrical activity at the myoneural junction and converts it to sound and visual display on a dial, to monitor muscle tension; 3) an electroencephalograph which displays brain wave frequency and amplitude, which we use to monitor mental tension (cerebral hyperactivity) and mental relaxation (a quiet mind). From the onset we were well aware that there was more to training than teaching the individual to use the instruments. We soon learned that regardless of the presenting symptoms, the patient does best, in learning to control his internal states, on the instrument that he likes best, whether or not it is directly related to the symptom. A patient with Raynaud's disease may control her symptoms best with EEG training rather than using, primarily, the temperature trainer.

Gardner Murphy, in his 1969 paper, suggests that psychiatric, psychological, and electrophysiological skills by the therapist will be required to most effectively enable the subject to become aware of and to modify his internal states. We conceptualize our work as biofeedback training with a kind of psychotherapy, that uses reinforcement and support during the training and therapeutic intervention when indicated. The patient is encouraged to practice at home, without the biofeedback equipment, since the use of the instrument, in the presence of the therapists, facilitates the personal interaction, which is crucial to the treatment process. During the interaction with the therapists, usually after the instrument training sessions, the patient tends to talk about problems that he has in his day-to-day living. It is at this time that psychotherapeutic intervention is possible. The instrument gives tangible evidence of progress and the patient has been rewarded by the praise (encouragement) of the therapists so that there is a positive atmosphere in which the psychotherapy is conducted. Thus, we do instrument training and psychotherapy in the office and let the patient carry over the experience himself into his everyday external environment.

The patients who were referred to us had been studied by several physicians, and had had various diagnostic procedures. The primary physician who undertakes the diagnosis and treatment of a psychosomatic problem, of necessity faces the fact that he must have thorough examinations, consultations, laboratory tests, etc., which in a nonverbal fashion convey to the patient that the doctor does not know what's wrong, must learn the nature of the difficulty, and even then cannot be positive about helping him. At the onset there is available to us an extensive history of the illness, so that we are able to deal directly with the patient without the need of taking a history or performing any tests. Thus, we discourage rumination about complaints, causes of problems, and negative statements. We instruct the patient that he is here to learn control of his internal states, and we discourage elaboration of his complaints. Drs. Norman Shealy and Thomas Beckner, of the Pain Rehabilitation Center in LaCrosse, Wisconsin, introduced us to the idea of discouraging patients in the recitation of their symptoms. We prefer to focus the patient's attention on ways that he can use the skills learned from biofeedback training to get well.

In the first session we insure that the patient experiences at least some success with one of the instruments, so that we can praise him. In every contact thereafter, we provide him with a positive experience. If the skin temperature decreases instead of increases, for instance, we emphasize the demonstration of autonomic control. We keep our explanations of the instruments and of control of internal states to a minimum, in keeping with the extent of the patient's curiosity. Further questions usually arise in subsequent sessions, at which time more detailed explanations can be made.

The use of biofeedback facilitates a change in the usual doctor/patient relationship that appears to us to be quite unique, since the patient becomes his own therapist; the paradigm of the doctor/patient, parent/child relationship is pushed aside, and the doctor becomes more of a colleague. Various forms of psychotherapy have been designed to play down or nullify the active doctor treating the passive patient. Biofeedback appears to be one of the most effective forms of treatment in producing this change in the doctor/patient relationship. The patient produces obvious change in the functioning of his own autonomic nervous system and becomes aware, therefore, that malfunctioning is produced by himself. The concept that symptoms just happen, that the doctor will take care of them, is no longer feasible. Instead, he is responsible to himself for results. He is able to take the initiative in diminishing or eradicating symptoms. One patient with chronic migraine finally stated: "It is very difficult for some people to admit that they are causing their own illness. Other people do the same work as I and don't have headaches." Prior to this time the patient blamed her symptom on the pressure of her job and the nagging of her alcoholic ex-husband. Once the individual has identified the cause and effect relationship to his symptom (his particular way of dealing with stress) whether verbally expressed, or not, he begins to assume responsibility for controlling the symptom with what he has learned in his biofeedback sessions. This experience is expanded to other areas of his lifestyle, and the particular symptom is left by the wayside, forgotten, often never again mentioned unless on questioning by the therapist. Those patients who have terminated with good control and symptom removal have been encouraged to "keep in touch" and to call on us when they feel the need for reinforcing their early learning experiences.

We do not function out of character, but we do keep in mind that we serve as an example in the way we relate to the patient and to each other. The entire atmosphere of the treatment situation is obviously relaxed and without pressure. We go so far with certain tense, compulsive patients as to chide them for being so early in arriving for their appointment. One such patient who was beginning to lose her symptoms came in ten minutes late, apologizing for any inconvenience this might have caused us, saying that she felt it would be best for her if she stopped first for coffee before her appointment. Obviously, the combination of biofeedback training and psychotherapy had radically changed her view of herself in relation to other people. When it became clear that one female patient had a stereotyped view of men, in general, and doctors, in particular, we made it a point to function in such a way as to illustrate that this view is not always correct. In this case, Dr. Gladman made the coffee and served it to the patient and to Mrs. Estrada.

In our brief experience with the clinical application of biofeedback, we have treated chronic headache (migraine and tension, usually mixed), chronic pain, Raynaud's disease, vascular hypertension, depression accompanied by various somatic complaints (weakness, palpitations, fatigue, etc.) and anxiety states. Symptom removal has occurred rapidly, but more significant to us is the overall change that appears in the patient when the instruments are mastered and the internal state is generally more calm and less vulnerable to stress. Paskewitz and Orne (1973) speculate that alpha feedback training develops the subject's "skill to disregard stimuli in the external and perhaps internal environment, that would ordinarily inhibit alpha activity" (i.e., inhibit the ability to quiet the internal state). One patient with Raynaud's disease reported that her constipation of longstanding had disappeared. In the process of overcoming frequent attacks of incapacitating headaches, using EEG training, a patient reported enjoying social functions which she had always experienced as unbearable. This substantiates Green, Green, and Walters' "psychophysiological principle." Our patients report functioning more to their satisfaction in relation to themselves and the people around them.

In our efforts to kindle interest in this mode of treatment there follow some brief case histories which we hope will illustrate the direct clinical application of some significant research findings. We have combined the art of medicine[2] with the research techniques. The personality of the therapist becomes an essential ingredient in the therapeutic process and a contributing factor to the ultimate outcome of treatment (Certcev & Calvo, 1973). In presenting examples of the types of problems we treat, it must be noted that no person in our series could be called typical. Even though presenting symptoms may be similar, each person with the symptoms is his own individual self and will solve his problem in his own way.

Case No. 1—The patient was female, aged thirty-eight, married, with four children. Diagnosis: Migraine headaches, at least two times a week for fifteen years (probably longer). The patient had been in psychotherapy before coming to us and continued in group therapy during our treatment. We saw her once a week for approximately three months, with sessions usually lasting thirty minutes. When she failed to move the temperature trainer in the first five minutes, we monitored the frontalis muscle with the EMG and praised her as she achieved a degree of relaxation. On the next visit we used the EEG and gave her feedback of white noise when she approached the alpha brain wave state. On subsequent visits she trained on the EEG, achieving a quiet state of mind as evidenced by a high percentage of alpha wave production. Her migraine disappeared in the fourth week, but she preferred to continue to come to make sure that symptoms would not return. She has been free of headaches for four months.

Case No. 2—The patient was female, aged forty-seven, married, without children. This patient had been severely phobic for approximately twenty-five years. Psychotherapy began in 1949, at which time she could not let her husband out of sight without developing severe anxiety. She had multiple

---

[2]Practice of the art of medicine allows the physician to use all his senses, thus combining intuition with science while at the same time forming a relationship with his patient which is based on trust, mutual respect, and direct communication.

somatic complaints which changed on every visit. She was very anxious in an automobile and could not be more than a few miles from home. Her symptoms gradually diminished in severity but did not disappear. Her basic complaint of anxiety remained, and there were recurring and changing somatic complaints. She continued sporadic office visits with Dr. Gladman, who rather facetiously suggested EEG training. She overcame her fear of the instruments after her husband tried it first. After four visits at weekly intervals she could produce 80–100% alpha with eyes open. "I never felt that I could control anything, while at the same time I have always needed to—now I know I don't have to be nervous." She reported enjoying a vacation trip in the mountains while free of symptoms. After another week or two she lost her ability to reach the "alpha state" and reported return of some symptoms. Further alpha training and support led to a stabilized, almost symptom-free state.

Case No. 3—Patient was female, aged eighty-three, with grown children. This patient was referred by her son (a psychologist) because of tension headaches of two years' duration following bilateral cataract removal. This case illustrates an intense personal interaction between therapists and patient, in which the therapists assume a parental role.

In the first visit she achieved some relaxation by the use of the EMG, and we gave her direct, explicit directions about changing her way of working around the house and caring for her husband. Both therapists gave her full, undivided attention. On the second visit she was able to generate a high percentage of alpha on the EEG, for which she was praised. Again, we gave direct suggestions while the patient was sitting quietly and comfortably in the treatment room. The headaches disappeared in the third and fourth week, while she gradually changed her way of functioning at home. On the fifth visit she reported finding an agency that would provide a person to come in daily to take care of her husband and housework. She also reported that her husband had remarked on seeing her smile for the first time in one and a half years. (This person listened to everything that was said, and made remarkable changes in her everyday approach to living). Completely free of headaches by the fifth visit, treatment was terminated on mutual agreement.

Case No. 4—This vignette illustrates the role of biofeedback in engaging a person who needed psychotherapy, but who had a number of years in one-to-one psychotherapy with limited success.

A forty-nine-year-old male, father of four children, obtaining a divorce, sought help on the premise that biofeedback was a new and different form of treatment. (The presence of the equipment introduces a new parameter, so that the therapists could relate in a relaxed and friendly way). We created a relaxed and friendly atmosphere without formality. This patient required a detailed introduction to the equipment with lengthy descriptions of the function of each (this to us is quite unusual). Because of his skepticism and curiosity, we introduced him to the literature on biofeedback. We cut short his complaints about previous treatment and involved him in controlling his own internal states. There followed a period of six weeks while the patient obtained mastery of his brain waves and skin temperature and formed a warm relationship with the therapists. He was helped to identify his view of himself as a helpless victim of external forces while at the same time he came to realize that he could control his internal and (later) external states. With mastery of his internal states, as evidenced by control of EEG, he discovered his ability to master his environment. "I don't have to put up with my relatives' attitude that I'm the village moron."

Case No. 5—This patient illustrates the psychophysiological principle and the value of psychotherapy done by an independent psychiatrist, in conjunction with biofeedback.

The patient, a forty-eight-year-old, married female with three sons, had suffered from Raynaud's disease for at least twenty years. She once made a suicide attempt approximately twelve years ago. Her therapist referred her for biofeedback because of severe vasospasm of the hands and feet (a sympathectomy had been recommended because of beginning necrosis of the toes). She was introduced to the temperature trainer and EEG at the same time. She soon learned to raise her skin temperature in her hands (later feet) while learning to produce alpha EEG in a quiet, eyes-open state. During the learning period, we noted changes in her attitude toward the youngest son, who was still at home, and toward her husband. She developed a sense of mastery— "I'm doing this myself—I can warm my hands." Concomitant, was the attitude—"I can buy what I need, I don't have to ask permission." Soon after learning to "quiet her mind" as evidenced by high alpha production, the patient stated that she had been constipated for years to the extent of using enemas, and now (in the fourth week of training) was having normal bowel movements.

Case No. 6—A fifty-five-year-old divorced female complained of "migraine" headaches of six years' duration, occurring every 24 to 36 hours and somewhat relieved by injection of ergot compound. She injected the medication herself when she felt a headache approaching. The obvious muscle spasm around her eyes led us to feel we were actually treating tension headaches. The patient was anxious about her job, her financial security, and one daughter. During the first four visits (weekly), she was only able to produce sporadic alpha waves and slight lowering of EMG readings displaying considerable physical tension and hyperactivity. She became increasingly aware of her tension and was told that she must find ways of being less tense on her job. She later devised ways of detecting and diminishing physical tension. After three months of weekly training she had quieted her cerebral activity as evidenced by high percentage of alpha production and had slowed the pace of her life. Her headaches have lessened in frequency and severity, and she expressed optimism that she could master them. The turning point seemed to occur when she stated during the ninth visit, "It is very hard for some people to admit that they are causing their own symptoms."

Our experience with the clinical application of biofeedback underlines the fact that it is indeed a holistic approach to the treatment of psychosomatic problems and is not simply symptom removal. In closing, we quote our colleague, Dr. Tod Mikuriya, "The realization of personal willful control over internal states is a powerful existential change in premises. Before the discovery, the individual sees himself as a particle in Brownian movement without any possibility of being released from the chronic compulsion of reacting to the environment. After the discovery of voluntary internal state control, the person now has vastly expanded his repertoire of options for dealing with his circumstances in an active, rather than passive way. This discovery of the power of voluntary internal state control also implies the assumption of responsibility for the cure of the stress-produced symptoms."

References

Certcev, D., & Calvo, J. The problems of psychotherapy in psychosomatic medicine. *Psychosomatics,* 1973, **14** (3), 142–146.

Green, E., & Green, A. Personal communication, August, 1973.

———. The ins and outs of mind-body energy. *Science Year, 1974.* Chicago: Field Enterprises Educational Corporation, 1973.

———. & Walters, E. Voluntary control of internal states: psychological and physiological. *Journal of Transpersonal Psychology,* **2** (1), p. 3.

Murphy, G. Experiments of self-deception. Paper presented at the First Annual Meeting of the Bio-Feedback Research Society, Santa Monica, California, October 20–23, 1969.

———. *Biofeedback and self-control.* Chicago: Aldine-Atherton, 1970.

Paskewitz, D., & Orne, M. Visual effects on alpha feedback training. *Science,* 1973, **181**, 360–363.

Pelletier, K. Neurological and clinical differentiation of the alpha and theta altered states of consciousness, a dissertation proposal. Research conducted in the laboratory of Joe Kamiya, Langley Porter Neuropsychiatric Institute, U.C. Medical Center, San Francisco, California, August, 1973.

Section III

He cures most in whom most have faith
—Claudius Galenus (Galen), circa 200 A.D.

TRANSCULTURAL PSYCHIATRY, more than any other branch of medicine, has brought to physicians an awareness of the extent to which prescientific healing is practiced throughout the world. We shall call the healers "shamans" for the sake of uniformity. Although some shamans utilize a primitive type of *materia medica* and surgery, most reenact the ancient ritual of casting out evil. Thus, it is no exaggeration to say that the practice of exorcism in one form or another is more prevalent the world over than is the practice of medicine.

There is no doubt that people have always believed in the power of faith, prayer, and suggestion to cure disease. More than 2000 years ago, the Greek physician, Hippocrates, known as the father of medicine, wrote, "Some patients, though conscious that their condition is perilous, recover their health simply through their contentment with the goodness of the physician."

Physicians have always been aware of occasional spontaneous remissions in serious disease, but until recently, they were ascribed to physical causes. Now, however, reputable doctors are taking a closer look at the possibility of spiritual factors and, perhaps, a transfer of mysterious forms of energy (Kirlian emanations?) from healer to patient. A year ago three medical doctors published a paper boldly entitled "Faith Healing" in a reputable medical journal—E. M. Pattison, N. A. Lapins, H. A. Dorr (*Journal of Nervous and Mental Disease,* 1973, 157:397–409)—in which they presented an impressive documentation of various types of pentecostal healing. (See also William A. Nolen, "In Search

235

of a Miracle," *McCall's,* 1974, **101,** 83, 101–107, taken from his book to be published by Random House, *Healing: A Doctor in Search of a Miracle.*)

In May 1974, the first world conference on spontaneous cancer cures was held at the Johns Hopkins medical center. Many known explanations were reviewed, such as immunological response, hormonal factors, effects of radiation, infection and fever, and of noncancer drugs. But in addition, three specialists, Mastrovito, Lewison, and Cole, discussed cures that were apparently brought about by faith and prayer (*Medical World News,* June 7, 1974, pp. 13–15). More recently, in a prestigious publication of the American Medical Association, there were articles by two physicians advising that doctors should take a spiritual history on their patients because healing miracles do occur (W. H. Hobbins, *American Medical News,* June 10, 1974, p. 14; J. E. Holoubek, same issue, p. 15).

And even more recently, F. J. Evans of the Institute of Pennsylvania Hospital reported that placebos, commonly known as "sugar pills," allayed pain under appropriate circumstances of rapport between patient and physician. Emphasizing the special "magic" of the doctor-patient interaction, Dr. Evans said, "The very fact that both patient and doctor believe that a powerful treatment is being administered is sufficient to produce a broad range of therapeutic responses in a large percentage of patients."[1]

The big three of psychic research looming on the medical horizon are biofeedback, Kirlian electrophotography, and meditation—with chemical alteration of consciousness and psychic healing close seconds. However, although testimonials abound in the hands of commercial exploiters, replicable research and detailed records are relatively sparse, though impressive enough to warrant accelerated effort.

Until a great deal more evidence is accumulated, we must proceed with patience and equanimity. Unfortunately, promoters of all kinds have joined the potential gold rush, so that legal and professional regulations and restraints have become matters of necessity and of grave concern. At the very least, nonmedical practitioners should be licensed, preferably to work under medical supervision as respected adjutants of the medical team, as is the case with acupuncturists in some states now.

Above all, physicians should study the new techniques themselves. The Bible contains more than forty references to spiritual healing, and the scientist

---

[1] Interview conducted with Dr. Evans in Roche, *Frontiers of Psychiatry,* 1974, 4:1–2, 11, "The Placebo: New Look at an Old 'Nuisance Variable.'"

embraces that faith in his religion. Perhaps the day is approaching when he will with equal devotion examine it in his laboratory.

Physicians may discover that psychic phenomena have a *purpose* in nature's scheme of things. That purpose may well prove to be a vigilance mechanism which, like the "fight or flight" mechanism, has a vital survival function necessary for the preservation of life. Thus, precognition and other forms of ESP may be a sort of "psychic radar," which, like our military distant early warning system (DEW), can prepare us to avoid or to counter impending disaster. Psychic healing (which predated "scientific" medicine) may have a similar life-preserving function.

And the same may be true of higher states of consciousness. We know that the ultraconscious state (also known as transcendence, peak consciousness, etc.) promotes mental and physical well-being, and induces an extraordinary degree of brotherly love and compassion—qualities that may ultimately prove to be as essential as technology in saving our planet from ecological and military ruin.

Seen in that light, psychic faculties may have been an early rather than a late development of nature—a conclusion that may explain their presence in primitive people, in certain animals, and in the preverbal stage of the parent-infant relationship.

E. Fuller Torrey

Psychic Healing and Psychotherapy

WITHIN THE PAST few years there has been a renewal of interest in psychic healing—that is, in the healing of physical and mental diseases using powers of the mind and body previously thought to lie beyond those powers. Within the past year there have been two symposia in New York City ("Psychic Healing: Myth into Science" and "The New Dimensions in Healing"), and psychiatrists participated in both. It is the purpose of this chapter to briefly review the claims made for psychic healing and to look at them in the light of known research on psychotherapy.

The claims made for psychic healing to date include a rather broad array. It has been said that injured mice can be healed faster by a psychic healer compared with control mice, that rats can be brought out of anesthesia faster than their controls, and that the enzyme levels and hemoglobin of humans can be affected (Chance, 1973). There have also been, of course, many individuals who claim to have extraordinary healing powers. The suggested mechanisms whereby these things occur, center around the transfer of a certain kind of energy from the healer to the patient. This energy is thought by some to be visible on photographic plates in Kirlian photography, a high voltage, high-frequency photographic technique adapted from Russian researchers and now in wide use in this country by researchers in metapsychiatry and psychic phenomena in general.

Some researchers using Kirlian photography have claimed that they were able to detect greater energy halos around the hands of psychic healers during healing sessions than at rest. This energy is said to be synonymous with the aura around the person's body. Along the same line, there is a report from two psychiatrists at Rockland State Hospital in New York that the energy given off from the fingertips of an acute untreated schizophrenic patient was minimal, whereas after five days on phenothiazine drugs, the amount of energy had markedly increased as the patient improved (*Medical World News,* 1973). This is consistent with other reports that individuals lose their auras when they become physically ill. Perhaps all the research in this field can best be summed up by a single observation by Stanley Krippner (Chance, 1973), head of the Dream Laboratory at Maimonides Medical Center in New York, who said: "We can't continue to hold on to our simplistic cause-and-effect notions of behavior" (p. 110).

Unfortunately, some of us are wedded rather happily to our cause-and-effect notions and I, for one, am not about to give them up on the basis of the research done in this field to date. I am willing, and think other psychiatrists should also be willing, to look at the research coming out of metapsychiatry with an open mind. We really cannot afford to do otherwise, since we have so little research data available on what constitutes the effectiveness of psychotherapy, the healing process which we claim to be using in our daily practices. Except for the rare individual psychiatrist like Jerome Frank (1963), there has been practically no attempt within psychiatry to identify and examine the components of the healing process of psychotherapy. Most of the work has been done by psychologists like Carl Rogers (1958), William Schofield (1964), A. E. Bergin (1963), C. B. Truax (1967), and R. R. Carkhuff (1965). Since our profession is so little prepared to counter the claims of psychic healing with hard data, we must remain open to these claims.

In looking at the results being claimed for psychic healing it is important to keep three questions in mind:
1. Is healing taking place?
2. Can it be explained using the natural laws of physics, chemistry, and biology along with proven psychological principles, or does it require the postulation of new laws and principles?
3. If new laws and principles are required, are they really significant or just incidental?

Keeping these questions in mind, a brief review follows on what has been learned about psychotherapy as a healing process.

Personality Characteristics

Perhaps the most striking thing that has emerged from resent research on psychotherapy is the importance of the therapist's personality in the healing process.

The research (Carkhuff & Truax, 1965) shows that certain personal qualities of the therapist—accurate empathy, nonpossessive warmth, and genuineness —are of crucial importance in producing effective psychotherapy. These three qualities of the therapist have been shown to relate significantly to a variety of positive patient personality and behavioral change indexes. Therapists who possess these qualities consistently and convincingly get better therapeutic results than those who do not possess them.

Four types of supporting research data have been brought forth (Truax & Carkhuff, 1967). The first is concerned with patient outcome in cases receiving high levels of the three personal ingredients of the therapist as contrasted with cases receiving low levels. The studies included individual therapy on fourteen schizophrenic inpatients, forty psychoneurotic outpatients, and eighty institutionalized male juvenile delinquents.

The findings on the forty psychoneurotic outpatients, for instance, showed a 90% improvement rate when the therapist provided high levels of the three therapeutic qualities, and only a 50% improvement rate when he or she provided low levels. Most of the research was done by trained raters who coded samples of tape-recorded psychotherapy using research scales designed to measure the three therapeutic qualities.

The second type of supporting research data focused on the three qualities themselves, contrasting patient change with control groups receiving no psychotherapy. The studies included 14 schizophrenic inpatients, 40 institutionalized female juvenile delinquents, and 24 college underachievers. The results with the college students, for instance, showed that 19 of the 24 had a higher grade point average in the semester after the counseling, compared with 11 of the 24 control students.

Truax and his co-workers also used these data to explain why past studies of psychotherapeutic outcomes have often failed. They maintain that such studies included all kinds of therapists, and did not differentiate between those with genuineness, empathy, and warmth, and those who lacked these qualities. Thus some therapists were helping their patients to get well whereas others were doing nothing or even making them sicker. The net result was zero.

The third type of supporting research data in the Truax study examined the respective roles of the therapist and patient in determining how high a level of these qualities was offered. One study used eight therapists and eight inpatients in a block design. This study and others showed that the levels of therapeutic conditions offered throughout counseling are due to the counselor rather than the client. In other words, it is the therapist who determines whether the genuineness, empathy, and warmth will be present or not. These qualities are either there or they are not, independent of the personality or type of problem of the patient.

Finally, converging evidence from research on learning and on parental influence was offered. It was shown, for instance, in a study of 120 third-graders and eight teachers that children learn to read faster under the teachers who offer high levels of the three qualities cited earlier.

None of this is to say that genuineness, empathy, and warmth are the only important personality characteristics of the therapist. Further research may identify others. The research does clearly point, however, toward certain human attributes as being relatively important in the therapist-patient relationship.

What this means for psychic healing is that the personality characteristics of the healer must be assessed as a variable. If a group of healers is identified who appear to get particularly good results, then their personality characteristics could be compared with those of a control group. It would then be possible to determine whether their healing power was related to personality or to possession of a special energy.

Patients' Expectations

Another important finding that has emerged from psychotherapeutic research in recent years is the importance of the expectations of the patients. Some of the strongest evidence (Egbert et al., 1964) comes from studies of patients facing surgery. In one such study, a group of surgical patients was warned before the operation about postoperative pain and was given breathing exercises for the pain. Another group was given neither warning nor exercises. The group that had been told to expect pain requested only one-half as much pain medication and left the hospital earlier than the control group by an average of almost three days. Clearly, patient expectations are a powerful therapeutic tool.

Turning to psychotherapy, one researcher (Friedman, 1963) studied 43 patients who were applying for psychotherapy. He found that a patient's expectations of help when he applied for treatment were significantly related to the degree of symptom relief he was able to obtain in the initial interview. The more the patient expected to be helped, the more he was helped. A similar study (Uhlenhuth & Duncan, 1968) using medical students as psychotherapists showed that a patient's optimism at the onset of treatment was directly related to the symptomatic relief achieved during the course of therapy.

In psychiatry, the effects of placebos have been compared with the effects of short-term psychotherapy (Gliedman, Nash et al., 1968). Fifty-six psychiatric outpatients, all diagnosed as neurotic, were given placebos as the only form of therapy. The outcome results compared favorably with the results obtained by short-term psychotherapy in a similar group. In another study (Frank, Nash et al., 1963), 109 psychiatric outpatients were given placebos (presented to them as "a new pill") and then followed for three years to see what the effect was. After one week on the pill, 80% of the patients reported improvement in their symptoms. And of those still taking it three years later, 66% reported continued improvement. Jerome Frank (1961) cites such experiments as confirming the hypothesis that part of the healing power of all forms of psychotherapy lies in their ability to mobilize the patient's hope of relief.

Probably the most impressive demonstration of the efficacy of patient expectation is voodoo death. This dramatic demise occurs when a person is hexed by another who is believed to be powerful enough to kill him (Cannon, 1942). The hexed person becomes sick and dies within a few weeks. He expects to die so he does die. The actual mechanism of death has been debated, but probably involves activation of the nerve to the heart, causing the heart to stop gradually. Deaths due to this kind of patient expectation have been reported by observers from South America, Africa, Australia, and the Caribbean. Voodoo deaths then, along with the other sources of evidence cited above, point to the great importance of patient expectations in determining a person's health status.

It has been demonstrated that a psychotherapist does a variety of things to raise the expectations of his patients. The impressive building and office which is utilized (the "edifice complex"), his ability to name what is wrong with the patient, his belief in himself, the impressive degrees on his wall, his reputation in the community, his distinctive dress, his use of mechanical, complex-looking gadgets, and other paraphernalia which identify him as a healer—all of these and more raise the expectations of the patient (Torrey, 1972). The important point here is that these may be utilized just as effectively by a psychic healer. We need to control for these variables when trying to assess the source of effectiveness of such healers.

Discussion

It can be seen from the above that, even within our rudimentary framework of research on psychotherapy, there is room to explain at least some of the claims now being made for psychic healing. The problem is that we have viewed our task too narrowly as psychotherapists, paying attention almost exclusively to the techniques of therapy and disregarding the other components of the healing process. We have spent our time arguing about whether it is better to have the patient lie down or sit up to free associate, or whether behavior therapy is useful for certain kinds of neurotics, or which psychotropic medication is best for anxiety. We have spent far too little time looking at the personality characteristics of the therapist and assessing the effect of increasing the patients' expectations.

And one reason why psychotherapists have not done these things is that they are threatening. We would like to think of ourselves as highly trained medical technicians, wisely selecting the best therapy for each illness in the classical medical tradition. After all, isn't that why we went to school for so many years? And isn't that what we paid all that money to learn? Now to turn around and say that most of that learning was irrelevant to the psychotherapeutic healing process, that untrained therapists with the proper personality characteristics or those who can raise the patients' expectations high enough can be *better* healers than we are, is too much to admit. However, until we start learning to do so, we will have no rational grounds for ignoring the claims of psychic healing.

In the light of what we now know, are there indeed parts of the healing process which cannot be explained using the natural laws of physics, chemistry, and biology along with the principles of psychology? It is too early to say. Researchers in the metapsychiatric field are themselves divided on the question. The Kirlian photographic phenomenon, for example, may ultimately be explained as a variant of static electricity on the body (as when you shuffle along a rug and touch somebody) or as electrons emanating from skin surface body chemicals which are slightly altered in disease states of the body. And even if it is ultimately shown that new laws and principles need to be invoked (and we are a long way from that conclusion yet), then there is still no assurance that the new phenomena would be of any real significance. In other words, even if it is ultimately shown that a previously unknown form of energy emanates from the fingers of effective healers, that would not necessarily make the energy important.

Finally, it is important to keep the current interest in psychic healing in the perspective of history and religion. Historically, this renaissance is occurring at a time of great antiscientific and antirational thinking among the younger generation. LSD, hashish, and parapsychology are all part of the same current ethos. That does not mean that the claims of psychic healing are not valid, but only that the claims may be more difficult to assess now than if they were being assessed at a different time in history. This can be seen in the reluctance among some with paranormal claims to submit their work to controlled scientific experiments. Too much of the work has been left at the anecdotal or impressionistic levels by people who should know better. The distrust of science and rational thinking may be warranted in their minds by recent past history, but their claims will never be taken seriously until they validate them empirically. Fortunately many of the better researchers in this field know this. The current ethos also means, of course, that questioning the claims of psychic healing, or any other aspect of metapsychiatry, leaves one open to the devastating epithet of being "an old rationalist."

It must be remembered that man has been searching for and creating gods, religions, and philosophies since time immemorial. As humans, we alone have the unique ability to be aware of and to contemplate ourselves simultaneously. Many animals think, but only man can think about his thinking, and furthermore talk about his thoughts. Our self-awareness, or consciousness of self, makes possible some of the grandest things of being human. It includes the ability to contemplate ourselves in relationship to the whole universe and to contemplate our own death. No other animal can do this. No other animal can ask: "What does it all mean?" "Why am I here?" "Why must I die?" "What will happen to me after death?" Because our brain has this peculiar ability, it also feels compelled to create answers to these questions that will satisfy us. Thus man has created gods to give him meaning, and life after death to quiet his fears. He has done this ever since he first emerged with his unique brain. Scientists have this need just as much as other people do, for scientists are human.

What this means is that we must be very careful that we don't fool ourselves. We must be prepared to ascertain the truth using all the empirical, rational means at our disposal. And we must be prepared to accept the answer either way. But we must be ever alert, for, as Albert Szent-Györgi once said: "The human brain is not only an organ of thinking but an organ of survival, like claw and fangs" (*Bulletin of Atomic Scientist* [May 1964], p. 2).

References

Bergin, A. E. "The Effects of Psychotherapy: Negative Results Revisited," *Journal of Counseling Psychology,* 10 (1963): 244–55.

Cannon, W. B. "Voodoo Death," *American Anthropologist,* 44 (1942): 169–81.

Carkhuff, R. R. and Truax, C. B. "Training in Counseling and Psychotherapy: An Evaluation of an Integrated Didactic and Experimental Approach," *Journal of Consulting and Clinical Psychology,* 29 (1965): 333–36.

Chance, P. "Parapsychology Is an Idea Whose Time Has Come," *Psychology Today,* 7 (Oct. 1973): 105–20.

Egbert, L. D.; Battit, G. E.; Welch, C. E.; Bartlett, M. K. "Reduction of Postoperative Pain by Encouragement and Instruction of Patients," *New England Journal of Medicine,* 270:16 (1964): 825–27.

"Finger-tip Halos of Kirlian Photography," *Medical World News* (Oct. 26, 1973), 43–48.

Frank, J. D. *Persuasion and Healing.* Baltimore: Johns Hopkins Press, 1961.

Frank, J. D.; Nash, E. H.; Stone, A. R.; Imber, S. D. "Immediate and long-term symptomatic course of psychiatric outpatients," *American Journal of Psychiatry,* 120 (1963): 429–39.

Friedman, H. J. "Patient-Expectancy and Symptom Reduction," *Archives of General Psychiatry,* 8 (1963): 61–67.

Gliedman, L. H.; Nash, E. H.; Imber, S. D.; Stone, A. R.; and Frank, J. D. "Reduction of Symptoms by Pharmacologically Inert Substances and by Short-term Psychotherapy," *AMA Archives of Neurology and Psychiatry,* 79 (1958): 345–51.

Rogers, C. R. "The Characteristics of a Helping Relationship," *Personnel and Guidance Journal,* 37 (1958): 6–16.

Schofield, W. *Psychotherapy: The Purchase of Friendship.* Englewood Cliffs, N.J.: Prentice-Hall, 1964.

Torrey, E. F. *The Mind Game: Witchdoctors and Psychiatrists.* New York: Emerson Hall, 1972.

Truax, C. B. and Carkhuff, R. R. *Toward Effective Counseling and Psychotherapy.* Chicago: Aldine, 1967.

Uhlenhuth, E. H. and Duncan, D. B. "Subjective Change with Medical Student Therapists: Course of Relief in Psychoneurotic Outpatients," *Archives of General Psychiatry,* 18 (1968): 428–38.

Lawrence L. LeShan

Toward a General Theory
of Psychic Healing

IN ATTEMPTING to understand the problems posed by the existence of the paranormal, we must probe into the nature of reality as we know it today. It is part of the faith of science that all phenomena that exist must exist under the category of natural law, and that none exist under the categories of magic or miracle. In following that faith and attempting to understand the paranormal in normal terms, it became necessary to change the question usually asked about this class of phenomena. Instead of asking "How do the 'sensitives' *do* it? How do they attain the paranormal information?"—questions that had not yielded results after long and careful work by serious men—I asked a new question: "What is going on between the sensitive and the rest of reality at the moment the paranormal event occurs?"

This question was put to some of the leading sensitives of our time in direct discussion and through a study of their written material. It became clear that at the moment they were acquiring the paranormal experience they viewed the cosmos as if it were constructed in a special way. I termed this way the "clairvoyant reality" and contrasted it with the way we view the nature of reality in our everyday commonsense life, which I termed the "sensory reality."

The clairvoyant reality is a coherent, organized picture of the way the world works. It is a complete metaphysical system. It implies that when one is using it, certain events (such as telepathy, clairvoyance, and precognition) are normal and explainable. Certain other events (such as being able to will or take action toward a goal) are paranormal in this system.

I then realized that two other groups of individuals had arrived at similar conclusions. The mystics and the Einsteinian physicists both agreed with the

247

clairvoyant that there are two valid ways of perceiving reality, and on what these two ways were. Except for tricks of language and a few comparatively minor disagreements, all were completely agreed on the nature and existence of the clairvoyant reality. It proved impossible to differentiate statements describing it that were written by mystics from those written by physicists.

In order to test this theory, I attempted to use it to learn how to accomplish one of the functions long described as paranormal, and to teach it to others. If the theory predicted that this paranormal function occurred in a certain psychological situation, and I organized that situation and found that the paranormal function occurred, then it would be a pretty good test of the theory. Psychic healing was chosen for this test, and by following the theory and its implications it became possible for me to learn to be a psychic healer and to teach it to others.

My first question was, Does the phenomenon of psychic healing really exist? With what we know today about hysterical symptoms and hysterical suppression of symptoms, do the phenomena described as "psychic healing" exist apart from these? Prior to my work in parapsychology, I had spent fifteen years working full time on a project in psychosomatic medicine, and so was aware at least of the scope of the problems involved.

A survey of the literature in this field made it plain that the phenomenon of psychic healing *did* exist. There was enough solid experimental work and enough careful evaluation of reported claims to make this clear. After I discarded the 95 percent of the claims that could have been due to hysterical change, suggestion, bad experimental design, poor memory, and plain chicanery, a solid residue remained. In these, the "healer" usually went through certain behaviors inside of his head, and the "healee" showed positive biological changes which were not to be expected at that time in terms of the usual course of his condition.

The "explanation," or theories of explanations, were another matter entirely. Generally speaking these seemed to be divided into three classes.

The largest group of healers described their work as "prayer" and believed that success was due to the intervention of God. A second group believed the healing was done by "spirits" after they had set up a special linkage between the spirits and the patient. The third group believed that they were transmitters or originators of some special form of "energy" that had healing effects.

With the group that involved God in the healing process I could find no quarrel. I could not, nor did I wish to, disagree with this explanation. Nevertheless, science must go further than this. We are concerned with the "how" of things: "How" does God work? The poet-philosopher Petrarch devised the rationale of science within a religious framework when he described the world as the "theater of God," the "Teatrum Dei," and said man could admire God by understanding His handiwork. Within this framework, I would work in harmony with those who used God as an explanatory force.

A serious difficulty with the use of the concept of God is that, with it, one can do little either to further one's understanding of a process or to increase his efficiency at it. To improve one's healing ability he can learn to pray better, but that is about all. For a scientific approach and a scientific society, more was needed.

The second group used "spirits" as an explanation. I have no particular opinion, one way or another, on the existence of discarnate entities who intervene in human affairs. Even after hundreds of hours spent conversing with mediums in trance during which the medium claimed to be someone who was dead, I still see no scientific way to determine if these spirits are (1) what they claim to be; (2) a multiple personality split-off; or (3) something else. At present we do not seem to have a way to test any of these hypotheses. . . .

In addition, "spirits" are notably difficult to work with scientifically. If you do not get results today, it is because the "spirits" were not in the mood! In any case, with the "spirit" explanation, I had to concentrate on "how" the spirits do it, how they can heal. I could not prove or disprove the spiritistic answer, but I could go on from there and study the "how" of the healing process, whether spirits existed or not.

The third group explained the healing on the basis of an "energy" which they either originated or transmitted. Certainly this sounded more promising scientifically than the other explanations. However, since no one has been able to define this energy further than by giving it a name presently acceptable to science, nor to find any of its characteristics, it did not seem very useful.

Furthermore, there is a very real problem about the use of a concept such as "energy" if it is accepted into one's thinking too early in the process of exploration. Such a concept has implications; it shapes our thinking in ways we are often unaware of. Energy does "work," for example. Is "work" done in the psychic healing process? Tempting as it is to answer "yes," one had better be careful about it. The Christian Science healers (and they often accomplish very serious results) would certainly not agree with this. In addition, energy "flows" or "travels" between "two things." Are there "two things" in the psychic healing process? If so, it would mean that we find our explanatory system in the sensory reality and not in the clairvoyant reality.

I could point out other implications of the use of a concept like "energy" that worried me, but these should do to show why I was so cautious about accepting it as an explanatory system early in the game. Rather than seeking the understanding of healing in the explanations of the healers, it seemed plain that another approach was needed.

I assembled a list of individuals who could be described as "serious psychic healers." These included all the individuals who I felt reasonably certain *did* accomplish results in this area, who worked consistently in it, and about whom there was either autobiographical or good biographical material. It consisted primarily of Olga and Ambrose Worrall, Harry Edwards, Rebecca Beard, Agnes Sanford, Edgar Jackson, the Christian Science group, Parahamsa Yogananda, Stewart Grayson, and Katherine Kuhlmann. A variety of other healers, ranging from Padre Pio to Mrs. Salmon and Sai Baba, were also studied in this way through the material which was available on them.

This group all described behaviors that they felt were related to the healing effect. When I listed these behaviors, I found that they fell into two classes. The first class were "idiosyncratic behaviors," that is, behaviors engaged in by one or a few of the healers. The second class consisted of "commonality behaviors," behaviors engaged in by all of the healers. The assumption was made that it was this second class of activities that was relevant to the healing effect.

At this point in time I had a set of behaviors, a series of activities, that all the serious healers engaged in when they were trying to heal someone. This series had been teased out of the larger mass of activities they described as related to the healing. I could reasonably assume that I had come as close as I could at the moment to the "pure method," to the activities really related to the healing process, and I could discard the other, idiosyncratic behaviors as culturally or personally conditioned and nonessential. Exactly what were these activities? How could I describe them?

I found that, from the viewpoint of the experience of the healer (what he believed and observed himself to be doing), they fell into two classes. From an experiential viewpoint, there seemed to be two separate types of healing here. In a brilliant flash of genius I named these "Type 1" and "Type 2"!

The healers themselves had not made this differentiation as far as I could tell. Some used both, slipping back and forth without apparently noticing that the two phenomena were qualitatively different. Some used only one of them. To my best knowledge, this was the first time they had been separately delineated in detail.

Type 1 seemed to me to be the most important type. Many healers, such as Edgar Jackson and the Christian Science group, used it exclusively.

In Type 1 healing, the healer goes into an altered state of consciousness in which he views himself and the healee as one entity. There is no attempt to "do anything" to the healee (in Harry Edwards's words, "All sense of 'performance' should be abandoned"), but simply to meet him, to be one with him, to unite with him. Ambrose Worrall put this simply and clearly: "I followed a technique I have of 'tuning in,' to become, in a metaphysical sense, one with the patient." Edgar Jackson defined intercessory prayers (prayers for a patient's recovery) as "a subject-object bridge." And Edwards wrote that in psychic healing the healer ". . . then draws 'close' to the patient, so that 'both' are 'one.' "

These are clear statements. Jackson put the entire matter in a larger frame of reference:

> Prayer as a specialized state of consciousness moves beyond the usual considerations of real or unreal, conscious or unconscious, organic or inorganic, subjective or objective to a place where he is dealing with the totality of being at one and the same time in a way that produces sensitivity to the whole.

What we have here began to become clear. The healer views the healee in the clairvoyant reality at a level close to that in which all is one. However, he is focused by love, by caring, by *caritas,* on the healee: this is an essential factor. In Agnes Sanford's words, "Only love can generate the healing fire." Ambrose and Olga Worrall have said, "We must care. We must care for others deeply and urgently, wholly and immediately; our minds, our spirits must reach out to them." Stewart Grayson, a serious healer from the First Church of Religious Science, said, "If this understanding is just mental it is empty and sterile" and "the feeling is the fuel behind the healing." Sanford wrote: "When we pray in accordance with the law of love, we pray in accordance with the will of God."

It is essential that there be a deeply intense caring and a viewing of the healee and oneself as one, as being united in a universe—the clairvoyant reality—in which this unity is possible. This seemed to be the heart of the Type 1 healing. It seemed only to take a moment, a moment of such intense knowledge of the clairvoyant reality structure of the cosmos that it filled consciousness entirely, so that there was—for that moment—nothing else in the field of knowing to prevent the healing results from occurring. "Become conscious for a single moment that Life and intelligence are . . . neither in nor of matter [and] the body will cease to utter its complaints." So wrote Mary Baker Eddy, and there seemed general agreement on the brief span of time of complete consciousness necessary for the biological effects to occur.

The healers used a wide variety of "techniques" to attain this altered state of consciousness. Some prayed, some attempted to look at the healee from God's viewpoint or to see him as he looked from the spirit world, and some were able to describe what they did without much of an explanatory system. All agreed, however, that there must be intense caring and a viewing of the healee within a framework in which healer and healee could become one entity in a larger context without either of the two losing their individuality. Indeed, both would have their uniqueness enhanced by becoming one, as do two people who fall in love.

Gradually a theory began to emerge. At one moment, the healer was operating in the metaphysical system of the clairvoyant reality to the degree that he "knew" it was true. This was a moment of such complete knowing that nothing else existed in consciousness. In some way this was transmitted to the patient. I could use the word "telepathy" or else could point out that—for a moment—the healer's assumptions about how-the-world-works were true and valid. As has been proved over and over again by mediums, mystics, and physicists using the clairvoyant reality to accomplish their own ends, this is a perfectly valid set of beliefs about reality. Since at this moment of intense knowing on the part of the healer it was valid and the healee was an integral and central part of the system, the healee knew it, too.

Knowing this at some deep level of personality, the healee was then in a different existential position. He was back at home in the universe; he was no longer "cut off"; he was now living the full life of the "amphibian" in both land and water. In a way, he was for a moment in what I might call "an ideal organismic position." He was completely enfolded and included in the cosmos with his "being," his "uniqueness," his "individuality" enhanced. Under these conditions there were sometimes positive biological changes.

There is a beautiful Haiku that Nikos Kazantzakis puts into the mouth of St. Francis that seems relevant here:

> I said to the Almond tree
> "Sister, speak to me of God"
> and the Almond tree blossomed.

The healers—and this is particularly true of those with a Christian approach —make this statement quite clearly. They view "wholeness" and "holiness" as having the same meaning, as they did in the original meaning of the words. In describing their healing technique, Ambrose and Olga Worrall wrote: "In true prayer our thinking is an awareness that we are part of the Divine Universe."

I felt that I understood what these healers were saying about their work. But why did it often produce results? How could positive biological changes occur under these conditions? I asked myself this question, and in answering it I looked first at the limitations of psychic healing.

George Bernard Shaw once said that the Shrine at Lourdes was the most blasphemous place on the face of the earth. He explained that while it contained evidence of cures in the form of mountains of crutches, wheelchairs, and braces, it did not have as evidence a single glass eye, wooden leg, or toupee. This implied a limitation of the power of God and *this* was the blasphemy.

Like most Shavian wit, there is a grain of biting truth here. Furthermore, in all the serious cases of psychic healing I was able to uncover, there was not a single case of the regrowth of an amputated limb or the resuturing of a severed optic nerve.

In addition, there is a very serious report by Alexis Carrel, who observed under a lens what happened to an open, visible cancer during a "miraculous healing" in the course of which it regressed and cleared up. Carrel (a very highly trained and reliable observer) reported that the cancer followed the usual, well-known course a cancer follows when it regresses. These include specific courses of development in the formation of scar tissue fibers, changes in blood distribution, etc. This cancer, said Carrel, followed this progression, but many many times faster than he had ever seen or heard of it happening before.

I began to see the light on a possible way of explaining the biological changes. None of us do anything as well as we potentially can. We can all learn to read faster, jump higher, discriminate colors more precisely, reason more accurately, and so on through practically any abilities you can name. One of these abilities is the ability to heal ourselves, our ability at self-repair and self-recuperation. This too usually operates far below potential.

What appeared to happen in Type 1 healing was that because he was momentarily in an "ideal organismic situation," the healee's self-repair and self-recuperative systems began to operate at a level closer than usual to their potential. Type 1 psychic healing was not a "doing something" to the healee, but a meeting and uniting with him on a profound level, a uniting that permitted something new to happen. The reason, then, behind Shaw's comment on the lack of wooden legs at Lourdes is that the regrowth of a severed limb is beyond the ability of the body's self-repair systems. The rapid remission of a cancer is not.

Henry Miller had once written something that was in a curious way very similar to the way I had begun to see this:

> The great physicians have always spoken of Nature as being the great Healer. This is only partially true. Nature alone can do nothing. Nature can cure only when man recognizes his place in the world, which is not in Nature, as with the animal, but in the human kingdom, the link between the natural and divine.

When man is "at home" in both realities, when he is fulfilling himself as an "amphibian," living in both—in Miller's terms of the "natural and the divine"—the healing of many wounds can occur. The healer does not "do" or "give" something to the healee; instead he helps him come home to the All, to the One, to the way of "unity" with the universe, and in this "meeting" the healee becomes more complete and this in itself is healing. I was reminded here of Arthur Koestler's words: "There is no sharp dividing line between self-repair and self-realization."

This fit very well with one of the analogies used in Christian Science to "explain" this type of healing. Christian Scientists point out that a rubber ball retains its usual shape of roundness (here the analogy for "health") so long as there is no pressure to deform it (here the analogy for "illness"). As soon as the pressure is released, it springs back to roundness. The pressure, they say, is being cut off from God, is the lack of the knowledge that one is a part of God, or, in our terms, the All. When this "pressure" is "released" through the healer setting up a metaphysical system where the healee is included in the All, brought "home" to it, the healee's body responds by a tendency to repair itself and work toward health.

A basic theory had emerged for Type 1 healing. Now would come the crucial test of the theory: a test that involved learning to meet and unite with another person (and training others to do this) according to the theory, and see if it provided positive physical changes. But I have gotten ahead of myself. Type 2 healing remains to be described, since the analysis of both methods was done at the same time.

Experientially, Type 2 is quite different from Type 1. The healer perceives a pattern of activity between his palms when his hands are "turned on" and facing each other. Some healers perceive this as a "flow of energy," some as a sphere of activity. The hands are so placed—one on each side of the healee's pathological area—so that this "flow of energy" is perceived to "pass through" the troubled area. This is usually conceived of by the healer as "healing energy" which "cures" or "treats" the sick area. In a large percentage of cases (I would estimate about 50 percent in my own experience) healees who do not know the literature and do not know the expected response perceive a good deal of "heat" in the area. Frequently there are surprised comments like "It feels like diathermy!" "It's like an electric blanket!" "Where is all that heat coming from?" A smaller percentage of naïve subjects (about 10 percent in my experience) report a sensation of a great deal of "activity" in the area. A very few report a sensation of "cold." These sensations are almost invariably felt only in an area in which there is a real physical problem. One can "turn on" one's hands to any degree and it is still almost unheard of to get a perceptual response from the healee when the hands are held on each side of a healthy area.

In Type 2 the healer *tries* to heal; he wants to and attempts to do so through the "healing flow." In both Type 1 and Type 2 he must (at least at the moment) care completely, but a fundamental difference is that in Type 1 he *unites* with the healee; in Type 2 he tries to cure him. Harry Edwards, writing of Type 2, explained his attitude:

> When the author is engaged in this work, only one thing exists and that is his hands through which the healing power flows. The healer's whole being is concentrated on his fingers—nothing else seems to exist. The desired result is the only thing that is his concern.

Some healers see themselves as the *originators* of this healing power; others see themselves as the *transmitters* of it. Frank Loehr has called them the "God Withiners" and the "God Beyonders," respectively. In either case, the procedure and the experience are essentially the same.

This much I learned from reading the works of the serious healers, but I could not understand what was going on. Even now I do not have the faintest idea what Type 2 is all about or how it "works." And it frequently does "work," that is, produces positive biological changes in the healee. I know how to "do it," to "turn on" my hands and teach others how to "turn on" theirs. It seems perfectly reasonable to me that we may be dealing with some kind of "energy." It also seems reasonable to me that Type 2 may be a sort of "cop out" on Type 1 in which healer and healee say, in effect: "We are both too frightened of all this closeness and uniting that is a part of psychic healing. Let's pretend with each other that all that is happening is a flow of energy is coming out of the hands and treating the problem. That way we will both be more comfortable." It also seems reasonable to me that the most fruitful explanation of Type 2 healing may be quite different from either of the above two hypotheses.

At a complete loss for a theory about Type 2, the time had come to test the theory of Type 1. Following the theory, the test I set up was to train myself to go into the state of consciousness indicated and see if—as the theory predicted—positive biological changes would occur in the healee's body. If this worked, the next step would be to try to train others to do this. The others would be individuals like myself who had never done this type of healing before, and who were not accustomed to having paranormal experiences of any sort. If the theory pointed out that certain activities had certain results and that when these activities were carried out the results occurred, it would at least prove the theory to be a fruitful one.

I had therefore to teach myself to go into an altered state of consciousness of a particular type. For at least a moment, I had to *know* that the cosmos was run on field-theory lines, that All is One, and to do this somehow "centered" about the uniting of another person and myself in the clairvoyant reality. The next question was *how* to do this.

The writings of the various mystical traditions are a vast resource of training techniques for problems of this sort. I experimented with a wide variety of these techniques, trying with each one to understand its purpose, to relate that purpose to my goal and then to my particular personality organization.

Any way of dividing up these techniques into classes is bound to be faulty. Not only is there a great deal of overlap, but all techniques have as one of their goals a tuning and training of the personality similar to the way an athlete tunes and trains his physical structure. However, bearing this in mind, some general classifications can be made. One of these is a division into meditation techniques, rhythm techniques (as the Dervish dances, the chanting of Mantras, and the Hassidic body movements), and assault-on-the-ego-techniques (such as fasting, the use of hallucinogenic agents such as LSD, and various methods of the *Via Ascetica,* the way of the ascetic). It was clear from what I knew about myself—and found out further in experimenting—that the meditation techniques were closest to my own easiest path.

These meditation techniques are all partially ways of learning to discipline the mind, to make it learn to do what you want it to do. No one who works at one of them for five minutes is left in the slightest doubt that his mind is as undisciplined as—in St. Teresa's phrase—"an unbroken horse. . . ."

One way of classifying meditation techniques is the threefold division into what has been called in the East the Inner Way, the Middle Way, and the

Outer Way. In the Inner Way, one concentrates on the spontaneously arising contents of one's own mind, upon the images and feelings that arise. In the Middle Way one strives for stillness of the mind; one withdraws from both internal and external perceptions. It has been called the Way of Emptiness. In the Outer Way one concentrates on and meditates on an externally given perception; one relinquishes spontaneity and disciplines the mind to stay with this perception until it blends with oneself. One contemplates one thing, following the statement of William Blake: "If the gates of perception were cleansed, all things would appear as they are, infinite."

These divisions are not clear-cut, and various meditation techniques cut across these arbitrary lines. A Zen Koan, for example, is both a meditation technique of the Outer Way and an assault-on-the-ego technique, in that what is being meditated upon cannot be dealt with by the ego operating in its usual manner. The Theraveda techniques in which one concentrates on a spontaneously generated rhythm of one's own (as the rise and fall of the chest in breathing) are a combination of rhythm and meditation techniques.

Another way of classifying mystical training technique is major avenues of approach: the body (as in Hatha Yoga), the feelings and intuition (perhaps the most widely used avenue; examples include Bhakti Yoga, the way of Meher Baba, and the monastic practicing his prayers, devotions, and deepening his ability to love), or the route of the intellect. From what I understood of myself, and of American culture generally, it seemed that the way of the intellect would be best and fastest for my purposes. In the East this is known as the Narodhi Samadhi. In the West it was the approach followed by the Habad school of Hasidism. It starts with an intellectual understanding of the structure of the two ways of being at home in reality, which I have described earlier as the sensory reality and the clairvoyant reality. From this point, one trains himself to perceive and "be" more and more in the clairvoyant reality through various (primarily meditation) techniques. For myself, I had thus chosen the meditation approach, the Outer Way, and the intellectual Samadhi.

The Outer Way (the Way of Forms or Way of Absorption) has been more commonly used in the West than the other two paths. In the West it is often called contemplation and we hear of the lives of the contemplatives, as the Christian followers of this path were called. In the East it has been called "one-pointing," or the Buddhist "bare attention." The clearest book on this subject I know of is Evelyn Underhill's *Practical Mysticism,* from which I learned much.

Using contemplation as a central exercise, I gradually devised a series of techniques which it seemed would, if practiced enough, lead me to the state of consciousness that appeared to be associated with the positive biological changes that occurred in successful psychic healing. It took me about a year and a half of experimentation and practice until I felt I could achieve this state.

At the end of this time I felt ready to try. If the theory was right and what was being stimulated was the individual's own self-repair systems, I did not see how I could do any damage. If the theory was invalid, nothing would happen. It seemed ethically legitimate to try it.

Once again—as when I discovered that physicists also believed in the clairvoyant reality—I found myself surprised at what occurred and surprised at my surprise. This time I was surprised that positive biological changes *did* occur to healees when I was able to go into the special altered state of consciousness. So deep are the prejudices ingrained in us about the nature of reality being that of the sensory reality that I—in spite of all the intellectual understanding and the intensive training program I had put myself through— still somewhere felt that it could *not* work, that it was all fantasy and that "reality *was* reality." I was surprised at positive results and surprised that I was surprised.

The results of the "healing encounters" I now began to have fell into five classes:

1. I went into the altered state of consciousness and nothing happened so far as the healee was concerned.
2. I went into the altered state and positive biological changes occurred in the healee's body.
3. I went into the altered state and positive psychological changes occurred in the patient.
4. I went into the altered state of consciousness and there were telepathic exchanges between the patient and myself.
5. I was unable to go into the altered state of consciousness.

There were all possible combinations also between numbers 2, 3, and 4. Further, again to my surprise, there was no particular relationship between these that I have been able to discover. A patient might consciously observe nothing psychological during the session and still have positive physical changes. He might observe a very strong "calming," "relaxing," or "tranquiliz- ing" effect with or without telepathic exchanges and with or without physical effects. The presence of one of these three factors appears at this time to have nothing much to do with the presence or absence of others.

In order to show the different types of results, I will describe some healing encounters which give a fairly accurate overall picture.

The general procedure followed in the healing encounters was simple. After enough general conversation so that we knew each other a little and felt reasonably relaxed together, I would ask the healee to simply get comfortable physically and to let his mind do as it pleased—not to cooperate in any particular way or to "try" to do anything, but to let happen whatever happened. I would then find myself a comfortable standing position (for no particular reason except that I concentrate more easily standing), close my eyes, and conceptualize this particular healee being in both realities at the same time. I would attempt to reach a point of being in which I would *know* that he not only existed as a separate individual inside his skin and limited by it, but that he also—and in an equally "true" and "real" manner—existed to the furthest reaches of the cosmos in space and time. When I *knew* for a moment that this was true and that I also coexisted with him in this manner— when, in fact, I had attained the clairvoyant reality—the healing work was done. Generally, I tried for two or three such moments in each encounter to "make sure," although this is probably more a statement about my own insecurity than it is about anything else.

Often I would use various types of symbols to help myself reach this point of knowing. For example, I might use the symbol of two trees on opposite sides of a hill with the tops visible to each other. From one viewpoint, they looked like two separate trees, but inside the hill, the two root masses met and were one. The two trees were really one and inseparable. Further, their roots affected the earth and the earth the rocks until I could know that in the whole planet and cosmos there was nothing that was not affected by them and affecting them. This sort of symbolization, different in each case, as the healee and I are different in each healing encounter, would often be useful in helping me reach the clairvoyant reality with the healee and myself centered in it. With practice, the situation often arose where no symbols were needed, where I could move immediately to the point of complete *knowledge* of both realities at once. Each healing encounter was different; symbols which would be useful in one would be empty and sterile in the next.

There is certainly something that the healee can do to increase the probability of a positive response to the healing. At present, however, I do not know what this is. In spite of experimentation (still continuing) on having the healee relax, meditate, or do half a dozen other things, I do not know at this time what the best activity (if, indeed, there is one best way for everyone) is for him to do. Curiously, belief in the efficacy of healing of this kind does not seem to be a factor. Our results seem to be as good with skeptics as they are with believers.

Sometimes, if the Type 1 healing described above goes well, I feel the palms of my hands begin to tingle and realize that I "want" also to do a Type 2 ("laying on of hands") healing with this person. When I have this impulse, I follow it, but never force it or try to do a Type 2 when it does not "feel" right to do so after a strong Type 1 encounter with the healee. The whole procedure rarely takes less than ten minutes or more than fifteen. There comes a certain point when it "feels" complete; there is the sense that whatever could be done has been done. It is then time to stop.

Frequently, I will go through this procedure and have a feeling of having been deeply into it, and as far as the healee is concerned all that has happened is that he relaxed for fifteen minutes in a comfortable chair. So far—in spite of a belief that in science the failures need study exactly as much, if not sometimes more than the successes—I have been able to find no clues as to why this happens with many healees, nor any ideas as to how to predict in advance which healees will respond in this way. The factors are certainly there, but so far I have not been able to analyze them.

With some healees, there is a positive physical response apparently associated with the healing encounter. Although coincidence has a long long arm and some of these cases are certainly "false positives" (that is, the positive physical response occurred for some other, unknown reason and the relationship in time to the healing encounter was coincidence), the successes have been frequent enough and impressive enough to persuade me that this research is worth continuing.

> A woman, well known to me, 75 years old, had had a painful arthritis and swelling of both hands for over a year. Although she could hold and use a pencil, or a knife and fork, it was impossible for her to bring her fingers closer than one inch from her palm. Attempts to do so, or pressure from outside the fingers, brought severe pain. Persuaded by members of her family to let me try psychic healing, she agreed and said she was not "against it," but did not believe in it. She asked what she should do during the time I was working. I replied that she should read a newspaper and she did so.
> I started with a Type 1 approach and in the course of about ten minutes felt that I had achieved the filling of consciousness with the field-theory viewpoint several times. I then moved into a Type 2 with her left hand only. It seemed to me that this was a strong

Type 2, as I had the perception of a good deal of energy between my palms, which were on both sides of her left hand.

After about five minutes of the Type 2 I felt that the experience was over and stopped. We chatted a moment and she told me she had felt nothing unusual. I asked the other members of her family to come back in (they had gone into the next room when I started the healing). Her husband asked her if there had been any effect. She replied, "No, it's just the same as it was," and to demonstrate this "flapped" the fingers of both hands. To everyone's surprise—certainly including hers and mine—they swung easily to the palm and out again. She now had full and painless movement in the fingers.

This has not changed in the full year since the healing encounter. She had been taking Prednisone (a Cortisone preparation) for three days before the healing, but up to one minute before the healing encounter, it had no apparent effect.

The following healing encounter occurred quite early in the work before I had set up the basic rule of *never* doing a Type 2 without a strong Type 1 first. By and large, Type 2 results (when done alone) tend to be transient; Type 1 results strongly tend to be permanent.

A woman known to me, aged thirty-six years, had intermittent, very large "cold sores" for over twenty years. Two or three times a year she would get one on her lip and it would take approximately thirty days to heal. She and her family knew the phenomena thoroughly and what to expect each time.

I held one hand on each side of her face, not touching the affected area, for about twenty minutes in a strong Type 2 healing. Afterwards she reported that during the twenty minutes she had been conscious of several periods of heat, and one of "tingling" in the lip area. About one half hour later she left my office to drive home (a drive of about an hour); en route she felt suddenly a strong "tingling" in the lip area, she looked at it in the rear-view mirror, and in her words, "I nearly had an accident, I was so surprised. I pulled off the road and sat for ten minutes watching the new skin regrow. The dead skin in the center did not seem to change, but new skin slowly grew over the whole raw pink area." When she arrived home, her son and her husband both reacted in surprise to the complete unexpected change and almost complete healing of the cold sore.

The next day it had returned about one-third the size it had been when she arrived in my office the day before, and disappeared over the next week.

A woman, aged thirty-eight years, had an overstretched cartilage of the knee. Her physician had termed it a "loose joint" and told her that if she was very careful and did not put any weight on it while it was in a bent position, it would recover in a year to eighteen months, or if she immobilized it in a cast, in four to six months. The knee joint was quite swollen, had no strength to bear weight when moving from a full bent (90-degree angle) position to a straight position, although once straightened she could walk on it, and was constantly painful. She came into the end of one of the training seminars I was holding and all ten people present did a Type 1 healing with her. She said afterwards that she felt very relaxed, calm, and "loved" during the ten-minute session. For me at least, it was a very strong Type 1 with full focus established several times. This was in the early afternoon. By that evening the swelling was reduced and the pain had lessened. On awaking the next morning there was no more sensation of pain in the area, its full strength had returned, and the swelling—according to her physician—was about half of what it had been. This lasted for several months, and the swelling gradually diminished to normal. In the following eighteen months, there has been no recurrence.

This case concerns a fifteen-year-old boy who broke his back on a trampoline. A letter dictated by his father, a surgeon, on November 1, 1971, and written by his mother, reads in part that the "period of detraumatization is over, and we must face the fact that 'medically' Chris is where he will be forever. That means: No feeling below the chest. Some feeling on the backs of the hands and the thumb and first finger. Movement of the lesser flexor muscles in the arm so that he has limited movement and strength in his arms—with supportive braces he may be able to use his arms to a limited degree. Indomitable inner strength and a smile that still knocks you dead."

On November 7, a group made up of students who had been at one of the healing seminars and were now working at an advanced workshop did a distance healing with Christopher. We had a letter about him and a picture, and the group—none of whom had ever met Christopher—were deeply involved. Chris, however, did not know of our existence or that anyone was going to do a psychic healing with him. He was in Denver and we were in Greenwich, Connecticut. An earlier healing had been held Friday evening, but it was on Sunday between 11:55 and 12:15 in the day that the group really "turned on" in a very strong long-distance, Type 1 healing. In the early afternoon (2—3 P.M.?) Denver time, Christopher suddenly called out that he could "feel" his legs. It soon became apparent that he could not only feel pressure sensations, but "could even tell which of his toes was being touched at any given time." The father said (to the woman who had written the letter to us, a close family friend) "that there is no explanation for this since the period of detraumatization was well

over and no hope was held for any further improvement or
restoration in Chris's physical condition."

However, all results must be evaluated cautiously. The most dramatic single
result I had occurred when a man I knew asked me to do a distance healing
for an extremely painful condition requiring immediate and intensive surgery.
I promised to do the healing that night, and the next morning when he awoke
a "miraculous cure" had occurred. The medical specialist was astounded, and
offered to send me pre and post healing X-rays and to sponsor publication in
a scientific journal. It would have been the psychic healing case of the century
except for one small detail. In the press of overwork, I had forgotten to do
the healing! If I had only remembered, it would have been a famous demonstration of what can be accomplished by this method.

Coincidence has a long long arm and the unexpected *does* often happen.
All reports of medical improvement by psychic healing (or by any other
therapeutic technique) must be interpreted with this in mind. It is also true,
however, that a technique must be evaluated in terms of its results, and not
in terms of a previously held theory. If the application of a theory produces
results in the predicted direction, its fruitfulness has been demonstrated and
previously held theories which imply that these results could not occur must
be abandoned or modified.

The third group of cases reported psychological effects only and no positive
effects. Almost invariably (and there were no negative or disturbing psychological effects) these were reported in terms like "I felt very calm and relaxed,"
"It was as if I were being tranquilized," "I felt so peaceful," "It was as if a
great wave of warm love came over me." Although this comprises a considerable group of healees, and is a definite and consistent phenomenon, in a pure
research sense these cases must be regarded as failures, since no physical
changes were observed. There is a difference between results of an experiment
from which one learns something new (it is hoped one learns something from
all results) and results that conform to one's predictions.

In the fourth group of cases there were strong indications of telepathy
exchanges between the patient and myself during the healing encounter. To
put this more accurately, I should state that there was a movement of images
and information *within* the Gestalt that had been formed and that included
the two of us.

A woman well known to me, aged twenty-eight, had an area of
psoriasis on the abdomen which had shown no signs of clearing up

over a five-week period, in spite of various prescribed topical
treatments. A Type 1 session was divided into two ten-minute
periods with a ten-minute rest period in between. In the first
period I visualized her as a part of the "All," and connected to it
through white bands (the love she felt and had felt for others
during her life) and by black bands (her perceptions of others and
events). (She is a writer with a very sharp, perceptive eye.) During
the rest period she reported first having had the sensation of waves
of heat pouring over her and then a pattern of alternating lighter
and darker waves of light intensity. I told her nothing of what I
had been conceptualizing. During the second period, I was able to
conceptualize her very strongly and one-pointedly in the same way
and began to merge the bands of black and white into grays—
symbolizing her relationships as "loveknowledge" (in Maslow's
sense) rather than love *and* knowledge separately.

At the end of the session she was obviously deeply moved, and
just wanted to sit quietly and not talk for a few minutes. Then,
after drinking some water, she said that it had seemed to her as if
she was surrounded by black and white clouds fanning out from
her like the spokes of a wheel. They presently began to revolve
around her, going faster and faster until the spokes of black and
the spokes of white began to merge and blur. She then said to
herself "They are outside of me. I'm inside. What would happen if
I let them in?" She let them in, and after the session said that
they were still inside and outside and she felt that they always
would be. On questioning, she would not say that it had been a
"good" or "bad" experience (although she now felt very good), but
that it had been an "ecstatic" experience and that she now felt "as
if I had just made love." She was deeply moved by the experience
and we talked in generalities for a half hour.

This is a person I know quite well and have much respect and
affection for. The next day she reported that there had
been—during the night—a period of intense itching of the
psoriasis and a sense that her entire abdomen was "breaking out"
with it. In the morning the area was—to her inspection—
unchanged. She said that she had since the session "a deep feeling
of calm and competence."

And another relevant example: An exceptional healing session
with a woman of sixty-five with multiple myeloma. I had met her a
few times fifteen years ago. Through a mutual friend she knew of
this work. I saw her at her house. A *very* strong Type 1 session.
During it, the main symbol system I used was to visualize "A
thousand Ilses," each a moment younger than the previous one,
each holding the next youngest in her arms and (a word I have not
used before) "approving" of her. From the future, older Ilses also
formed a line following the same procedure. A gap was in the

future part of the line, and I placed myself in it. At this point, the Gestalt solidified very strongly, went from black and white into full and rich color (unusual for me) and really filled the total field of my consciousness. To my surprise, the imagery took on a life of its own and one of the younger girls—in middle adolescence—left it and with a wicker basket over her arm went into a brightly lit field gathering flowers near some trees. This seemed only good, so I let it happen and simply lived with and participated in the picture for some time.

Afterward I asked Ilse what her experience had been. She replied that three things had happened. First, she felt a great deal of pleasant heat throughout her entire body and now felt very good and relaxed. Secondly, she had two strong images. The first concerned an incident at twelve that she felt had changed her entire life. In the town in Northern Germany where she had been raised there were two kinds of pretty girls: those with black hair, blue eyes, and white skin like her sister's, and those with blond hair, fair skin, and blue eyes. "And there I was with mud-colored hair, slate gray skin, and these washed out pale blue eyes." When the nurses dressed up her sisters, they "did not even bother to put a bow in my hair, it was hopeless." One day her mother had gone downtown and she went to her mother's room for something. She caught sight of herself in her mother's full-length mirror. "I realized that I was not pretty, but that I *approved* of myself. Since then I have always *approved* of myself and it has made a great difference in my life." (The word "approve" was both times spoken with real emphasis.)

The second image was of herself, as a young girl "gathering flowers in a bright, sunlit field with trees. I was putting them into a wicker basket on my arm."

After the session it was apparent from both our feelings that there was a deep and warm relationship. We sat talking as two people who have had a long, caring relationship for some time. When I left, she spontaneously kissed me on the cheek, which, for a person of her personality and background as I understand it, was a highly atypical action.

In the fifth group, I was simply unable to go into the altered state of consciousness with the patient healee.

There are experientially two separate phenomena here. In the first, the patient actively does not want the healing. This is a clear experience that one of my students in psychic healing has described as "feeling as if you were running into a rubber wall." Often a person has been "persuaded" by family or friends to try this type of healing and does not want to. The feeling that results when the healer tries is unmistakable; it just cannot be done. Put bluntly, it is impossible to "unite" with someone who does not want to unite with you.

The second class of those with whom I could not go into the altered state of consciousness is not so easy to define. Sometimes it was probably due to a fatigue state or distraction of my own that I could not transcend. At other times, it may have been due to something in the healee or to the "mix" our two personalities formed. We know so little about the best (and worst) healer-healee pairings that at this stage all we can do is be aware of our ignorance and our wish to overcome it. The experience in these cases was simply that I could not move into the world of the One; the symbols I used remained empty and just images, the world of the many remained the world I was in.

As it became clear that the first stage of testing the hypothesis of "how" psychic healing worked checked out, the time for the second stage drew closer. This was to determine if it could be taught to others. In the past, the ability to "do" psychic healing had always been regarded as "a gift of grace" or due to a special personality organization. Although I had never done any psychic healing before, it was possible that I had the special personality organization (or "gift of grace") and the reason I had never done it was because I had never tried to. From this viewpoint, the theory and self-training might be irrelevant to the results. I might, for all I knew, have been a "natural" healer and had this ability activated by my interest. The only way to test this was to see if the theory could be used to train others. If it worked there, if following the procedures indicated by the theory could lead others to the ability, I could be reasonably sure that the theory was valid and had not worked the first time merely by coincidence.

The first training seminar was held in September, 1970. I let it be known at the annual convention of the Association for Humanistic Psychology that I was interested in holding such a training seminar. With ten participants (mostly psychologists and others who were interested in the human potential movement), I went off to a private Florida estate which had been offered by Margaret Adams, the owner. The three and a half days scheduled was a very short time, but most of the participants learned to do Type 1 healing. Later seminars were scheduled for five days, and although the pace was still terribly exhausting, it proved possible to teach the majority of participants how to go into both Type 1 and Type 2 states during this time.

Participants were selected for the seminars on the basis of several qualifications. A strong ego structure was needed, as the exercises used are often quite powerful types of meditation, and the time available is too short to allow for members going on "trips" with them. Second, a good ethical approach to life is, from my point of view, important. And third, I selected the kind of people I felt I would like to be associated with in a new field. In the first five seminars I generally also ruled out people who had had a number of psychic experiences or who had ever been involved in psychic healing. The reason for this was that I was less interested in training those already in this area than I was in trying to see if individuals who had never been so involved could be trained. It is important to note, however, that the very act of applying for a seminar in itself was a selection system. Academic or formal qualifications were not considered as standards for acceptance, as I believe that they mean very little. I tend to agree with a patient of mine who once observed that she knew a lot of Ph.D.s and M.D.s who were educated far beyond their intelligence!

The procedure at all the seminars was structurally similar. First came a theoretical discussion of the concept of the sensory reality and the clairvoyant reality. (All students were asked to read my monograph on the subject *before* we started so we did not start from scratch.) A series of exercises composed the bulk of the seminar. These were designed to accomplish three purposes:

1. To strengthen the structure of the ego—a sort of personality calisthenics.
2. To loosen the individual's usual concepts of dealing with space, time, the location of the self, etc., and to make him emotionally aware that there were alternative valid ways of conceptualizing in these areas.
3. To move in a step-by-step progression until one arrived at the altered state of consciousness theoretically associated with psychic healing.

At the end of this series, the group did Type 1 healing on each other and had a good deal of practice at this. On the last day, a small group of individuals with medically described physical problems would come in, one at a time, and the group would hold healing encounters with them. At one point or another, depending on the fatigue level of the group, a short series of exercises leading to Type 2 healing would be held.

Five days is a very short time for this procedure, but it proved feasible. The pace was exhausting, three sessions a day with each session ending when the group was too tired to go on. The pace was so intense and the pressure so heavy that it was necessary to hold the sessions in a residential setting and in a non-urban atmosphere so that the contact with nature could refresh the participants. At present, I and some of the advanced students who received training in teaching the seminar are experimenting with other forms of structure, such as several intensive weekends in a row.

Overall, this general format proved successful. As I learned more and more how to put the exercise series together and how to pace the progress, and as I learned from the contribution of those involved, the seminars improved, and more and more of the participants learned how to go into the altered states. At the seminar in September, 1971, all the students became quite proficient at this, continued to practice it after the seminar and—working together—became an amazingly strong healing circle. It was this group that, at a three-day follow-up advanced seminar, was involved in the case of the boy with the broken back described above.

It was clear from these results that if one followed the implications of the theory, a training method for psychic healing could be devised. If one then went through the training, it was possible for most people to become fairly effective at psychic healing, and further practice improved this ability. This seemed the most important type of test I could devise of the validity (or fruitfulness) of the theory. Other tests of the more usual "experimental" type have been devised, . . . but the healing approach seems to me to be the most critical test of the general theory of the paranormal implied in the concept of the clairvoyant and sensory realities.

There is still, of course, a tremendous amount we need to learn about psychic healing. We do not know its limits or in what types of physical problems it is most effective. We do not know its implications for emotional problems, or how it can best be integrated with standard medical and psycho-therapeutic procedures. We know little about how to select the best candidates for training, or how to set up the best healer-healee pairings. We need to know much more about training, about the comparative effectiveness of group and individual healing, and about how to form healing groups. We have no adequate theory for Type 2 healing, and we have only impressions about the comparative effectiveness of the two types or if, indeed, they are more than experientially different. We have no idea how to predict which healing encounters will be associated with positive biological changes and which will not. We are very much at the beginning of this work.

References

Bergin, C. R. The effects of psychotherapy: negative results revisited. *Journal of Counseling Psychology,* 1963, **10,** 244–255.

Cannon, W. B. Voodoo death. *American Anthropologist,* 1942, **44,** 169–181.

Carkhuff, R. R., & Truax, D. B. Training in counseling and psychotherapy: an evaluation of an integrated didactic and experimental approach. *Journal of Consulting Psychologists,* 1965, **29,** 333–336.

Chance, P. Parapsychology is an idea whose time has come. *Psychology Today,* October 1973, 7, 105–120.

Egbert, L. D., Battit, G. E., Welch, C. E., & Bartlett, M. K. Reduction of postoperative pain by encouragement and instruction of patients. *New England Journal of Medicine,* 1964, 270:16, 825–827.

Frank, J. D. *Persuasion and healing.* Baltimore: Johns Hopkins Press, 1961.

———, Nash, E. H, Stone, A. R., & Imber, S. D. Immediate and long-term symptomatic course of psychiatric outpatients. *American Journal of Psychiatry,* 1963, 120, 429–439.

Friedman, H. J. Patient-expectancy and symptom reduction. *Archives of General Psychiatry,* 1963, 8, 61–67.

Gliedman, L. H., Nash, E. H., Stone, A. R., Imber, S. D., & Frank, J. D. Reduction of symptoms by pharmacologically inert substances and by short-term psychotherapy. *Archives of Neurology and Psychiatry,* 1958, 79, 345–351.

Medical World News. Finger-tip halos of Kirlian photography. October 26, 1973, 43–46.

Rogers, C. R. The characteristics of a helping relationship. *Personnel and Guidance Journal,* 1958, 37, 6–16.

Schofield, W. *Psychotherapy: the purchase of friendship.* Englewood Cliffs, N.J.: Prentice-Hall, 1964.

Torrey, E. F. *The mind game: witchdoctors and psychiatrists.* New York: Emerson Hall, 1972.

Truax, C. B., & Carkhuff, R. R. *Toward effective counseling and psychotherapy.* Chicago: Aldine, 1967.

Uhlenhuth, E. H., & Duncan, D. B. Subjective change with medical student therapists: course of relief in psychoneurotic outpatients. *Archives of General Psychiatry,* 1968, 18, 428–438.

*Stanley R. Dean and
Denny Thong*

Transcultural Aspects of Metapsychiatry: Focus on Shamanism in Bali

CULTURE MAY BE defined as the sum total of social behavior patterns resulting from learned arts and skills, such as language, religion, customs, mores, technology, family structure, and group relations. Cultural psychiatry is the study of cultural influences—as distinct from biological and intrapsychic influences —upon the psychopathology and psychotherapy of a given people in a given period. And transcultural psychiatry is simply the global extension of such studies beyond any one culture. It is closely related to anthropology, sociology, and religion.

Such interfaces were not always recognized. In 1901 a French sociologist, Émile Durkheim, issued a dictum that was accepted as dogma for several years: "Whenever a social phenomenon is directly explained by a psychological phenomenon, we may be sure that the explanation is false [p. 5]."

We have come a long way since then. In this era of accelerated communication, acculturation, and travel, transcultural psychiatry has emerged as one of the major branches of our field. It coalesces with metapsychiatry when cultural influences of a mystical nature affect the mental outlook of a group (Dean, 1973). Prime examples are the psychogenic culture-bound reactive syndromes, and their treatment by indigenous healers, otherwise known as shamans, witch doctors, *bomohs, dukuns,* and so forth.[1]

Such syndromes are usually associated with primitive societies—but, as a matter of fact, they may crop up in closely knit ethnic groups and cults anywhere in the world. While there may be regional differences, they all share

---

[1]For the sake of uniformity I shall use the terms "shaman" and "shamanism" to represent all the others.

a common belief in such esoteric concepts as spirit possession, sorcery, hexing, voodoo, trance states, and exorcism. They resemble, for the most part, our psychiatric concepts of acute schizophrenic episodes. The symptoms are similar: transient attacks of depersonalization, dissociation, agitated depression, echo reactions, and automatism—usually against a background of paranoid, hysteriform, psychosomatic structuring wherein the mechanisms of denial, projection, massive regression, and a magical-animistic world view are the principle ego-defensive reactions.

In Bali the syndrome in question is known as *bebainen*. It will be described separately. Here, for purposes of comparison, are a few examples from other regions:

Amok (Malay)—sudden attacks of frenzy, rage, and violence, at times indiscriminately homicidal, and followed by amnesia.

Latah (Malay, Philippines, Africa, Siberia, Lapland, North America)—compulsive echolalia and echopraxia, i.e., repetitive imitation of words, sounds, and actions, often obscene.

Windigo (Canadian Indians, especially Cree and Ojibway tribes)—attacks of agitated depression with oral-sadistic (cannibalistic) fears and impulses.

Piblokto (Eskimo women)—attacks of screaming, crying, and running naked through the snow, sometimes with suicidal or homicidal tendencies.

Susto (Latin America)—panic reactions due to fear of the evil eye, black magic, and spirit possession.

Koro (China and Southeast Asia)—a phobia that the penis will retract into the body and cause death; to prevent that calamity, a stick may be tied to the penis. Less commonly, women have similar fears about their breasts.

The psychodynamic interpretation of these exotic syndromes is beyond the scope of this paper, but has been extensively reported by Yap (1967), Kiev (1972), Weidman and Sussex (1971), Torrey (1972), and Wittkower and Weidman (1969), to name but a few. From a practical viewpoint, certain broad generalizations are needed to provide an understanding of folk psychiatry *vis-à-vis* more academic concepts.

First of all, it may be assumed that no *specific* type of psychotherapy has ever been devised—or is ever likely to be devised—for mental illness. Literally thousands of methods have been advocated, and their protagonists have claimed success for each of them. This affords pause for reflection. One can only conclude that a common denominator underlies all of them. It is that common denominator and not any particular school of thought that determines the success or failure of treatment.

The entire gamut of psychotherapy—from the native witch doctor at one extreme to the academically trained psychiatrist at the other—hinges upon two constants: the therapeutic personality (charisma) of the therapist, and the expectant faith of the patient, both of which apparently involve a suprasensory, suprarational level of mentation (the ultraconscious), as yet little understood (Dean, 1971). A close third is cognitive congruence—empathic communication that is reciprocally understood and accepted by both healer and patient. This implies the use of culture-specific techniques and strategies in treatment, and perhaps even a common ethnic background for therapist and patient. For example, a preliterate Bushman is a poor candidate for psychodynamic insight therapy, but might respond to occult rituals, whereas the reverse would be true in a more sophisticated setting.

To these constants may be added such variables as the therapeutic environment: reinforcing status symbols (titles, reputation, testimonials, diplomas, publications); the use of medicinals (potions, herbs, and incense on the one hand; sophisticated synthetics on the other); props and various tools of the trade (amulets, masks, and other regalia of the shaman versus the couch, the notebook, and batteries of tests of the psychiatrist).

Finally, no account of the therapist-patient relationship would be complete without mentioning the growing belief among some psychic investigators that a mysterious transfer of energy takes place between the healer and the patient. This ancient idea has gained considerable momentum in recent years as a result of the alleged discovery through Kirlian photographic techniques of emanations or energy fields emitted by all forms of life (Dean, 1973).

Viewed in these perspectives, it is no surprise, as Torrey has pointed out, that a common bond unites the psychiatrist and the shaman (Torrey, 1972). Their differences are extrinsic rather than intrinsic. It follows that the merit of any treatment should be judged by its effectiveness, not by its label, subject of course to enlightened professional and legal safeguards.

The above is an oversimplification because of limitations of space. My purpose at this writing is merely to crystallize an idea already shared by many: that indigenous healers be considered in the psychiatric scheme of things; and that future applicants for psychiatric training be judged on the basis of therapeutic personality as well as grades.

Focus on Bali

In an antecedent paper (1972), Denny Thong and I described the observations of one of us (S.R.D.) and the experiences of the other (D.T.) in psychiatry in Bali. Though a relatively small island among the hundreds that make up the Indonesian archipelago to the east of Djakarta, Bali is known and loved the world over. Its idyllic setting, attractive inhabitants, numerous temples, colorful religious ceremonies, and exotic ritual dances have earned it such sobriquets as Morning of the World, Temple of Heaven, and Island of the Gods.

Bali covers an area of 2000 square miles, and has a population of about 2.5 million, which, unlike the rest of Indonesia, is predominantly Hindu. With more than 1000 people to the square mile, it is second only to Djakarta in density of population. Because of that fact and its important role in tourism, the government has designated it as a province, the smallest of twenty-six, with a governor at its head.

Bali is divided into eight districts *(kabupaten)*, each of which is subdivided into smaller communities *(ketjamatan)*, and finally into villages *(bandjars)* consisting of fifty to 250 families. The village chief *(Klian bandjar)* plays an important role, not only in village problems, but in family matters as well.

The Balinese people are normally tranquil, dignified, and controlled. But under stress they lose their composure and become susceptible to seizures, trances, and other forms of altered consciousness. Habitual decorum is also cast aside at public celebrations and, paradoxically, at cremation ceremonies. Such manifestations are usually transient and regarded as normal. They are even mimicked in their colorful ritual dances.

But in such a large population there are also thousands of mental cases that require special treatment. To supervise their care, at the time of our study in 1971, there was only one self-trained psychiatrist, Denny Thong, formerly a general practitioner. He directed a 150-bed government hospital in which he was able to accommodate almost double that number by the simple expedient of sleeping two to a bed. To a Balinese accustomed to sharing sleeping quarters with entire families, that was no great hardship.

From personal observation it was evident that the psychiatric needs of the populace were quite adequately met. How was that possible? The answer is: with the aid of hospital-based and village-based shamans, known locally as *baleans*. [2] Dr. Denny proudly called them his "psychiatric aides," and was frank to admit that it would have been impossible to manage his psychiatric case load without them. *Baleans* successfully handled the great bulk of

---

[2]The spellings used here were furnished by Dr. Denny Thong. Minor variations are found in the older literature; for example, *balian* was preferred by Jane Belo (1960), and by Bateson and Mead (1942).

indigenous mental problems, leaving the more serious cases for Dr. Denny.

The Balinese recognize two main types of mental illness: *bebainan* and *buduh.* These are further classified according to symptoms, e.g., *nengil* (mute), *gadungan* (grandiose), and so forth. It is only since 1968 that Dr. Denny has used modern classification.[3]

Bebainan, ascribed to demons *(kala)* or to small, evil spirits sent by enemies *(bebai),* is a culture-bound reactive syndrome ethnogenic to Bali. It is thought to be caused by vengeful persons or evil spirits, together or alone. Such an illness (and the less common *latah*) is the special field of the medicine man *(balean).* *Buduh,* on the other hand, is said to be caused by sins in a previous existence *(karma)* or by current emotional problems. It encompasses the major global psychoses, and is usually referred to a physician.

Bebainan is by far the most common derangement. It usually has a very acute onset. The patient suddenly begins to cry, seems terrified, tries to run away, and fights off any attempt to restrain him. The struggle continues until the patient falls limply or convulsively to the ground in a state of utter exhaustion, after which recovery usually occurs spontaneously. However, if the attack is unduly prolonged or keeps recurring, the family or the entire *bandjar* holds a conference, and the patient is referred to a suitable *balean.*

There are various specialists among *baleans.* One who practices a type of exorcism is the most favored. He attempts to cast out the evil spirit by prayer and purification *(kebathinan).* He pits his will against the will of the demon *(kala, bebai)* in a determined dialogue that sounds very much like haggling over a bargain. Sometimes coconut oil and holy water are used in this ritual. If the *balean* is successful, an agreement is reached, whereupon the *bebai* cries out and confesses its guilt. This results in an abrupt cure, leaving the patient with complete amnesia for the attack. It might be well to remind the reader at this point that exorcism, the symbolic battle between good and evil, has been the mainstay of primitive medicine since ancient times, and is still practiced in one form or another in many parts of the world. It is deeply rooted in the mind of man, and helps to explain the recent furor over Peter Blatty's book, *The Exorcist,* and the movie made from it.

Other *baleans* practice a primitive type of *materia medica* as recorded in the *lontars.* These are instructions inscribed on dried palm leaves that have been carefully preserved and handed down from generation to generation.

---

[3]In 1971, of 260 patients, 131 were diagnosed schizophrenia, and 78, acute schizophrenic episodes corresponding to the culture-bound reactive syndromes. There were 9 manic-depressive psychoses, 12 senile psychoses, 13 psychoneuroses. The remainder were divided among organic psychoses, socio-psychopathies, and epilepsy.

Sections on the treatment of mental illness *(usada)* include the following procedures:

1. *Tutuh* (nose-drip method): A concoction is prepared from pepper and other pungent ingredients. It is then forced into the nostrils of the patient in order to produce a copious nasal discharge.
2. *Dusdus* (inhalation method): This is the same as *tutuh* except that the concoction is heated over a fire and the patient ordered to inhale as much of the smoke as possible.
3. *Lukat* (bathing method): The patient is bathed on certain propitious days and offerings are simultaneously made to the deities; or the patient is held under a waterfall, if need be for hours at a time; or his head is repeatedly forced under water in a river or the sea; or he is made to walk across a stream on a bamboo pole, which is suddenly pulled from under him.

Still other *baleans* specialize in foretelling the future and evoking the past during meditation or trance-like states. This allegedly enables them to tell a patient exactly what penance, sacrifice, ritual, or other specific procedure he must follow in order to effect a cure. In addition, herbs and other medicinals may be prescribed.

It is obvious that a *balean,* like his medical counterpart in our society, plays a highly important and respected role in Bali. He is found in every town and village. He may be a high-ranking, educated official or a charismatic individual with no formal education; but in either case he must possess the essential features of a therapeutic personality and reputed supernatural powers. In some instances these attributes have existed since childhood, and have led him to be selected for special training by local *baleans* and village elders. Others have had a call—a subjective ultraconscious experience (Dean, 1971) believed to indicate that one had been specially selected by the gods for the mission of healing.

In most cases the *balean* is successful. But should his treatment fail, or a doctor's care be too long delayed or inadequate, further disposition of the patient will depend on his overall behavior. If he is quiet and not too troublesome, he may be cared for at home or be left to fend for himself as best he can. In almost every hamlet and town, vagrant psychotics, rejected by their families, can be found roaming the streets, ragged, dirty, and often sick, foraging for food and shelter. Asuni (1971) and Prince (1969) have described similar conditions in Nigeria, and they no doubt exist in other parts of the world. As yet very few projects are under way to provide professional care for these unfortunates. It is a problem that deserves greater attention from health organizations than it has so far received.

If, on the other hand, the patient is seriously disturbed, he may be impris-
oned pending hospitalization; or he may be restrained by tying or the use of
stocks *(blagbag)*. The exact method is carefully prescribed, for it is believed
to have therapeutic value in addition to providing restraint. The confinement
may take place in the home, in a public place such as the village square, or
in a cemetery, this last in the hope that the evil spirit possessing the patient
will be frightened away by rival spirits residing in the cemetery.

The patient's limbs may be confined in stocks or his hands may be tied by
one or more of several methods: in front, in back, or around a pole, together
or separated by a length of wood (see Figure). If stocks are used, the wood
is usually taken from a *dapdap* tree (L. *Erythrina lithosperma*) because of its
sacred properties and in order that its relative softness may minimize pain. In
many instances a short period of *blagbag* may suffice. But in chronic cases it
may be resorted to continuously or intermittently for long periods of time.

Only if all else fails will the patient be brought to a doctor—and then
reluctantly because going to a doctor is an admission that one is *buduh*,
something to be ashamed of, whereas being *bebainan* carries little more

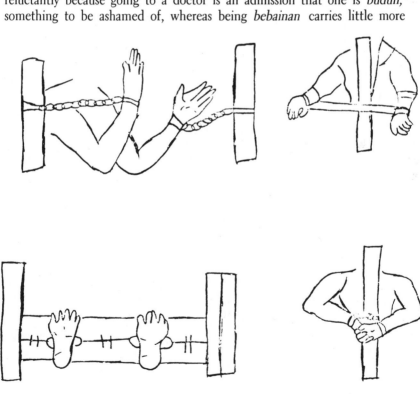

stigma than having a cold. Admitting a patient to a mental hospital is even more complicated, involving considerable red tape, months of waiting, and expense.

Discussion

Shamanism and its counterparts are prevalent throughout the world. It is no exaggeration to say that more people consult shamans than physicians. The extent to which psychiatry should or should not recognize shamanism as an adjunctive form of therapy has become the subject of considerable controversy. At one extreme, Torrey assigns absolutely equal importance to both of them within their particular cultures, and categorically advocates their close collaboration. He believes that adherence to an exclusive intrastructured school of psychotherapy without regard for ethnocentric cultural pathogenesis is bound to be self-defeating in the long run (1972).

At the other extreme Cerrolaza (1972) rejects all multidisciplinary collaboration, and warns against "antipsychiatrists" who would discredit and undermine the very foundations of psychiatry. "The villain," he admonishes, "is the psychiatrist himself, for he was the one to start the invasion of fields not related to his professional training. . . . Therefore the end result of the egalitarian principle may be to debase psychiatrists and to promote the paramedical members of the team to a superior rank[4] [p. 306]."

For most experts, however, the truth lies somewhere between those two extremes. There are realistic indications and contraindications for various types of parapsychiatric collaboration. Our judgment should be influenced by a sense of perspective and flexibility rather than by categorical imperatives.

America is no longer the melting pot it used to be. Ethnic groups tend to congregate in relatively homogeneous communities. Sparked by Black assertiveness, our Mexican, Indian, Cuban, Puerto Rican, and other ethnic minorities exhibit pride in their cultural heritage, so intense as to defy complete acculturation. Especially tenacious is their attachment to elements of folk medicine and faith healing. Our Cuban compatriots wish to retain their *santeros;* Mexicans, their *curanderos;* Puerto Ricans, their *espiritistas;* Indians, their medicine men; other Americans, their evangelical, spiritual, or psychic healers. There is a growing sentiment that they should be permitted

---

[4]In a subsequent personal communication Dr. Cerrolaza concedes that paramedical aides "can be as competent as we are in certain areas provided they are enlisted according to appropriate criteria."

to do so under a system of enlightened supervision. Already a step has been taken in that direction in New York City (Lubchansky & Stokes, 1970); and in Miami, Florida, Dr. Hazel Weidman (1973), an anthropologist on the medical faculty, urges that medical anthropology, mediated through trained culture brokers, be added to medicine's community health services. Others are bound to follow, for society can learn the following lessons from shamanism:

1. It removes the stigma from mental illness. There is no onus upon the patient, since blame is assigned to the evil spirit rather than to the victim.
2. The illness is accepted as an integral part of community experience, likely to affect anyone at any time, and no more unusual than everyday physical illness. It is so stereotyped as to appear almost psychotomimetic, at times reaching the dimensions of a *folie en groupe.*
3. The healer is a peer with whom the patient can identify, for he too experiences trances, hallucinations, and other supernatural manifestations. Therefore, his participation is accepted as a matter of fact. Belief in the supernatural, although universal, is especially dominant in the thinking of primitive societies. They accept the fact that the shaman is an agent of the gods, as well as a healer in his own right, and the effectiveness of treatment is greatly enhanced by that dual faith.
4. Empathic communication (cognitive congruence) between shaman and patient exists at the very onset, whereas it must be painstakingly developed, often over a long period of time, in the psychiatrist-patient relationship.
5. The Balinese world is one of sharing. Within his village a man belongs to his family, his caste, his community, and his gods. Every occasion for joy or sorrow is treated as a shared event among family, friends, and divine guardians. Rarely does a Balinese experience oppressive loneliness. Therefore, because treatment occurs in a community continuum, there is minimal disruption of family and community ties, and the patient stands a better chance of rehabilitation.

Some of the preceding statements may seem strangely familiar to Western minds—and not without reason, for there is a surprising analogy between ancient practices and modern concepts. Within recent years an increasing parallelism has developed between the two extremes. Witness the current thrust toward community psychiatry, crisis intervention, encounter groups, peer-directed therapeutic social clubs (such as Alcoholics Anonymous, Synanon, Recovery, Inc.,) and the proliferation of training programs for paraprofessional psychiatric aides, and even for indigenous community mental health workers (Dean, 1971).

Psychiatrists and other behavioral scientists are also beginning to pay more attention to mystical levels of consciousness and other psychic phenomena. Several panels on those subjects have been presented at recent meetings of the American Psychiatric Association. They created widespread interest that has resulted in mobilizing other professionals who are mindful of the important interface between psychiatry and mysticism. One result will be the formation of the American Metapsychiatric Association (AMPA), now in its preliminary stages (Dean, 1973).

Only the nonmedical healer, despite his ubiquity, continues to be set apart. Yet the function of the physician and doctor-priest was once inseparable. Jules Masserman (1966), stressing that ancient affinity, advocated greater collaboration between them. Ari Kiev stressed the importance of research in what he called "prescientific psychiatry" in the light of modern concepts (1959). Elsewhere in this paper similar references are cited (Yap, 1967; Torrey, 1972; Weidman, 1973). Sooner or later the question will have to be decided whether or not the nonmedical healer should play an adjunctive role in the psychiatric armamentarium. Wintrob and Wittkower (1969) have put it this way:

> Whether he likes it or not, the psychiatrist in countries progressing through transitional stages of their development has to tolerate the role and function of the nature healer and may, in the interest of his patients, be forced to cooperate with him [p. 13].

But if shamanism has its virtues, it also has its faults. Its advantages must be carefully weighed against the following disadvantages:

1. Shamanism abounds in testimonials, but maintains no accurate records.
2. There is no adequate follow-up.
3. Noninnovative, formulistic rituals are employed.
4. There is a tendency to adopt a "panacea complex" and to disparage other techniques.
5. There is a risk of bungling by inept amateurs.
6. There is a danger of delaying adequate professional help in serious cases.
7. Shamans are chiefly concerned with symptom removal, and this may result in antitherapeutic suppression of important intrapsychic pathology.
8. Patients are treated without adequate screening, referral, or diagnosis.
9. Shamans are usually not subject to legal, professional, or other regulatory restraints as are licensed professionals.

If these shortcomings can be modified or corrected, it is entirely within the realm of probability that cooperation between professional and paraprofessional healers can be ethically condoned. Psychiatry and shamanism could then have a meeting if not yet a marriage. The psychiatrist could become a sharer as well as a spectator of the past.

References

Asuni, T. Vagrant psychotics in Abeokuta. *Journal of the National Medical Association,* 1971, **63**, 173–180.

Bateson, G. & Mead, M. *Balinese character: A photographic analysis.* New York: New York Academy of Sciences, 1942, Special Publications II.

Belo, J. *Trance in Bali.* New York: Columbia University Press, 1960.

Cerrolaza, N. The nebulous scope of our current psychiatry. Paper presented at the annual meeting of the Canadian Psychiatric Association, Montreal, Canada, June, 1972.

Durkheim, E. *Les régles de la methode sociologique.* Paris: Felix Alcan, 1901. In I. Galdston (Ed.), *The interface between psychiatry and anthropology.* New York: Brunner-Mazel, 1971.

Dean, S. R. Metapsychiatry: The interface between psychiatry and mysticism. *American Journal of Psychiatry,* 1973, **130**, 1036–1038.

_____. Metapsychiatry and the ultraconscious. *American Journal of Psychiatry,* 1971, **128**, 154–155.

_____. The role of self-conducted group therapy in psychorehabilitation: A look at Recovery, Inc. *American Journal of Psychiatry,* 1971, **127**.

Dean, S. R. & Thong, D. Shamanism versus psychiatry in Bali. *American Journal of Psychiatry,* 1972, **129**, 91–94.

Kiev, A. *Transcultural psychiatry.* New York: The Free Press, 1972.

_____. Prescientific psychiatry. In S. Arieti (Ed.), *American Handbook of Psychiatry.* New York: Basic Books, 1959.

Lubchansky, I., Egri, G., & Stokes, J. Puerto Rican spiritualists view mental illness: the faith healer as a paraprofessional. *American Journal of Psychiatry,* 1970, **127**, 312–321.

Masserman, J. H. *Modern therapy of personality disorders.* Dubuque, Iowa: W. C. Brown, 1966.

Prince, R. Indigenous Yoruba psychiatry. In A. Kiev (Ed.), *Magic, faith and healing.* New York: The Free Press, 1969.

Torrey, E. F. *The mind game: witchdoctors and psychiatrists.* New York: Emerson Hall, 1972.

Weidman, H. H. Implications of the culture-broker concept for the delivery of health care. Paper presented at the annual meeting of the Southern Anthropological Society, Wrightsville Beach, N.C., March, 1973.

Weidman, H. H. & Sussex, J. N. Cultural values and ego functioning in relation to the atypical culture-bound reactive syndromes. *Transcultural Psychiatric Research Review,* 1971, 8, 13–18.

Wintrob, R. & Wittkower, E. D. Witchcraft in Liberia and its psychiatric implications. In S. Lesse (Ed.), *An evaluation of the results of the psychotherapies.* Springfield, Ill.: C. C. Thomas, 1968.

Wittkower, E. & Weidman, H. H. Magic, witchcraft and sorcery in relation to mental health and mental disorder. In N. Petrilowitsch and H. Flegel (Eds.), *Social psychiatry.* New York: S. Karger, 1969.

Yap, P. M. Classification of the culture-bound reactive syndromes. *Australian & New Zealand Journal of Psychiatry,* 1967, 1, 172–179.

Elmer and Alyce Green

Mind Training, ESP, Hypnosis, and Voluntary Control of Internal States

IN ORDER TO sharply delineate the main points of this note, it is convenient first to summarize the subjects of discussion and our understanding of them as follows:

1. Through hypnosis and through various training programs, including biofeedback, many persons can become aware of normally unconscious processes.
2. Awareness of normally unconscious processes is sometimes accompanied by spontaneous (and sometimes volitional) ESP phenomena.
3. Commercial mind-training courses promising ESP powers are using hypnosis as the major method and, advertising to the contrary, do not give biofeedback or brain-wave training, nor are the subjects necessarily in an alpha brain-wave state.
4. Commercial mind-training "teachers" generally deny that they use hypnosis, and by denying or ignoring the risks associated with hypnotic "programming" are inducing in some persons a form of paranoid neurosis or psychosis, often related to obsession or "possession."
5. Hypnotic programming for ESP bears a similarity to some of the methods used for development of trance mediumship, especially the "possession by spirits" of low grade mediumship.
6. Awareness of normally unconscious processes can be safely taught under the guidance of a counselor, without hypnotic programming, by methods which allow each person to develop according to his own inner needs.
7. Mind-training procedures should be voluntarily modified by those interested in the subject to eliminate psychic hazards. If this is not done, government agencies may summarily ban many research and training

programs that otherwise, if carefully developed, might become valuable adjuncts to our education and health systems.

8. The major problems are (a) to determine what techniques are safe as well as efficient for the extension of awareness, (b) to establish standards of qualification and responsibility of teachers, and (c) to offer the benefits of awareness training programs to the public through non-profit institutions.

Many psychologists in the last few years have become interested in research possibilities that a few years back were considered beyond the realm of science, namely, voluntary control of normally unconscious psychological and physiological processes. The first medical approaches to this subject in the West, starting in about 1910, sprang from the researches and developments of Autogenic Training and Psychosynthesis, beginning with Johannes Schultz in Germany and Roberto Assagioli in Italy, respectively (Schultz & Luthe, 1959; Luthe, 1969). At about the same time, Edmund Jacobson (1938) was beginning to develop in the United States his training program known as Progressive Relaxation. In other parts of the world, new interpretations of yoga were developing, such as the Integral Yoga of Aurobindo (1955). His *Synthesis of Yoga,* for instance, is concerned with a program for enhancement of consciousness and for control of normally unconscious processes. The newest development along this line of self-regulation of mind and body, and perhaps the most applicable to Westerners in general, has resulted from research in the area of biofeedback training (Green, Green & Walters, 1970; Barber et al., 1971; Kamiya et al., 1971).

The programs mentioned above deal with one's power to modify and control, through volition, one's own mental, emotional, and physiological states, without hypnotic programming by another person; and in all of these developments (except perhaps Progressive Relaxation, which deals primarily with problems of muscle tension) parapsychological events sometimes occur. These events are not, however, the goals of training. The primary goal is self-mastery, and in Psychosynthesis and in Integral Yoga the primary goal is self-mastery coupled with the development of awareness of what, in Zen, is called the True Self. Unless this aspect of Self is developed, it is said, psychic powers become an "ego trip." The attainment of psychic powers may follow safely *after* a degree of self-mastery (ego mastery) is achieved, but if paranormal development comes first, psychological problems develop. Aurobindo's way of saying this focuses attention on what he calls the Overmind level of one's being. After achieving awareness of that, he says, one can explore in "astral" dimensions with a measure of safety. Otherwise, it is possible to become involved in psychic (psychological) entanglements and not be able to find one's way through layers of mental and emotional confusion back to one's center. The ancient Christian advice concerning these matters was to seek first the kingdom of Heaven, which was within, it was said, and other things would follow in due course.

These considerations seem to have an especially important meaning today because we are bombarded by newspaper advertisements of entrepreneurs who (for a fee) will develop psychic powers in us, through hypnosis. It is denied that hypnosis is the technique employed, because hypnosis is a "bad word." Instead, it is called "conditioning," "programming," "brainwave training," "alpha training," etc., but nevertheless, it *is* hypnosis. On this professionals agree, although they do not always agree on how hypnosis works (Marcuse, 1959; Hilgard, 1965; Gill & Brenman, 1959). The "countdown" induction procedure used in commercial mind-training "programming" is a classical hypnotic technique.

Hypnosis is an extremely powerful tool for control of physiological and psychological states. It is well-known that through hypnosis, painless surgery can be performed, people can be made to see things that are not there, and not see things that are there, but it is not generally realized, even by professionals, that through hypnosis, parapsychological sensitivity can be enhanced. Frederick Myers, in 1901, clearly summarized the major findings of hypnosis experimentation in the last century and showed that hypnosis and parapsychology are not necessarily two separate subjects (1954).

More recently, Beloff (1964), in an analysis of the paranormal, ventured the opinion that "hypnotism may not be just a psychological phenomenon but may have a certain paranormal component as well [p. 236]." The points being made here are that hypnosis *can* involve the paranormal, and the paranormal is being invoked by hypnosis in some of those who take commercial mind-training courses, opinions of noninvestigators notwithstanding.

The question might now be raised, "So what? What difference does it make?" This question can be answered in at least three ways, depending on whether one looks at commercial mind-training (1) from a traditional *psychological* point of view, that is, treat the various phenomena that result from the program as figments of the imagination; (2) from a *psychosomatic* point of view, in which the power of mind over events inside the skin is accepted, but parapsychological events are considered to be figments of the imagination; or (3) from a *parapsychological* point of view, in which the phenomena of hypnosis are seen as consistent with research data from various psychological, psychosomatic, and parapsychological studies.

But before these points of view can be considered, it is necessary to identify some of the phenomena that are claimed by commercial mind-training teachers and by many of their students, namely:

(a) A person can "go down" into his own "unconscious," and while in that deep "level," can program his own physiological and psychological processes so that various diseases in him that have not yielded to standard medical treatment can be brought under control, at least temporarily.

(b) While at his deep "level," a person can become aware of physical, emotional, and mental states and diseases in other people, and can correctly diagnose ailments.

(c) While at his "level," a person can learn to manipulate the physical, emotional, and mental natures of other persons, sick or healthy, and thereby modify their behavior.

(d) While at his "level," a person can learn to manipulate nature so that coincidences, "accidents," or lack of accidents, can come under his control. This is, essentially, a promise of psychokinetic powers.

Now from a traditional *psychological* point of view, the above ideas are sheer nonsense, some would say "sheer madness." From that point of view, the tens of thousands who have taken mind-training courses, and who are convinced of the reality of some or all of the above claims, have been programmed into a serious delusional system and can be expected sooner or later, if rationality is not reestablished, to develop, in consequence, some degree of neurosis or psychosis.

From a *psychosomatic* point of view, it might be acceptable to hypothesize that one could learn to manipulate certain normally unconscious psychological processes whose physiological correlates are thereby brought under control, that is, item (a) above might be accepted, but items (b) through (d) would be considered to be belief in sheer nonsense, which, if persisted in, would probably lead to mental or physical breakdown.

From the *parapsychological* point of view, none of the items listed above is at variance with data accumulated in the last fifty years indicating that such events are possible or at least worthy of hypothesis testing, even though not statistically probable.

In an attempt to evaluate mind-training, all scientists are not equally qualified. Scientists who subscribe exclusively to the traditional psychological or the psychosomatic views are in main those who either (a) have not studied the paranormal data and literature, (b) have had no spontaneous paranormal events in their own lives (that they admit, at least), (c) have not developed their own existential sensitivities and knowledge, or (d) all or some combination of the above. A probable example of this type of "scientist" is E. U. Condon, the former head of the National Bureau of Standards. According to McConnell (1970), Condon made the following pronouncement:

> Flying saucers and astrology are not the only pseudo-sciences which have a considerable following among us. There used to be spiritualism, there continues to be extrasensory perception, psychokinesis, and a host of others. . . . Where corruption of children's minds is at stake, I do not believe in freedom of the press or freedom of speech. In my view, publishers who publish or teachers who teach any of the pseudo-sciences as established truth should, on being found guilty, be publicly horsewhipped, and forever banned from further activity in these usually honorable professions. [p. 26]

Opinions from such scientists, who apparently have no adequate existential or experiential base, or who have not done their homework in the field of parapsychology, or who may (in some cases) have unconscious fears of the subject, are not appropriate here. The following is written, therefore, for those who can consider the parapsychological hypothesis without doing violence to their belief structure.

To continue then from the parapsychological viewpoint, the main questions that must be raised about commercial mind-training programs are (1) judged by professionals rather than entrepreneurs, what is actually happening to students in regard to psychological, psychosomatic, and parapsychological events and accomplishments? (2) what are the dangers of hypnotic programming for the purpose of enhancing psychic development? (3) what is the level of responsibility of program organizers and associated teachers? (4) what mind-training techniques are safe as well as efficient in bringing a person to a level of psychic development that is not inappropriate for him? (5) what is the most responsible way of presenting mind-training and its various benefits to the public? and (6) how is the mind-training movement to be regulated in the interest of public welfare? Concerning these questions, the following comments might be made.

Hypnotic programming as used in the commercial courses has several defects, namely: (a) Many people are psychically catapulted, so to speak, into existential realms in which they cannot protect themselves from dangers arising either from within their own unconscious, or from psychic manipulation by other persons, or from "extrapersonal" sources (dangers inherent in so-called "astral" dimension). There is not time here to review the history of spiritualism since 1849 and the psychic disasters that often resulted from dabbling in the area of trance mediumship, but mental hospitals, even today, contain many people who "hear voices." These people usually cannot turn the voices off, cannot separate fact from fiction, have lost their "reality testing" powers, and often are obliged to act out "against their will" instructions they are "given." (b) Commercial mind-training students are often "programmed" in ways not appropriate to their own needs, nor at their own proper rates. What is proper for one can be disastrous for another. This hazard arises because, apart from the dangers of hypnotic penetration into "astral" levels of being, (c) many mind-training teachers are incompetent to work with people in matters where psychological and physical health are at stake. For example, former salesmen who have had a few courses in hypnotic programming are not qualified to work in this very delicate area of the human psyche with its psychosomatic correlates. (d) And most seriously, psychic submission may be enhanced in "astral" dimensions rather than powers of self-volition. This is the consensus of Eastern teachers who, it must be conceded, reflect much experimentation and experience over the centuries with training methods for self-mastery. It is admitted that psychosomatic *self*-regulation, achieved by any volitional method, is slow compared to submitting oneself to hypnotic instruction, i.e., turning the control of one's mind over to another person, but it is also maintained by the most accomplished teachers that the power of psychic self-determination is the *sine qua non* for safety in astral dimensions.

Concerning safety in "astral" dimensions, possibly the greatest specific danger associated with hypnotic submission in commercial mind-training programs lies in the developing, or obtaining, of psychic "advisors." They are the male and female assistants who "know everything," who at the deep "level" of mind advise the student, and sometimes tell him what to do.

In the *mediumistic* version of the parapsychological paradigm, these advisors, however constructed or found, may serve as masks for "entities" who may attempt (now that the student has become amenable to suggestion at the unconscious level) to control the student's mental, emotional, and physical behavior. The mediumistic concept will clearly be rejected by mind-training teachers because, if accepted, it would imply that these teachers might be responsible for serious problems in the lives of some of their trainees. The physical frontiers of our planet have presented many dangers to humans; can it be safely assumed that the inner frontier has no corresponding perils? Is it realistic to accept the assurances of commercial mind-training instructors that dangers that may be associated with "territorial invasion" by humans on "astral" levels are not possible? For those who accept the possibility of "enti-ties," is it safe to assume that only good, nice, and safe beings (like humans?) are functioning in "astral" dimensions? This would be a truly Ptolemaic assumption.

Regarding the hazards associated with the all-knowing advisors found at the deep "level," some time ago we pointed out to an acquaintance that friends of his who were students of one of the mind-training programs might consider being on guard against the possibility of mediumistic-like "possession" through the agency of the advisors. The upshot of this was that these students challenged their advisors, asked them to get out of their "psychic space." Eventually we received a letter saying:

> You may be interested in knowing that after I told my two close friends . . . the warning about the assistants . . . they both went down to their workshops and told their assistants to leave. In both cases a strong but eventually successful test of wills or something took place, with the assistants becoming very ugly and hostile in the process. However, they were finally forced to leave. . . . The wife later told me that before I had talked to them about it, she had been having increasing trouble getting to sleep at night or going down to her levels because of the appearance of hostile and ugly faces in her mind. It had become a serious problem. Afterwards she told me that since her assistants left she was no longer bothered by the faces, that they had disappeared. So perhaps it was fortunate for them that you gave your warning.

Along this same line, one of our friends in the Bay Area, a counselor on psychological and religious problems, reports that at least a dozen of his clients are suffering from paranoid neuroses as a result of taking mind-training courses. Another acquaintance, a psychiatrist who took one of the commercial courses himself, reported to us that four of the thirty who went through the program became psychotic. Two of them had to be hospitalized. In part, he attributed this result to the psychic peculiarity of the instructor. Other stu-dents with whom we have discussed the "instructor effect" have reported similar events. Apparently a kind of psychic "transference" phenomenon can occur, a kind of "psychic pollution" can take place due to the unconscious receptivity of the subject to "extrasensory projection" by the hypnotist.

Another point: mind-training teachers often maintain that no harm can be done to another person by themselves or by their students, because they are programmed with the idea that if these "powers" are used for ignoble or selfish purposes they will be lost, but this is likely to be nonsense. Posthypnotic suggestions are notorious for their impermanence, so if real psychic "powers" are developed in students, it can be assumed that hypnotically-imposed restrictions on the use of such powers will not be long-lasting.

The examples given above indicate that whether one chooses to examine commercial mind-training methods from either the traditional psychological point of view or from the parapsychological point of view, there is risk involved for students. We do not presume to be able to answer all the questions raised, but when over 100,000 persons have already been processed through such mind-training programs (including 2000 high school girls at a school in Philadelphia in October, 1972), some questions should be asked. In view of the hazards associated with hypnotic programming in commercial mind-training courses, the present writers believe that hypnosis as a technique for inducing self-awareness and parapsychological faculties is not adequately safe and should be discarded.

Does this mean that there is no use for hypnosis? Not at all, no more than there is no use for surgery. But even as surgery has particular use in acute situations, where something must be done or else unbearable pain, or permanent damage, or death may occur, so also with hypnosis. For *chronic* situations, however, those which are characteristic of most psychosomatic diseases, nonhypnotic volitional training programs such as those employing biofeedback are more desirable. For exploring in psychic domains, new and safe training methods are being developed by Dialogue House and Psychosynthesis, for example, and through research in brain-wave training. Other safe methods also exist, as is well known, such as the various forms of yoga meditation. In all of these methods, both old and new, accent is placed on learning to handle psychological and physiological problems through voluntary control at a rate consistent with one's capacity for self-protection.

Spiritual teachers concerned with the development of inner awareness have always excluded hypnosis as a technique, both in the East and in the West, not because it was not understood, but because it *was* understood. Self-development and programming by another were considered antithetical. There is no logical reason to assume that things are now different merely because we are in the twentieth century and people are in a hurry, wish to have immediate results, and perhaps even hope to get something without effort. Hypnotic programming (like LSD) has convinced many people that an inner terrain exists, and in this way it has been instrumental in drawing attention to an important dimension of human life, but it is also important that we now look at the entire area of "inner exploration" and, in as balanced a way as possible, evaluate the many programs that are being offered for penetration into hitherto arcane dimensions of the psyche. Commercialism should not enter into such a vitally important matter. Commercialism often results in (a) false and misleading use of scientific terms, such as "alpha and theta brainwave training," and distortion of what is actually accomplished by such training, (b) exaggerated claims for "powers" that can be obtained by anyone who pays the price and takes the course, (c) stressing of powers not appropriate to certain persons, such as the ability to diagnose and treat diseases, and (d) undue emphasis on large enrollment in courses in order to earn more money, rather than to be of service. Large enrollment interferes with one-to-one contact between teachers and students so that whatever problems arise are unlikely to be properly handled, even if the teacher has the necessary skill.

In short, commercialism in the mind-training field does not lead in the direction of high responsibility and service, and this raises the very important question about the manner in which regulation can best be established in the mind-training movement. We are of the opinion that if responsible control is not established quite soon by those already involved, government agencies will step in and provide regulation in the interest of public welfare.

In our estimation, a list of positive guidelines to follow in establishing an "ideal training method" might include the following items:

1. Make it possible for each person to discover "himself" at a proper rate, that is, penetrate into the unconscious at a rate consistent with his ability to keep his feet on the ground, keep his reality-testing powers intact. This means that those for whom psychic unfolding would lead to destructive neuroses or psychoses should obtain only those insights and awarenesses which, in the usual therapeutic sense, would help integrate and bring under control various discordant sections of the personality.

2. The student should be shielded by the training method from imperfections of the teacher that might otherwise become part of the student's "psychic atmosphere" and hinder his progress.

3. Teachers should be ranked or evaluated according to their level of insight and awareness so that as each student progresses existentially, he has a properly qualified *human* advisor with whom to talk.

4. The student should be passed on from teacher to teacher, so to speak, as rapidly as his experiences require more advanced advice or suggestion (not analysis or programming).

5. Training centers for self-awareness should be located within access of anyone interested in participating in the program and should be established on a *nonprofit* basis.

References

Assagioli, R. *Psychosynthesis.* New York: Hobbs, Dorman, 1965.

Aurobindo (Sri). *The Synthesis of Yoga.* Pondicherry, India: Sri Aurobindo Ashram Press, 1955. Can be obtained from the California Institute of Asian Studies, San Francisco, California

Barber, T. X. et al. (Eds.). *Biofeedback & Self-Control, 1970, An Aldine Annual.* Chicago: Aldine-Atherton, 1971.

Beloff, J. *The Existence of Mind.* New York: Citadel Press, 1964.

Gill, M., & Brenman, M. *Hypnosis and Related States.* New York: John Wiley & Sons, 1959.

Green, E., Green, A., & Walters, E. Voluntary control of internal states: Psychological and physiological. *Journal of Transpersonal Psychology,* Vol. II, 1970.

Hilgard, E. Hypnosis. *Annual Review of Psychology,* Vol. 16. Palo Alto: Annual Reviews, 1965.

Jacobson, E. *Progressive Relaxation.* Chicago: University of Chicago Press, 1938.

Kamiya, J., et al. (Eds.). *Biofeedback & Self-Control, An Aldine Reader.* Chicago: Aldine-Atherton, 1971.

Luthe, Wolfgang (Ed.). *Autogenic Therapy,* Volumes I–VI. New York: Grune and Stratton, 1969.

Marcuse, F. L. *Hypnosis, Fact and Fiction.* Baltimore: Penguin Books, 1959.

McConnell, R. A. *ESP Curriculum Guide.* New York: Simon & Schuster, 1970.

Myers, F. W. H. *Human Personality and Its Survival of Bodily Death.* New York: Longmans, Green, 1954.

Schultz, J. H., & Luthe, W. *Autogenic Training: A Psychophysiologic Approach in Psychotherapy.* New York: Grune and Stratton, 1959.

Carl Simonton

The Role of the Mind in Cancer Therapy

I BECAME INVOLVED in cancer research in 1966. By 1969, I was very disappointed and disturbed. I had gone into medicine with the hope of being able to help people obtain better health, and I had addressed myself to cancer research with the hope of making some major breakthrough in the field of cancer therapy. As I got further into medicine, I discovered that it was very difficult to help people in the way that I had hoped to help them. On every hand I was being shown that it was impossible, or at least nearly impossible, to make any major breakthroughs in the field of cancer research therapy. I am sure most physicians go through some degree of this when they find out that the good they are able to do is much less than they had hoped it would be. While the young physician is under all the pressures of current concepts and limitations both from the system itself and the people who teach him, at the same time he feels a tremendous responsibility to make right decisions. He *must* always be right, for fear that in being wrong he may endanger someone's health or life. This fear causes him to accept the medical teachings that are given to him. He hesitates to think much on his own for fear his wrong thinking may cause further ill health, or ultimately death on the part of a patient. This feeling is largely generalized in our thinking, and during these focal years we have a tendency to be very closed-minded because of this tremendous, overwhelming fear.

Much of my thinking along these lines was changing during 1969, when I happened to hear a speech by a very prominent immunotherapist in Portland. He was speaking on a relatively unaccepted theory at that time, a theory that everyone has cancer many times during his or her lifetime and that there are two basic factors that cause clinical cancer to manifest itself; first, that particularly resistant cancer cells develop or particularly strong cancer cells invade the body; and, second, that the body's "immune mechanism," or host resistance, breaks down to some degree and allows these abnormal cells to grow into a size which is detectable. The same basic host defense mechanism is the one that destroys all abnormal cells presented to the body—bacteria, viruses, and the like.

He went on to talk about how he had developed the concept of taking terminal leukemic patients who had failed on all other forms of chemotherapy, making a solution of a concentrate of their abnormal white cells, and applying this solution to a prepared area of the skin in the hope of evoking an immune reponse that would in turn attack the leukemic cells causing the disease in the body. He indeed went ahead and developed this and achieved a 50% remission rate in these leukemic patients, which was extremely unusual for patients with this extent of disease. He then published his results, and other investigators immediately attempted to reproduce these results. But there is one essential difference between the initial investigator's approach and that of those attempting to reproduce his work, and that is that the idea was his idea to begin with—an idea about which he was very enthusiastic—a quality which is lacking in the approach of subsequent investigators.

The initial investigator had taken more pains to explain to the patients and their families the basic mechanisms and the expected results; he had taken a very much more intensified approach. The subsequent experiments by other investigators showed approximately one-half as good results as his initial work had shown. After these less favorable reports were published, subsequent investigators were even more skeptical of the possible good of such forms of therapy, and further investigation showed a corresponding decrease in response of the patients treated. So the results went from 50% remission by the initial investigator to approximately 25% remission with a mixed group of investigators, and down to a 5% to 10% remission rate on subsequent trials. As I listened to this I could see the similarities between this and the way in which so many initial investigators had worked on a drug for years and had shown us very good initial response, whereas subsequent investigators trying the same drug had achieved much less favorable results. Even further down the line, more people tried it, and their results were even less convincing. Most people explain this away on the part of the honesty and objectivity of the investigator; but it seems much easier to correlate it with interest, excitement, and enthusiasm—as well as belief—on the part of the investigator.

About the time that I heard this lecture I had become interested in the fact that approximately 2% to 5% of patients who have very extensive cancer have unexpectedly good results. I had decided to look into this and evaluate the patients that had such good responses to see if I could find a common denominator among them. I started tracking down patients in the greater Portland area. I talked with the patients, families of patients, and a large number of older physicians in the area, to evaluate their experiences. Very early in the course of my investigation, after I had accumulated relatively few cases, it became very clear to me that there was one strong factor that seemed to run through each history that I read, and that was the attitude on the part of the patient—his attitude toward the disease and his basic attitude toward life. I continued to accumulate more and more cases, and I continued to find this high correlation between attitude and response. It then behooved me to learn how to teach attitude—the will to live, or whatever you want to call it—to my patients.

I then went on a very unusual search—a search to find out how to teach attitude, or the will to live. Some of the experts teaching attitude, I soon found out, are in the sales field. Here you can tell the attitude of the salesman by his results in income. The methods centered largely around postive thinking and imagery.

During the time of exploring these areas, I came upon the terms "autogenic" and "biofeedback." The principles of biofeedback were just coming into their own. I found two allies; one was a pediatrician, and the other a neurologist, both at the university. Here we had access to all the gadgetry we needed, and as we started to apply the biofeedback principles to ourselves, amazing things started to happen. In attempting to obtain the desired EEG or EMG results, we found that relaxation was not as easy as we had supposed, but we did eventually gain some control over our blood pressure, temperature, and other physiological processes of the body. As we talked to other investigators who were working in these areas, it seemed that it would be equally as easy (or difficult) to gain control over the immune mechanisms, which are an exceedingly big factor in cancer.

While we were experimenting with biofeedback, I happened onto my first mind control course. I was extremely skeptical, for I thought their claims were ridiculous, and I also thought it was far too expensive. I met the instructor for the Portland, Seattle area, a young man of 23. My misgivings were increased, but I went ahead and took the course; and in spite of the instructor's youth and lack of credentials and all my skepticism, taking the course was like being shot from a slingshot. Everything really seemed to start happening. It was as though all the work I had gone through to learn to teach attitude to patients had been put together in this class. I completed the course on April 4, 1971, with a basically clear idea of how I was going to incorporate my previous month's work into medicine.

The following Monday I started the process with my first patient. In addition to the medical treatment, I explained what my thinking was. I told him how, through mutual imagery, we were going to attempt to affect his disease. He was a sixty-one-year-old gentleman with very extensive throat cancer. He had lost a great deal of weight, could barely swallow his own saliva, and could eat no food. After explaining his disease and the way radiation worked, I had him relax three times a day, mentally picture his disease, his treatment, and the way his body was interacting with the treatment and the disease, so that he could better understand his disease and cooperate with what was going on. The results were truly amazing. When I explained to my colleagues what I was doing, they said to me jokingly, "Why do you even bother to turn on the machine?" My response to that was, "I just don't know enough yet." That patient is now a year and a half post-treatment, with no evidence of cancer in his throat. He also had arthritis, and he used the same basic mental process and eliminated that.

This same man also had trouble with impotence. He had been impotent for over twenty years. It took him ten days of relaxing and mentally picturing this problem and the solution in his mind's eye, and he was able to resume intercourse with his wife. He now states he is able to have intercourse two or three times a week. So when he called me and told me about resolving his impotence, I had him explain how he did it, just in case I should need the techniques later on in my own life.

It was immediately after that that I was drafted. This was initially very upsetting to me, because I was concerned that I couldn't go on with my work in the military. These fears were unfounded, because I was sent to Travis Air Force Base, where there was a brand new department I was allowed to head. When I explained my basic approach to my commanding officer, he saw this as primarily attending to the psychological needs of the patient and was most receptive to my ideas.

At this time, I would like to tell you some of the results we have achieved at Travis Air Force Base. The first case is that of an Air Force navigator. He was a nonsmoker who had a squamous carcinoma in the roof of his mouth and also one that was larger in the back of his throat. The cancer in the roof of his mouth should have had a cure rate of 30% to 50%; the one in his throat one of about 5% to 40%. Collectively, however, the estimated cure rate would probably be around 5% to 10%, since it definitely worsens the situation to have two cancers arising at the same time.

I should emphasize that he was an extremely positive patient. He was also very cooperative, and after one week of treatment the tumor was beginning to shrink. After four weeks of treatment the ulceration had no growth evidence of tumor, and so it was doing essentially the same thing—showing a very dramatic response. It was generally outside my experience to get such dramatic response in two separate tumors in such a short time.

After one month there was one small ulceration, healing nicely, and about ten weeks after treatment the roof of his mouth was essentially normal in appearance. The truly beautiful thing was that the lesion in the throat showed the same response as the one in the mouth, and on routine examination it was impossible to tell where the throat tumor had been. Only three months after he had been taken off flying status, this gentleman had unanimous clearance from the head and neck tumor board to go back on flying status and resume his profession.

The second case is very unusual. This one involved a wart. The gentleman had had this wart treated for a year, and it had become progressively worse on all types of medical management. He was brought back from Vietnam for amputation of the finger because of pain. He also had a very large wart on the thumb of the opposite hand that we were not planning to treat initially; we were going to watch and see if the immune mechanism would be stimulated by treatment of the first wart.

The patient was extremely receptive, and as we started treating the wart on the index finger, we began to get a similar response on the untreated thumb, except that it lagged behind by about one to one and a half days. After one month of treatment, there was essentially no evidence of any warty tissue either on the treated index finger or the untreated thumb.

The next case is that of a large anal carcinoma in a psychotic black woman, fifty-five years old. She had a very extensive tumor, and she had large, clinically positive inguinal nodes that had not been biopsied. The tumor successively decreased in size at one week of treatment and at two weeks of treatment. At three weeks of treatment, most of the gross tumor was gone. At the completion of treatment after a four-and-a-half-week period there was no gross evidence of tumor, and the enlargement of the lymph nodes had nearly completely disappeared without treatment. Another interesting fact is that she had received a very high [x-ray] dose in this area, and the skin did not break down. To be able to give such a high dose locally with so little local reaction by normal tissue is also outside my previous experience. At about four weeks post-treatment, there was marked healing of the ulcerated areas, with little central ulceration remaining. Two weeks after that it was virtually totally healed, with no evidence of tumor.

The first fifty patients we treated at Travis were divided into attitude groups, going from double negative to double positive. Five members of the department graded these patients individually, and then we averaged the results. Next, we classified the results from poor to excellent. We found a direct line of correlation between poor attitudes and poor responses, with good attitudes correspondingly showing good responses. One exciting point here is that only four out of fifty patients had a poor response, and this includes all patients that came through the door for treatment, including very extensive disease. Out of the fifty, thirty-seven (or 74%) had either good or excellent responses; and 12% had excellent response.

When I was presenting this initially to General Reynolds, our hospital commander, his first question was about the nature of the disease and the seriousness of the disease in these twelve excellent responders. This is summarized in my paper; but briefly, eight of the twelve had less than a 50% chance for cure, and four of the twelve had better than a 50% chance for cure. Now, as you can see, we are talking only about response of the patient during treatment, and it is too early to make any implications as to possibilities for cure.

One case I would like to mention is that of a twenty-six-year-old pre-med student with Hodgkin's disease, which is cancer of the lymph nodes. He had been treated approximately two years previously and had now developed recurrent disease in previously treated areas—which presents, technically, a difficult management problem. He was in the middle of exams and wanted to wait two weeks before starting his radiation therapy, to which I was very agreeable. I merely asked him to start on his relaxation and mental imagery before he returned for the treatments. He was receptive to these ideas and left for his exams, agreeing to take time three times a day to work on his disease. When he returned two weeks later, he was excited. The disease had been getting progressively worse over a three months' period, and now he came back with the disease getting better. The lymph nodes had decreased in size, and his symptoms of fever and chills had subsided. We then discussed whether we wanted to start treatment immediately or wait and evaluate the situation in another week. We decided on the latter course, and one week later he returned, with the lymph nodes still getting progressively smaller. At this time, the regimen has been continued for four months, although he has had his ups and downs.

One example of a very rough period for him was when his brother, who uses drugs extensively, dropped in on him and was very negative about this type of approach. The brother did a great deal to disrupt his home life, and during this period of time his disease flared up. He has had two other episodes that were very stressful during which the disease did exacerbate; but at this time, now four months since we began, his lymph nodes are approximately one-half the size they were when I originally saw him. How far we will be able to go with this, I don't know; we are doing it one week at a time.

Another case I would like to share with you is that of a thirty-five-year-old lady who had a cervical carcinoma—a carcinoma of the uterus. She developed a very bad infection at the time diagnosis was made, and this is a very bad sign in my experience. As you know, patients developing serious wound infections go on to a very rapid downhill course. I was very pessimistic when I examined this lady with the gynecologist. He had previously examined the patient, and at this re-examination in my presence he made the statement that the tumor appeared somewhat smaller than it had two weeks previously. That surprised me but I took it with a grain of salt. I had her come back to my department approximately two weeks later. When I examined her then, the tumor had decreased by at least 50% of its volume.

This astounded me, and I immediately asked her if she had any idea why the tumor had decreased so markedly in size. Her statement was that she had heard that drinking grape juice could help tumors, and she had been drinking four glasses of grape juice a day. I could tell by the way she said it that she didn't really believe that this was what had caused the tumor to go down, but I didn't question her any further on the subject.

On a subsequent day, when I was getting ready to begin her treatment, I started to explain to her what I wanted her to do regarding her relaxation and imagery. She looked at me and said, "My, that sounds like meditation!" I said that it certainly could be considered meditation, and asked her why she made this statement. Her answer was that approximately a year previously she had begun reading Edgar Cayce's work and had started meditating on a regular basis, and it had changed her life. I then asked if she had been meditating regarding her tumor, to which she answered that indeed she had been, and she felt that that was why the tumor had gone down. When I asked her why she had told me it was the grape juice, she said she was afraid to tell me that she thought it was the meditation for fear I would ridicule her for doing it, and she felt very strongly about it.

Well, we continued with her treatments and had an excellent response. We were very excited to have found someone meditating on her own and having a tumor go away without any treatment, only the meditation, in a way that made sense to me.

Now the last case I am going to present I have chosen in order to show some of the problems that stand in the way of the patient's recovery. At the time I first saw this nineteen-year-old patient with advanced Hodgkin's disease, he was very near death. He had had the disease for two years and had been on almost every drug available. He was presented to me with an involvement of both kidneys, obstruction of his intestinal tract, and bleeding from the mouth and nose. He was barely conscious, and the first thing he said to me was, "I think I'm going to die." As I looked back at him, I said, "You are right—unless something changes."

One interesting thing I have discovered is that when patients are in this sort of semiconscious state they are, by and large, very receptive. I actually welcome patients who come to the department in this condition since their conscious resistance to what I am trying to do seems to be very much less. This patient was no exception, and we began to see a rapid change in his general condition. He recovered sufficiently to go home, but he was only home a little over a week when he was back in the hospital again. During this stay in the hospital, I got to know a great deal about the patient. When I asked him how badly he wanted to get well, he told me that he really didn't want to. He was so used to being sick after having been sick for two years that he could not even mentally see himself being well. He also stated that he enjoyed the sympathy he got from other people. He said, "My life is basically what I want. If I could just stay moderately sick and not be severely ill, it would be fine."

As we talked about his childhood, he mentioned to me that he had had several homosexual experiences and that these had been discovered by his parents. He had been teased a great deal by his whole family, and as a result his self-image was very poor. He felt that he was basically evil and did not deserve to live. We were able to work through a number of these problems, but it was only with great difficulty.

One of the most interesting stories that he related to me was his great feeling of lack of love and affection from his parents. He told me about how, when his older brother developed a kidney infection and was placed in a hospital, he had received a lot of attention from all the people around him. My patient was extremely jealous and so longed for this love and attention that at one time during this period he attempted to throw himself in front of a car while he was out playing, hoping to break his leg so that he could go to the hospital and get some attention.

Gaining intellectual insight into these problems is very valuable, but it is a long way from there to getting a patient well. We had this boy's family in and worked with them on several occasions, and it was dramatic to see the changes that occurred in the attitude of the whole family. I had not been aware previously of the many home situations where so little love is expressed outwardly and where such poor communications exist. I had come from a very loving home myself, and it was difficult for me to imagine that situations like this could exist. Since then it has become obvious to me that entire home situations must be changed in order to prevent the perpetuating of disease.

I have been pleased with the reception that presentations of my work have had at different places. I presented this material to the Bay Area Kaiser physicians, after which they even asked me if it would be possible for me to treat some of their lung cancer patients. This was a much warmer reception than I had anticipated. I was also pleased at my reception by the Santa Clara County Psychiatric Society when I presented my work to them.

The most difficult person for me to convince as to the validity of my work, however, has been my father. He is a Southern Baptist minister and thought for a while that I was practicing some pagan religion. He has been intermittently very ill for the past four years, being very near death on several occasions. He has severe lung disease, gall bladder disease, high blood pressure, and heart disease. It has become obvious to me that, in general, he has not been dealing with his stress very well.

During a recent serious episode of complete heart block, when his heart rate was approximately thirty beats a minute, he was approached by the cardiologist, who had him watch his television monitor and mentally picture his heartbeat in a relaxed state to see if he could affect the rate. He became very excited by the fact that he was able to affect his heart rate, and he suddenly realized that this was very similar to methods I had been talking about with him for the previous two years.

When he returned home he telephoned me and related this experience. He was now receptive to the idea of my coming to him and teaching him my complete basic approach to disease. The results have been extremely gratifying; he is now off his high blood pressure medicine, his general health is improving dramatically, and he states that he feels better than he has in two years.

One topic I am frequently required to address is that of medical or scientific proof. Before I began this study and had only the ideas, most of my colleagues told me that I would never be able to prove anything because there were too many variables involved. As I have accumulated more and more results, I still find that the question of scientific proof is a very difficult one. About a week ago I came across an article which meant a great deal to me, and I would like to share it with you.

The article was about a psychiatrist who was doing some rather unorthodox work with schizophrenic patients approximately twenty years ago and was obtaining some very good results. Because of the nature of his techniques, however, his colleagues were reluctant to listen to him. He wrote approximately ten articles on the subject, but their standard response was, "Well, you really haven't proven anything." So he continued his work and wrote about ten more articles, and people continued to say the same thing. He began to wonder just what it is that constitutes scientific proof. He did still more work and published more papers, with the same result. He became determined to investigate thoroughly this question of scientific proof.

Being the editor of a psychiatric journal, he decided to hold a symposium on the subject. He wrote letters to several leading scientists, asking for their participation in a study to determine what constitutes scientific proof. The first reply came from a man who sent a very short note: "The question," he wrote, "is much too difficult for me." He went on to say, briefly, that he doubted that he could make a significant contribution to so complex an issue.

This answer was more than the humility of a great man; it was more than the reflection of scientific honesty. It was at the root of a great man's whole philosophy of being. The letter was signed, "Albert Einstein."

References

Abse, D. W., Wilkins, M. M., Kirschner, G., Weston, D. L., Brown, R. S., and Buxton, W. D. Self-frustration, night-time smoking and lung cancer. *Psychosomatic Medicine, 34,* 395, 1972.

Andervont, H. B. Influence of environment on mammary cancer in mice. *National Cancer Institute, 4:* 579–581, 1944.

Bacon, C. L., Rennecker, R., and Cutler, M. A psychosomatic survey of cancer of the breast. *Psychosomatic Medicine, 14:* 453–460, 1952.

Bahnson, C. B. Psychophysiological complementarity in malignancies. *Annals of the New York Academy of Science, 164,* 319, 1969.

———. Second Conference on Psychophysiological Aspects of Cancer. *Annals of New York Academy of Sciences, 164,* 1969.

———. The psychological aspects of cancer. Paper presented at the American Cancer Society's 13th Science Writer's Seminar, 1971.

Bahnson, C. B. and Kissen, David M. Psychophysiological aspects of cancer. *Annals of the New York Academy of Sciences, 125,* 1966.

Bahnson, C. B. and Bahnson, M. B. Ego defenses in cancer patients. *Annals of the New York Academy of Science, 164,* 546, 1969.

Barrios, Alfred A. Hypnosis as a possible means of curing cancer. Unpublished manuscript, 1961.

_____. Hypnotherapy: A reappraisal. *Psychotherapy: Theory, Research, and Practice, 7,* 1970.

_____. Self-programmed control: A new approach to learning. Paper presented at the VI International Conference of Hypnosis, Uppsala, Sweden, 1973.

Bennett, Graham. Psychic and cellular aspects of isolation and identity impairment in cancer: A dialectic of alienation. *New York Academy of Sciences Annals, 164,* 352, 1969.

Booth, G. General and organic specific object relationships in cancer. *Annals of the New York Academy of Science, 164,* 568, 1969.

British Medical Journal. Editorial: The nervous factor in the production of cancer. *20,* 113, 1925.

Burrows, J. *A practical essay on cancer.* London, 1783.

Butler, B. The use of hypnosis in the case of cancer patients. *Cancer, 7,* 1, 1954.

Cutler, Max. The nature of the cancer process in relation to a possible psychosomatic influence. *The Psychological Variables in Human Cancer,* University of California Press, 1954.

Dorn, H. F. Cancer and the marital status. *Human Biology, 15,* 73–79, 1943.

Dunbar, F. Emotions and bodily changes: *A survey of literature-psychosomatic interrelationships 1910–1953;* 4th edition. New York: Columbia University Press, 1954.

Dunham, L. J. and Bailar, J. C. World maps of cancer mortality rates and frequency ratios. *Journal of the National Cancer Institute, 41,* 155, 1968.

Eliasberg, W. G. Psychotherapy in cancer patients. *Journal of American Medical Association, 147,* 525, 1951.

Evans, E. *A psychological study of cancer.* New York: Dodd, Mead, & Co. Inc., 1926.

Everson, T. C. and Cole, W. H. Spontaneous regression of cancer. *Philadelphia, 7,* 1966.

Ewing, J. *Causation, diagnosis and treatment of cancer.* Baltimore: Williams & Wilkins Co., 1931.

Ferracuti, F., Lotti, G. and Rizzo, G. Contributo all studio della psicologia del canceroso terminale. *Bollettino di Oncologia, 27,* 3–53, 1953.

Ferracuti, F., and Rizzo, G. Psychological patterns in terminal cancer cases. *Education & Psychology. Delhi, 2,* 26–36, 1955.

Fisher, S., and Cleveland, S. E. Relationship of body image to site of cancer. *Psychosomatic Medicine, 18,* 304–309, 1956.

Freud, S. Psychogenic visual disturbance according to psychoanalytical conceptions. In *Collected Papers.* Vol. 5. London: Hogarth Press, 1949.

Friedman, S. B., Glasgow, L. A. and Ader, R. Psychosocial factors modifying host resistance to experimental infections. *Annals of New York Academy of Sciences, 164,* 381–392.

The psychological variables in human cancer: A symposium presented at the Veterans Administration Hospital, Long Beach, Calif., Oct. 23, 1953 (Gengerelli, J. A., and Kirkner, F. J., eds.). Berkeley: University of California Press, 1954.

Greene, W. A., Jr. Psychological factors and reticuloendothelial disease. I. Preliminary observations on a group of males with lymphomas and leukemia. *Psychosomatic Medicine, 16,* 220–230, 1954.

————. The psychosocial setting of the development of leukemia and lymphoma. *Annals of the New York Academy of Science, 125,* 794, 1966.

Greene, W. A., Jr., Young, L. and Swisher, S. N. Psychological factors and reticuloendothelial disease. II. Observations on a group of women with lymphomas and leukemias. *Psychosomatic Medicine, 18,* 284–303, 1956.

Greene, W. A., Jr., and Miller, G. Psychological factors and reticuloendothelial disease. IV *Psychosomatic Medicine, 20,* 124–144, 1958.

Groddeck, G. *The book of the IT.* New York and Washington, D.C: Nervous and Mental Disease Publication Co., 1928.

Hagnell, O. The premorbid personality of persons who develop cancer in a total population investigated in 1947 and 1957. *Annals of the New York Academy of Science, 125,* 846, 1966.

Hedge, A. R. Hypnosis in cancer. *British Journal of Hypnotism, 12,* 2–5, 1960.

Hoffman, F. C. *The mortality from cancer throughout the world.* Newark, N. J.: Prudential Press, 1915.

————. *Some cancer facts and fallacies.* Newark, N. J.: Prudential Press, 1925.

Hughes, C. H. The relations of nervous depression toward the development of cancer. *St. Louis Medicine and Surgery Journal,* 1885.

Hutschnecker, A. *The will to live.* New York: Thomas Y. Crowell Co., 1953.

Kavetsky, R. E., Turkewich, N. M. and Balitsky, K. P. On the psychophysiological mechanism of the organism's resistance to tumor growth. *Annals of the New York Academy of Sciences, 125,* 933, 1966.

Kissen, D. M. Personality characteristics in males conducive to lung cancer. *British Journal of Medical Psychology, 36,* 27, 1963.

———. Psychosocial factors, personality and lung cancer in men aged 55–64. *British Journal of Medical Psychology, 40,* 29, 1967.

———. Relationship between lung cancer, cigarette smoking, inhalation and personality and psychological factors in lung cancers. *Annals of the New York Academy of Science, 164,* 535, 1969.

Kissen, D. M. and Eysenck, H. G. Personality in male lung cancer patients. *Journal of Psychosomatic Research, 6,* 123, 1962.

Kissen, D. M., Brown, R. I. F. and Kissen, Margaret. A further report on personality and psychological factors in lung cancers. *Annals of the New York Academy of Science, 164,* 535, 1969.

Klopfer, B. Psychological variables in human cancer. *Journal of Projective Techniques, 21,* 331–340, 1957.

Kowal, S. J. Emotions as a cause of cancer; eighteenth and nineteenth century contributions. *Psychoanalyt. Rev., 42,* 217–227, 1955.

La Barba, R. C. Experimental and environmental factors in cancer. *Psychosomatic Medicine, 32,* 259, 1970.

LeShan, L. and Worthington, R. E. Some psychologic correlates of neoplastic disease: preliminary report. *Journal of Clinical & Experimental Psychopath, 16:,* 281–288, 1955.

———. Loss of cathexes as a common psychodynamic characteristic of cancer patients. An attempt at statistical validation of a clinical hypothesis. *Psychol. Rep., 2* 183–193, 1956.

———. Personality as a factor in the pathogenesis of cancer. A review of the literature. *British Journal of Medical Psychology, 29,* 49–56, 1956.

———. Some recurrent life history patterns observed in patients with malignant disease. *Journal of Nervous Mental Diseases, 124,* 460–465, 1956.

———. A psychosomatic hypothesis concerning the etiology of Hodgkin's disease. *Psychol. Rep., 3,* 565–575, 1957.

———. Psychological states as factors in the development of malignant disease: A critical review. *Journal of the National Cancer Institute, 22,* 1959.

———. An emotional life history pattern associated with neoplastic disease. *Annals of the New York Academy of Sciences, 125,* 780–793, 1966.

———. A basic psychological orientation apparently associated with malignant disease. *The Psychiatric Quarterly, 35,* 314, 1961.

———. An emotional life-history pattern associated with neoplastic disease. *Annals of the New York Academy of Science, 125,* 807, 1966.

LeShan, L. and Gassmann, M. Some observations on psychotherapy with patients with neoplastic disease. *American Journal of Psychotherapy, 12,* 723–734, 1958.

Lombard, H. L. and Potter, E. A. Epidemiological aspects of cancer of the cervix; hereditary and environmental factors. *Cancer, 3,* 960–968, 1950.

Macdonald, I. Mammary carcinoma. *Surgery Gynecology and Obstetrics, 74,* 75, 1942.

MacMillan, M. B. A note on LeShan and Worthington's "Personality as a factor in the pathogenesis of cancer." *British Journal of Medical Psychology, 30,* 41, 1957.

Marcial, V. A. Socioeconomic aspects of the incidence of cancer in Puerto Rico. *Annals of the New York Academy of Science, 84,* 981, 1960.

Meerloo, J. The initial neurologic and psychiatric picture syndrome of pulmonary growth. *Journal of American Medical Association, 146,* 558–559, 1951.

———. Psychological implications of malignant growth; survey of hypotheses. *British Journal of Medical Psychology, 27,* 210–215, 1954.

Miller, F. R. and Jones, H. W. The possibility of precipitating the leukemia state by emotional factors. *Blood, 8,* 880–884, 1948.

Mitchell, J. S. Psychosomatic cancer research from the viewpoint of the general cancer field. *Psychosomatic Aspects of Neoplastic Disease, 215,* 1964.

Orbach, C. E., Sutherland, A. M. and Bozeman, M. F. Psychological impact of cancer and its treatment. *Cancer, 8,* 20, 1955.

Paget, J. *Surgical Pathology,* 2nd Ed. London: Longman's Green, 1870.

Parker, W. Cancer, *A study of ninety-seven cases of cancer of the female breast.* New York, 1885.

Parker, C. M., Benjamin, B., Fitzgerald, R. G. Broken hearts: a statistical study of increased mortality among widowers. *British Medical Journal, i,* 740, 1969.

Peller, S. Cancer and its relations to pregnancy, to delivery, and to marital and social status, cancer of the breast and genital organs. *Surg., Gynce. & Obst., 71,* 1–8, *71:* 181–186, 1940.

———. *Cancer in man.* New York International Univ. Press. 556, 1952.

Pendergrass, E. Presidential Address to American Cancer Society Meeting, 1959.

———. Host resistance and other intangibles in the treatment of cancer. *American Journal of Roentgenology, 85,* 891–896, 1961.

Quisenberry, W. B. Sociocultural factors in cancer in Hawaii. *Annals of the New York Academy of Science, 84,* 795, 1960.

Raef, Yehia. Psychosomatic aspects of cancer research—a literature survey. *National Federation of Spiritual Healers.,* n.d.

Rennecker, R. E. Countertransference reactions to cancer. *Psychosom. Med., 19,* 409–418, 1957.

Revici, E. A new concept of the pathophysiology of cancer with implications for therapy. New Haven: Yale Univ. Press, n.d.

Reznikoff: Psychological factors in breast cancer—a preliminary study of some personality trends in patients with cancer of the breast. *Psychosomatic Res., 2,* 56–60, 1957.

Sacerdote, Paul. The uses of hypnosis in cancer patients. *Annals of the New York Academy of Sciences, 125,* 1011–1012, 1966.

Schmale, A. H. and Iker, H. The psychological setting of uterine cervical cancer. *Annals of the New York Academy of Science, 125,* 807, 1966.

Schneck, J. M. *Hypnosis in modern medicine.* Springfield, Ill.: Charles Thomas, 1959.

Simonton, O. Carl. Meditation and cancer. Tape of science of mind symposium: Scientific approach to spiritual healing. *Science of Mind Magazine,* 1973.

Simonton, O. Carl and Tatera, Bernard. The role of increased fractionation and patient attitude in radiation therapy. Unpublished report, Air Force Base Medical Center, California, 1973.

Snow, H. The reappearance (recurrence) of cancer after apparent extirpation. London: J. & A. Churchill, 1870.

––––––. Clinical notes on cancer. London: J. & A. Churchill, 1883.

––––––. Cancer and the cancer process. London: J. & A. Churchill, 1883.

Solomon, G. F. Emotions, stress, the central nervous system, and immunity. *New York Academy of Science Annals, 164,* 335–343, 1969.

Solomon, G. F. and Moos, R. H. Emotions, immunity and disease. *Archives of General Psychiatry, 11,* 657, 1964.

Stephenson, J. H. and Grace, W. J. Life stress and cancer of the cervix. *Psychosom. Med., 16,* 287–294, 1954.

Surman, O. S., Gotlieb, J. K., Hochet, T. P. and Silverberg, E. L. Hypnosis in the treatment of warts. *Arch. Gen. Psychotherapy, 28,* 439–441, 1973.

Tarlau, M. and Smalheiser, I. Personality patterns in patients with malignant tumors of the breast and cervix; exploratory study. *Psychosom. Med., 13,* 117–121, 1951.

Tromp. S. W. Psychosomatische faktoren und der Krebs (insbesondere der lunge und der mamma) *Medizinische,* 443–447, 1955–March 26.

Trunnell, J. B. *Theories of the origin of cancer.* Paper read at the Texas Conference on Psychosomatic Implications in Cancer, Dallas, Sept. 1956.

Wainwright, J. M. A comparison of conditions associated with breast cancer in Great Britain and America. *American Journal of Cancer, 15,* 2610, 1931.

Weitzenhoffer, A. M. *Hypnotism: An objection study in suggestibility.* New York: John Wiley and Sons, 1953.

West, P. M. Origin and development of the psychological approach to the cancer problems. *The Psychological Variables in Human Cancer,* University of Calif. Press, 1–16, 1954.

West, P. M., Blumberg, E. M., and Ellis, F. W. An observed correlation between psychological factors and growth rate of cancer in man. *Cancer Res., 12,* 306–307, 279, 1952.

Wheeler, J. I., Jr., and Caldwell, B. M. Psychological evaluation of women with cancer of the breast and of the cervix. *Psychosom. Med., 17,* 256–268, 1955.

Section IV

NORMAL WAKING consciousness is but one special type of consciousness, while all around it, separated from it by the narrowest of margins, are other forms of consciousness of entirely different kinds. These range from sublimity at one end of their spectrum to madness at the other.

We know that the ultraconscious experience can make the mind or break it. But we don't know why nor how. Undoubtedly heredity, predisposition, and psychodynamic influences play a part, but many factors still remain unknown. When the answer is found, we shall have the key to mind and consciousness with their remarkable capacity for awareness—and, perhaps, to the enigma of life itself.

Altered states of consciousness (ASC), whether drug-induced or otherwise, are multipotential experiences with many factors influencing the outcome. They may be psychedelic (mind-expanding) or psycholytic (mind-destroying). One may precede the other, they may merge together, or stand alone. Or the experience may be as evanescent as a dream, which is in itself a psychotomimetic event. In altered states of consciousness we may indeed find William James's "snakes and seraphs" abiding side by side.

W. H. Belk, a businessman and scholar with a profound knowledge of religion and parapsychology, stated that most psychics he has known were egocentric, narrow-minded, schizoid to some degree, and had suffered a head injury or other serious illness at some point in their lives.[1] But he also agreed

---

[1] This is from an undated letter to Dr. Berthold Schwarz sometime in the fall of 1966. Also see W. H. Belk, *A Cosmic Road Map and Guide Analysis,* Charlotte, N. C.: Belk Foundation, 1974.

that many normal and sensible people in all walks of life can experience transitory hallucinations and other distortions of ordinary consciousness without harm. In fact, some have even been elevated by such occurrences to a level where the world became transfigured and acquired an undreamed of beauty and relevance.

Scientific replication of physical disease is an essential factor in discovering its cause and cure. The same is true of mental illness. Whatever else may be said of LSD and other psychotomimetic drugs, they are important elements in the scientific replication of mental pathology, especially in schizophrenia, the greatest menace of them all.

A gifted young friend of mine, who broke down under the impact of his genius, wrote a poem before the night closed in that could serve as a challenge to all of us:

> There was a time when music flowed
> Like a dark volcanic wine
> Through the cool and caverny recesses
> And crypts of my secret soul—
> Then over earth and over sky
> A distant thunder rolled,
> And finned thoughts flashed through that stream,
> Weird fish that darted blind—
> And in the cavern of my mind
> An awful night held sway,
> The entrance blocked by giant pines
> With all their roots uptorn—
> Where was the hand of God to roll
> Those monstrous trunks away?
> Where was the hand of God to still
> The terror yet unborn?[2]

I can find no better way to end my discourse than with this promise: We shall never cease looking for the answer. We shall never go back to our armchair until we find it.

---

[2]Dean, S. R., "Schizophrenia: a major public health problem. *Connecticut Medicine,* 1959, 23:328–331.

Stanislav Grof

Varieties of Transpersonal Experiences: Observations from LSD Psychotherapy

UNTIL RECENTLY the theoretical structures of psychiatry and psychology were based on the observations of a rather limited range of mental phenomena and human experiences. Very little systematic and serious attention was given to a variety of phenomena that have been described over centuries within the framework of the world's great religions, as well as temple mysteries, mystery religions, initiation rites, and various mystical schools. There has been a tendency in contemporary science to label such experiences simply as psychotic and to consider them manifestations of mental illness, because similar or identical experiences can frequently be observed in schizophrenic patients. Such classification has in the past almost precluded unbiased scientific study of these phenomena and acceptance of their possible relevance for the understanding of human personality and the nature of man. When such study was attempted, it focused frequently on peripheral aspects, and inadequate and often superficial explanatory hypotheses were offered by the investigators. This can be best illustrated by Freud's attempts to explain religious phenomena; obviously underestimating the paramount role of firsthand visionary experience for the development of religions, he equated religion with symbolic rituals and tried to explain it in terms of unresolved conflicts of the child's psyche and in terms of infantile sexuality (Freud, 1952).

In this situation, only some rather exceptional individual investigators have been able to do pioneering work in exploring certain territories of the human mind as yet uncharted by occidental psychiatry and psychology. William James' (1902) book on the varieties of religious experiences and Marghanita Laski's (1962) book on ecstasy have become classics in the field. Roberto Assagioli, the founder of psychosynthesis (1965), has recognized the experiences mentioned above and integrated them into a comprehensive system of personality theory and psychotherapy. Abraham Maslow (1969) laid the foundations of a new concept of psychology and of the nature of man based on observations of spontaneously occurring peak experiences. In his approach, these experiences are considered as supranormal, rather than pathological phenomena, and have important implications for the theory of self-actualization (Maslow, 1964). The most famous and systematic attempt to revise our concepts of the dimensions of human personality was made by Carl Gustav Jung, the founder of analytical psychology (Jung, 1959). Within his system, the narrow concept of the human unconscious as described by Freud has been considerably expanded to encompass the collective and racial unconscious and a variety of transindividual, primordial, experiential patterns, the archetypes.

The last decade has been a period of rather dramatic changes in the field of psychology and psychiatry, both in theory and in practice. The experimentation with psychedelic substances as well as their widespread abuse has confronted the professionals with a variety of observations and experiences for which the existing theoretical frameworks appeared to be too narrow and inadequate. At the same time revolutionary psychotherapeutic techniques have been developed, such as Gestalt psychotherapy, bioenergetics, encounter groups, marathon groups, etc. These new techniques have been able to induce in a relatively short time a variety of experiences that were only infrequently and exceptionally observed in conventional psychoanalytically oriented psychotherapy; some of them bear a striking similarity to the phenomena occurring in psychedelic sessions or those described within the framework of various religious and mystical systems. In addition, a variety of laboratory techniques have been developed by which similar experiences can be produced with a reasonable degree of consistency. Such techniques include, for example, sensory deprivation or sensory overload, use of alpha and theta feedback for voluntary control of internal states, new modifications of hypnosis, use of various kinesthetic devices, etc. The picture of this period of transformation and fermentation in psychology ad psychiatry would be incomplete without mentioning the striking increase of interest in ancient religious systems and Oriental spiritual disciplines among mental health professionals as well as laymen.

In the last five years these previously isolated efforts of individual investigators started to converge, and the foundations were laid for a new interdisciplinary approach to the study of consciousness. The annual Conferences on Voluntary Control of Internal States held at Council Grove, Kansas, made it possible for researchers from various scientific disciplines interested in the study of altered states of consciousness to get together for exchange of information and to make the first attempts at preliminary formulations in this new scientific field. Two new journals were established focusing primarily on publications in this area, the *Journal for the Study of Consciousness* and the *Journal of Transpersonal Psychology*. Several of the major professional meetings have had in recent years sections dedicated specifically to lectures and panel discussions on so-called transpersonal psychology. Recently Anthony Sutich announced the birth of a new organization specializing in this field, the Association for Transpersonal Psychology.

However, in spite of the fact that the terms *transpersonal experiences* and *transpersonal psychology* have been used quite frequently in a number of papers and professional discussions, no systematic effort has been made, to my knowledge, to define and describe transpersonal experiences. In this paper I would like to make such an attempt using the observations from my LSD research.

For more than fifteen years, experimental research in psychotherapy with LSD and other psychedelic substances has been the major area of my professional interest. During these years, I have personally conducted over 2000 psychedelic sessions and, in addition, had the privilege of access to records from over 1300 sessions run by several of my colleagues in Europe and in the United States. The majority of the subjects in these sessions were patients with a wide variety of emotional disorders, such as severe psychoneuroses, psychosomatic disorders, borderline psychoses and various forms of schizophrenia, sexual deviations, alcoholism, and narcotic drug addiction. Another rather large category of these subjects was that of "normal" volunteers—psychiatrists, psychologists, students, and nurses who asked for psychedelic sessions for training purposes; painters, sculptors, and musicians seeking artistic inspiration; philosophers and scientists from various disciplines interested in insights that the psychedelic experiences have to offer; and priests and theologians willing to explore the mystical and religious dimensions of these experiences. A small fraction of the sessions were conducted with patients suffering from a terminal disease and facing impending death, in particular with cancer patients (Grof et al., 1971).

During the early years of my LSD research when I worked in the Psychiatric Research Institute in Prague, most of the subjects received repeated medium dosages of LSD (100–250 μg) within the framework of analytically oriented psychotherapy (the psycholytic approach). In psycholytic treatment, the LSD sessions are given after 2–3 weeks of preparatory psychotherapy. A psycholytic series can consist of 15–80 LSD sessions usually with an interval of 1–2 weeks between sessions. Intensive psychotherapeutic help is offered to the patient during the drug sessions as well as in the intervals between the sessions. This method represents an intensification and acceleration of dynamic psychotherapy. According to the nature of the emerging unconscious material, Freudian, Rankian, or Jungian approaches might be used in various stages of the treatment. Since 1967 when I came to the United States, I have been using mostly high dosages of LSD (300–500 μg) in a special set and setting, aimed at facilitating a religious experience (the psychedelic approach). In the latter approach, the use of eyeshades, stereophonic earphones, and music of special selection was an important part of the treatment procedure.

I have spent many hours studying and analyzing the material from the LSD sessions obtained in this research. In several papers (Grof, 1970a, b, c, 1971) and in a book that is in press (Grof, in press), I have tried to conceptualize some of the clinical observations that seem to facilitate the understanding of the LSD reaction and that have a bearing on the theory of psychotherapy and on personality theory. In these papers I have mentioned and briefly described a variety of transpersonal experiences that are without doubt the most interesting phenomena observed in psychedelic sessions. Because of the general nature of these previous publications, a systematic and detailed discussion of transpersonal experiences was not included.

A Definition of Transpersonal Experience

It seems appropriate to introduce a discussion of transpersonal experiences by an attempt at their definition and description. Transpersonal experience is then defined as an experience involving *an expansion or extension of consciousness beyond the usual ego boundaries and the limitations of time and space.*

In the "normal," or usual, state of consciousness, the individual experiences himself as existing within the boundaries of his physical body (the body image), and his perception of the environment is restricted by the physically determined range of his exteroceptors; both his internal perception and his perception of the environment are confined within the usual space-time boundaries. In psychedelic transpersonal experiences, one or several of these limitations appear to be transcended. In some cases, the subject experiences loosening of his usual ego boundaries, and his consciousness and self-awareness seem to expand to include and encompass other individuals and elements of the external world. In other cases, he continues experiencing his own identity but at a different time, in a different place, or in a different context. In yet other cases, the subject experiences a complete loss of his own ego identity and a complete identification with the consciousness of another entity. Finally, in a rather large category of these psychedelic transpersonal experiences (archetypal experiences, encounters with blissful and wrathful deities, union with God, etc.), the subject's consciousness appears to encompass elements that do not have any continuity with his usual ego identity and cannot be considered simple derivatives of his experiences in the three-dimensional world.

Since the concept of normal or usual consciousness was introduced in the above discussion, it seems appropriate to mention the relationship between so-called altered states of consciousness and so-called transpersonal experiences. Although there is considerable overlap between these two categories of experiences, they do not appear to be identical. The term "altered states of consciousness" encompasses transpersonal experiences; there are, however, certain types of experiences that can be labeled altered states of consciousness, but do not meet the criteria for being transpersonal. For example, a vivid and complex reliving of a childhood memory occurs in an altered state of consciousness, but is not necessarily a transpersonal experience.[1] The same is true, for example, for various fantasy plays and symbolic experiences resulting from the use of the technique of induced affective imagery. Similarly, a primarily aesthetic experience involving visions of colors, ornamental patterns, and geometrical structures in psychedelic sessions would have to be labeled an altered state of consciousness, but would not meet the criteria of transpersonal experience as defined above.

Description, Discussion, and Some Clinical Examples

In the following text, transpersonal experiences occurring in psychedelic sessions with LSD and other substances will be described, briefly discussed, and some of them illustrated by clinical examples. The question naturally occurs as to what extent the definition and description of transpersonal experiences from psychedelic sessions can be applied to transpersonal experiences occurring under different circumstances. All the experimental and clinical evidence indicates that the psychedelic drugs are most likely only catalysts, or

---

[1]Even reliving of childhood memories in psychedelic sessions can, however, involve transpersonal elements; in the process of working through a traumatic incident from the past, the subject frequently has to re-experience the roles of *all* the participants involved in such a situation.

unspecific amplifiers, activating deep levels of the human unconscious. In this sense, they are truly "mind manifesting" agents and can be seen as important tools for investigation of the human mind. From the phenomenological point of view, it does not seem to be possible to distinguish the experiences in psychedelic sessions from similar experiences occurring under different circumstances, such as instances of so-called spontaneous mysticism, experiences induced by various spiritual practices, and phenomena induced by new laboratory techniques. The multilevel nature and the intensity of the psychedelic experiences make it possible to examine the complex mutual interrelationships among various categories of transpersonal experiences and to study various natural experiential patterns. There seems to be good reason to believe that the description and eventual classification of transpersonal experiences from the data of psychedelic research will be relevant to similar efforts with data on transpersonal experience obtained under a variety of nondrug conditions.

Perinatal Experiences

Several rather important types of transpersonal experiences can be referred to as perinatal experiences, because many LSD subjects associated them with or related them to the circumstances of biological birth. From a logical point of view, they should still be considered personal experiences because they reflect the early biological history of the individual. There are, however, several reasons for labeling them as transpersonal experiences. They are related to early periods of development which are traditionally considered beyond the possibility of memory recording or recall. Vivid and complex pictorial reliving of a past event (as compared to a mere recall) is in itself beyond the usual realm of personal experience. In addition, biological and emotional reexperiencing of various facets of the birth trauma represents only one important aspect of the perinatal experiences. The LSD subjects experiencing various perinatal patterns describe quite consistently that they are accompanied by other important categories of transpersonal experiences, such as the experience of spiritual death and rebirth, encounter with the archetypal images of the Terrible Mother and the Great Mother, elements of the collective and racial unconscious, identification with other persons or groups of persons, etc. In the following text, the perinatal transpersonal experiences will be described in a sequence corresponding to the stages of delivery from which they can be logically derived. The hypothetical significance of perinatal experiences for personality theory and psychopathology was outlined in previous publications and expressed in the concept of the so-called Basic Perinatal Matrices (BPM) (Grof, in press).

Experience of Cosmic Unity

This important transpersonal experience seems to be related to the primal union with mother, the original condition of the intrauterine existence during which the child and his mother form a symbiotic unity. The LSD subjects frequently related this experience to the "good womb," an intrauterine experience in the absence of any noxious stimuli. In such a situation the conditions for the child are optimal, involving security, satisfaction of all needs, and undifferentiated ecstatic feelings. The basic characteristics of this experience are transcendence of the subject-object dichotomy, exceptionally strong positive affect (peace, tranquility, serenity, bliss), a special feeling of sacredness, transcendence of time and space, experience of pure being ("eternity now and infinity here"), and a richness of insights of cosmic relevance. This type of tension-free melted ecstasy can be referred to as "oceanic ecstasy." With eyes closed, the cosmic unity is experienced as an independent complex experiential pattern. With the eyes open, it results in an experience of merging with the environment and unity with the perceived objects. It is basically this experience that is described by Walter Pahnke's mystical categories (Pahnke & Richards, 1966) and to which Abraham Maslow refers as "peak experiences" (Maslow, 1969). In psychedelic sessions, it seems to be closely related to the "good womb" experiences, "good breast" experiences, and to happy childhood memories. It also appears to be a rather important gateway to a variety of other transpersonal experiences, such as ancestral memories, elements of collective and racial unconscious evolutionary memories, archetypal experiences, etc.

Experience of Cosmic Engulfment

This experiential pattern appears to be related to the very onset of delivery. The previous harmony and equilibrium of the intrauterine existence is disturbed, at the beginning by various alarming signals of a biochemical and physiological nature, later by mechanical muscular contractions. This situation is subjectively experienced as an imminent threat of a vital danger. There is a high amount of anxiety, but its source cannot be identified and the atmosphere of insidious danger can result in paranoid ideation. Not infrequently the subject, from the adult level, reports experiencing evil influences coming from members of secret organizations, inhabitants of other planets, noxious radiation, gases, etc. Intensification of this experience typically results in the vision of a gigantic and irresistible whirlpool, a cosmic maelstrom sucking the subject and his world relentlessly to its center. A frequent experiential variation of this dangerous engulfment is that of being swallowed and incorporated by a terrifying monster (such as a giant dragon, python, octopus, whale, or spider). A less dramatic form of the same experience seems to be the theme of descent into the underworld and encounter with various monstrous entities.

Experience of "No Exit" or Hell

This experience can be logically related to the first clinical stage of delivery, when the uterine contractions encroach on the fetus and cause his total constriction, but the uterine cervix is still closed and the way out is not yet open. This experience is usually characterized by a striking darkness of the visual field and rather sinister and ominous colors. The subjects feel encaged and trapped in a claustrophobic, no-exit situation and experience incredible psychological and physical tortures. Typically this situation is totally unbearable and at the same time appears to be endless and hopeless; no possibility of escape can be seen either in time or in space. Typically the subjects feel that even suicide would not terminate it and bring relief.

The experience of agony usually has many biological concomitants (such as concerns about the heart beat, problems with respiration, feelings of general oppression, profuse sweating, etc.) and is usually accompanied by fear of death. This immediate and profound encounter with death has two typical consequences: the opening of areas of religious experiences intrinsic to the human personality make-up and unrelated to previous education and background; and a painful existential crisis where all values in human life and the meaning of life itself are seriously questioned.

This experiential pattern can be experienced on several different levels; these levels can be experienced separately, simultaneously, or in an alternating fashion. The deepest level is related to various concepts of hell—a situation of unbearable suffering that will never end, as it has been depicted by various religions of the world. In a more superficial version of the same experiential pattern, the subject looks at the situation in this world and sees our planet as an apocalyptic place full of terror, suffering, wars, epidemics, accidents, and natural catastrophes. Existence in this world appears to be completely meaningless, nonsensical, and absurd, and the search for any meaning in human life completely futile. The world and human existence are seen as though through a negatively biased stencil; the subject appears to be blinded to any positive aspects of life. In the most superficial form of this experiential pattern, the individual sees his own concrete life situation in terms of circular patterns and as completely unbearable and full of insoluble problems.

Agonizing feelings of metaphysical loneliness, alienation, helplessness, hopelessness, inferiority, and guilt are a standard part of these experiences. The symbolism that most frequently accompanies this experiential pattern involves the crucifixion and the suffering of Christ ("Father why hast Thou forsaken me?") and his visions in the Garden of Gethsemane; the Biblical story of the expulsion from Paradise; images of hells from various religions; the concept of the Dark Night of the Soul; Greek mythological figures from Hades (Sisyphus, Tantalos, Ixion, Prometheus, etc.) as well as the Buddha's concept of suffering as expressed in his Four Noble Truths.

The most important characteristic that differentiates this pattern from the following one is the unique emphasis on the role of the victim and the fact that the situation is unbearable, inescapable, and eternal—there is no way out either in space or in time.

Experience of the Death-Rebirth Struggle

Many aspects of this experiential pattern can be understood if we relate it to the second clinical stage of delivery. In this stage the uterine contractions continue, but the cervix stands wide open, and the gradual and difficult propulsion through the birth canal occurs. There is an enormous struggle for survival, mechanical crushing pressures, and a high degree of suffocation. In the terminal phases of delivery, the fetus can experience immediate contact with a variety of biological material such as blood, mucus, fetal liquid, urine, and even feces.

From the experiential point of view, this pattern is rather complex; it involves a variety of phenomena on different levels which can be arranged in a typical experiential sequence. The most important characteristic of this pattern is the atmosphere of a titanic fight. Condensation and explosive release of immense energy is experienced, and the subject describes feeling powerful currents of energy streaming through his whole body. Visions typically accompanying these experiences involve various dynamic geometrical images in rich colors, exploding volcanoes or atomic bombs, launched missiles, gigantic fires, dramatic scenes of war, destruction, power plants, hydroelectric stations, high-voltage electrical power lines and flash discharges, cosmic fire-works, etc. A mitigated form of this experiential pattern would involve scenes of wild battles, revolutions, and exploratory adventures (such as the conquest of new continents or the space race).

Another important aspect of this experiential pattern is excessive sexual excitement frequently mixed with intense aggression. These experiences can be accompanied either by imagery of abstract figures with a sexual and sensual undertone or rather complex scenes of wild orgies, lascivious carnivals, rhyth-mical sensual dances, harems, etc. Very frequent are visions of sadomasochistic orgies, with enormous discharges of aggressive energy, such as visions of bloody murders, tortures and cruelties of all kinds, executions, fanatical religious mobs mutilating themselves and others, atmospheres of wild battles and bloody revolutions.

Several important characteristics of this experiential pattern distinguish it from the previously mentioned no-exit experience. The situation here is not hopeless, and the subject is not helpless; he is actively involved and has the feeling that his striving has a certain direction and goal and that his suffering has a certain meaning. In religious terms, this situation, therefore, would be closer to the concept of purgatory than to that of hell. In addition, the subject does not play exclusively the role of helpless victim; he is an observer and at the same time can identify simultaneously or alternately with both sides. Frequently he can hardly distinguish whether he is the aggressor or the victim. Whereas the no-exit situation represents sheer suffering, the experience of the death-rebirth struggle represents the borderline between agony and ecstasy and the fusion of both. It seems appropriate to refer to this type of experience as "volcanic ecstasy" in contrast to the "oceanic ecstasy" of cosmic union.

Two additional aspects of the death-rebirth struggle should be mentioned in this connection, both belonging to the final stages of this struggle and immediately preceding the experience of rebirth itself. The first of these is often described as passing through a purifying and rejuvenating fire that destroys whatever is rotten and corrupted in the individual and prepares him for the experience of rebirth. The second is scatological in nature and involves rather disgusting encounters with various forms of repulsive biological materi-al, such as feces, urine, sweat, menstrual blood, products of putrefaction, etc. Here, not only visual and tactile elements are involved, but also olfactory and gustatory perception; the subject experiences eating feces, drinking blood or urine, sucking on open putrefying wounds, etc. It is interesting to mention in this connection the far-reaching parallels between these psychedelic experi-ences and elements of various mystical religions, temple mysteries, and initiation rites. The test by fire and the test by revulsive material are rather frequent elements of the latter. For example, the sequence of situations in the initiations of the Hermetic tradition involved a shattering encounter with imminent death, test by fire, test by oily and muddy material, and temptation by sexual seduction (Schure, 1961).

The religious symbolism of the experiential pattern of the death-rebirth struggle is related to religions that glorify or use bloody sacrifice as part of their ceremonies. Rather frequent are visions of scenes from the Old and the New Testament (the crucifixion, Moses and the tablet with the Ten Commandments, Abraham and Isaac), scenes of worshipping Moloch, Baal, Astarte, or Kali, images of ceremonies from various pre-Columbian cultures involving sacrifice and self-sacrifice, such as in the Aztec, Mayan, or Olmec religions, etc. Visions of religious rituals and ceremonies involving sex and/or wild rhythmic dances are also frequent illustrations of the rebirth struggle; they involve a wide range of scenes related to the cult of Cybele, various phallic sects, and the tribal religions of the aborigines. A frequent symbol associated with the purifying fire is the image of the legendary bird Phoenix; the scatological aspect of the rebirth struggle is symbolized occasionally by scenes such as Hercules cleaning the stable of Augeas, the Harpies contaminating the food of Fineus, etc.

A typical cluster of physical manifestations regularly accompanying the above pattern of experiences seems to confirm the relation of these experiences to the biological birth trauma. Examples of these physical manifestations are: enormous pressure on head and body, problems with breathing, torturing pains in various parts of the body, cardiac distress, profuse sweating, alternating chills and hot flashes, nausea and projectile vomiting, as well as great, generalized, aggressive tension discharged in tremors, twitches, jerks, and complex twisting movements.

Death-Rebirth Experience

This experiential pattern seems to be meaningfully related to the third clinical stage of delivery. In this stage, the agonizing experiences of several hours culminate, the propulsion through the birth canal is completed, and the extreme intensification of tension and suffering is followed by sudden relief and relaxation. Physiologically, after the umbilical cord is cut, the blood ceases to circulate in the involved vessels, and a new pathway is opened through the pulmonary area. The physical separation from the mother has been completed, and the child starts its existence as an anatomically independent individual.

The death-rebirth experience represents the termination and resolution of the death-rebirth struggle. Suffering and agony culminate in an experience of total annihilation on all levels—physical, emotional, intellectual, moral, and transcendental. This experience is usually referred to as an "ego death"; it seems to involve an instantaneous destruction of all the previous reference points of the individual. The ego-death experience can be accompanied by images of various deities, such as that of the goddess Kali, Moloch, Huitzilopochtli, Shiva the Destroyer, or experienced in identification with the death and resurrection of Christ, Osiris, Dionysus, etc.

After the subject has experienced the very depth of total annihilation and "hit the cosmic bottom," he is struck by visions of blinding white or golden light and experiences freeing decompression and expansion of space. The universe is perceived as indescribably beautiful and radiant; the general atmosphere is that of liberation, redemption, salvation, love, and forgiveness. The subject feels cleansed and purged and talks about having disposed of an incredible amount of "garbage," guilt, aggression, and anxiety. He feels overwhelming love for other fellowmen, appreciation of warm human relations, friendship, and love. Irrational and exaggerated ambitions as well as cravings for money, status, prestige, and power appear in this state absurd and irrelevant. The appreciation of natural beauties is enormously enhanced, and an uncomplicated and simple way of life in close contact and harmony with nature seems to be the most desirable of all alternatives. Anything of natural origin is experienced with utmost zest by all the widely opened sensory pathways. Brotherly feelings for all fellowmen are accompanied by feelings of humility and a tendency to engage in service and charitable activities.

The experience of rebirth is frequently followed by what is usually described as an experience of "cosmic union" and seems to be closely related to the "good womb" and "good breast" experiences and happy childhood memories. The individual tuned in to this experiential area usually discovers within himself genuinely positive values, such as a sense of justice, appreciation of beauty, feelings of love, self-respect, and respect for others. These values, as well as motivations to pursue them and act in accordance with them, seem to be on this level an intrinsic part of the human personality. They cannot be satisfactorily explained in terms of reaction formations to opposite tendencies or as sublimation of primitive instinctual drives. The individual experiences them as intrinsic parts of the universal order. In this connection, it is interesting to point to the parallels with Abraham Maslow's concept of metavalues and metamotivations (Maslow, 1969). Typical symbolism for this experiential pattern are visions of radiant sources of light experienced as divine, of a heavenly blue color, of a rainbow spectrum, or of peacock feathers. Rather frequent are nonfigurative images of God, such as the Cosmic Sun or Brahma, or personified representations of God and various deities. The subjects can see the traditional images of the Christian God as an old man sitting on a throne and surrounded by cherubim and seraphim in radiant splendor; they can experience union with the Great Mother or Divine Isis, see the Greek gods on Mount Olympus drinking nectar and eating ambrosia, etc. Other visions involve gigantic halls with richly decorated columns, huge marble statues, and crystal chandeliers; beautiful natural scenery, such as the starry sky, mountains, the ocean, flourishing meadows, etc. From the biological and physiological point of view, this experience is accompanied by a feeling of perfect and harmonious physical functioning.

Embryonal and Fetal Experiences

It was mentioned above that the LSD subjects experiencing the oceanic feelings of cosmic unity frequently refer in this connection to intrauterine existence. In addition, it is not infrequent in psychedelic sessions to experience concrete episodes that are identified as specific occurrences during intrauterine development. They are mostly instances of psychotraumatization resulting from disturbing stimuli of a physical or chemical nature. The reports of such relivings cover a wide range from attempted abortions through consequences of maternal disease or dietary trespassing to almost anecdotal descriptions of parental sexual intercourse experienced in advanced stages of pregnancy. Similarly as in the case of childhood memories and birth memories, the authenticity of these recollections is problematic. It seems, therefore, advisable to refer to them as experiences rather than as memories. Occasionally, however, it was possible to get surprising confirmation by independent questioning of the persons involved. Data from the sessions of professionals (such as psychiatrists, psychologists, and scientists from other disciplines) who experienced episodes of intrauterine existence in their LSD training sessions show that they were quite regularly astounded at how convincing and authentic these experiences appeared to be.

The following clinical example can be used to illustrate the problems involved in trying to verify the authenticity of relived intrauterine experiences in LSD sessions:

In one of the LSD sessions of a psycholytic series, the patient
described a rather authentic intrauterine experience. He was aware
of the fetal body image with his head being relatively bigger than
an adult's. He felt immersed in fetal liquid and fixed to the
placenta by the umbilical cord. There were two sets of heart
sounds with different frequencies and frequent sounds that he
identified as related to peristaltic movements of the intestines. On
the basis of cues that he was not able to identify, he diagnosed
himself as a rather mature fetus just before delivery.
  Suddenly he heard strange noises coming from the outside. He
felt they were distorted by the abdominal walls and the fetal liquid
and had a strange echoing quality. He could hear laughing and
yelling human voices and sounds reminding him of carnival
trumpets. He started thinking about an annual flower mart held
every year in his native village two days before his birthday.
  After having put together the mentioned pieces of information,
he concluded that his mother must have attended the mart in an
advanced stage of pregnancy. The mother confirmed independently
that she left home in spite of strong warnings from her mother
and grandmother to participate in the mart. This had precipitated
the delivery of the patient.

In general, intrauterine experiences are associated with other types of
transpersonal experiences. Positive experiences are related to feelings of cosmic unity and images of various blissful deities. Episodes of disturbances seem
to be accompanied by visions of demons, wrathful deities, and archetypal evil
appearances. A rather frequent concomitant of the embryonal and fetal experiences are phylogenetic (evolutionary) experiences. This liaison occurs even in
unsophisticated subjects, who do not know anything about Haeckel's biogenet-
ic law according to which the fetus in its embryonal development repeats, in
a condensed way, the history of its species.

Ancestral Experiences

In experiences of this type, the subject feels that he is exploring his genetic
lineage and reliving episodes from the lives of his ancestors. Sometimes such
experiences are related to the relatively recent history of the maternal or
paternal family, but occasionally they reach back many centuries. Thus a
Jewish subject can experience episodes from tribal life in Biblical times, a
person of Scandinavian origin can relive scenes from the adventurous cruises
and wild conquests of the Vikings, or an American Negro can witness events
from the early history of slavery. Ancestral experiences are usually rather

complex, and they represent a mixture of elements ranging from identification with individual ancestors through feeling the psychological atmosphere in the families, clans, and tribes, to insights into cultural attitudes, beliefs and prejudices, traditions, and customs. Sometimes the subject can acquire illuminating insights into the friction points and incompatibilities between the maternal and paternal lineage and can understand how he has introjected them as his own intrapsychic conflicts.

A very important characteristic of ancestral memories that distinguishes them from the following category (collective and racial experiences) is the convinced feeling of the subject that he is confronted with real elements from his individual history, reading his own genetic code.

Careful unbiased study of ancestral experiences can occasionally reveal that they contain specific information that was not known or accessible to the subject. One of several unusual coincidences observed during my LSD research can be used as an illustration of the complexity of this problem for the researcher:

> A female patient treated by psycholytic therapy because of her severe cancerophobia and borderline psychotic symptomatology had in the advanced stage of treatment four consecutive LSD sessions that consisted almost exclusively of scenes and sequences that took place in Prague of the seventeenth century. This time was a rather crucial period in Czech history; after the lost battle of the White Mountain in 1621, which marked the beginning of the Thirty Years' War in Europe, the country ceased to exist as an independent kingdom and came under the hegemony of the Hapsburg dynasty. In an effort to destroy the feelings of national pride and defeat the forces of resistance, the Hapsburgs sent mercenaries to capture the country's most prominent noblemen. Twenty-seven outstanding members of nobility were then beheaded at a public execution on a scaffolding erected on the Old Town Square in Prague.
>
> During her sessions, the patient had an unusual variety of images and insights concerning the architecture of the experienced period, typical garments and costumes, as well as weapons and various utensils used in everyday life. She was also able to describe many of the complicated relations existing at that time between the royal family and the vassals. The patient had never specifically studied this historical period, and special books had to be consulted in order to confirm the reported information. Many of the experiences were related to various periods of life of a young nobleman, one of the twenty-seven members of nobility beheaded by the Hapsburgs. In a rather dramatic sequence the patient finally

relived with powerful emotions and in considerable detail the
actual events of the execution, including the terminal anguish and
the experience of agony.

    I spent a considerable amount of time in an effort to verify the
historical information as well as to understand her experiences in
psychodynamic terms as symbolic disguise for her relevant
childhood experiences or present life situation. The experiential
sequences did not seem to make sense from this point of view, and
I finally gave up and forgot this incident after the patient's LSD
experiences moved into other areas. Two years later, when I was
already in the United States, I received a long letter from the
patient with the following unusual introduction: "Dear Dr. Grof,
You will probably think that I am absolutely insane when I share
with you the results of my recent private search." In the text that
followed, the patient described how she happened to meet her
father, whom she had not seen since she was three years old when
her parents divorced. After a short discussion, her father invited
her to have dinner with him, his second wife, and their children.
After dinner, he told her that he wanted to show her his favorite
hobby, which she might find of special interest.
    During World War II, it was required by the Nazis that every
Czechoslovakian family present to the German authorities its
pedigree demonstrating the absence of persons of Jewish origin for
the last five generations. Preparing such a pedigree because of
existential necessity, the patient's father became absolutely
fascinated by this procedure. After having completed the required
five-generation pedigree for the authorities, he has continued this
activity because of his private interest, tracing the history of his
family back through the centuries. This was made possible by a
rather complete system of birth records kept in the archives of
parish houses in the European countries.
    After dinner, the father showed to the patient with considerable
pride a carefully designed, ramified pedigree of their family,
indicating that they were descendants of one of the noblemen
executed after the battle of the White Mountain. After having
described this episode in the letter, the patient expressed her belief
that highly emotionally charged memories can be imprinted in the
genetic code and transmitted through centuries to future
generations. The information obtained from her father only
confirmed her previous suspicion, which was based on the
convincing nature of the relived memories.
    After my initial amazement in regard to this most unusual
coincidence, I was able to discover a rather serious logical
inconsistency in the patient's account. One of the experiences she

had in her "historical" LSD sessions was the reliving of the
terminal anguish of the nobleman during his own execution.
Physical death terminates, of course, the biological hereditary line;
a dead person cannot procreate and pass the memory of his
terminal anguish to future generations. Before completely
discarding the information contained in the patient's letter,
however, one fact deserves serious consideration—none of the
remaining Czech patients, who had a total of over 1600 sessions,
had ever even mentioned this historical period. In this patient, four
consecutive LSD sessions contained almost exclusively historical
sequences from this time. The most unusual coincidence of these
experiences with the results of her father's genealogical quest make
this clinical observation a problem rather difficult to interpret
within the framework of the traditionally accepted paradigms.

Collective and Racial Experiences

In advanced LSD sessions of a psycholytic series or in high-dose psychedelic
sessions, the subjects frequently experience episodes from various cultures in
the history of mankind. This can be associated with rather total and complex
insights concerning religion, social structure, moral code, art, and other aspects
of the cultures involved. These experiences can be related to any country of
the world and any historical period; they seem to be independent of the
subject's own racial background, cultural tradition, and even previous training,
education, and interests. Thus an Anglo-Saxon can experience the history of
the Afroamericans, a Jew, elements of the Japanese or Chinese tradition, or
a person of Slavic origin scenes from the Central American pre-Columbian
cultures.

These experiences frequently contain detailed information about various
cultural aspects that can be verified by study of archaeological sources; occasionally this can concern rather unusual and specific data definitely beyond
that known by the subject previously. Such information can, for example,
involve details of the mummification of Egyptian pharaohs or the esoteric
significance of the pyramids, technical aspects of the Zoroastrian "Towers of
Silence," symbolism of the Hindu sculptures and religious ceremonies, etc.

The subject experiences these elements as insights into the history of mankind, as cultural identification, or as illustrations of the cosmic drama; he does
not have the feeling of exploring his own individual history that is essential
for ancestral experiences.

Phylogenetic (Evolutionary) Experiences

In this type of experience, the subject identifies with his animal ancestors on various levels of development; this is accompanied by a realistic feeling that the subject is exploring his own evolutionary pedigree. The identification is rather complex, complete, and authentic; it involves the body image, a variety of physical feelings and physiological sensations, specific emotions, and a new perception of the environment. Occasionally the subjects report insight into zoological or ethological facts that by far exceed the level of their education in natural sciences. In addition, the experiences involved appear to be qualitatively different from human experiences and frequently even seem to transcend the scope of human fantasy and imagination. The subject can have, for example, an illuminating insight into what it feels like when a snake is hungry, when a turtle is sexually excited, or when a salmon breathes through its gills. Identification is most frequent with other mammals, with birds, reptiles, amphibians, and various species of fish. Occasionally, the subjects report identification with much less differentiated forms of life, such as coelenterates or even unicellular organisms. Evolutionary experiences are sometimes accompanied by changes in neurological reflexes and certain abnormal motor phenomena that appear to be related to the activation of archaic neuronal pathways.

"Past Incarnation" Experiences

This is probably the most fascinating and obscure category of transpersonal experiences. The subjects report experiencing in a vivid, dramatic, and convincing way scenes or fragments of scenes that happened at another time and place in history. These scenes usually involve one or several other persons (or less frequently animals) and are accompanied by powerful emotions. The feelings and emotions accompanying these situations are for the most part distinctly negative (physical pain, hatred, anguish, aggression, jealousy, greed, despair, etc.) and only exceptionally positive. They are accompanied by a feeling that these episodes are a reliving of events that actually happened in one of the subject's past lives (in one of his previous incarnations). The opening of this area of experiences is sometimes preceded by the emergence of complex nonverbal instructions about the phenomenon of reincarnation and the law of karma as a perennial law mandatory for each individual. Reliving of these scenes is usually experienced by the subject as "burning of bad karma." The full conscious reliving of all the painful emotions involved in the destructive karmic scene followed by mutual forgiveness results in a feeling of paramount achievement and indescribable bliss. This is sometimes accompanied by an interesting phenomenon—a subjective experience of a gigantic karmic hurricane, blowing through centuries and tearing the karmic bonds. According to the insights of LSD subjects, the laws of reincarnation seem to be independent of the subject's biological lineage and the genetic transfer of idioplasma. The assignment of an individual spiritual entity to a particular physical body and a specific life seems to bypass biological hereditary lines and violate genetic laws.

Precognition, Clairvoyance, and "Time Travel"

This category of LSD experiences involves those ESP phenomena that are characterized by temporal extension of consciousness. Occasionally the subjects report, particularly in advanced sessions of an LSD series, convincing anticipation of events that will happen in the future. Sometimes they see complex and detailed scenes of future events in the form of vivid clairvoyant visions. Some of these experiences show various degrees of similarity with actual happenings occurring later. Objective verification in this area seems to be a particularly difficult task. The possibility of the *déjà vu* phenomenon and of the subject's distortion in the perception of later events are just two of the major pitfalls involved.

Another interesting phenomenon of this category is the experience of "time travel." The individual has a convincing feeling that he can transcend the limitations of time at will and travel to any specific time period in a way not dissimilar to that described in science fiction about time machines. The subjective feeling of a free decision distinguishes these experiences from elemental and uncontrollable reliving of episodes from childhood, ancestral history, or from elements of the racial and collective unconscious. It is usually combined with a similar voluntary manipulation of the location of the events involved.

Ego Transcendence in Interpersonal Relations

This type of experience is characterized by various degrees of loss of ego boundaries and by merging into union and oneness with another person to the point of experiencing dual unity. In spite of the subjective feeling of total merging with the interpersonal partner, the subject always retains simultaneously the notion of his own identity. In psychedelic sessions, this dual unity can be experienced with the therapist, sitter, or other participating persons. It can also occur as a purely subjective experience independent of the actual persons present during the session. Typical examples in this case are the experience of unity with a sexual partner (with or without the element of genital union), the mother-child union, and the experience of oneness in the disciple-guru relationship. This type of experience is typically accompanied by profound feelings of love and of *sanctity* of the relationship involved.

Identification with Other Persons

Unlike the preceding type of experience, the subject experiences complete identification with another person and loses to a great degree the awareness of his own original identity. This identification is total and complex; it involves the body image, the full range of emotions and psychological attitudes, facial expression, gestures and mannerisms, postures, movements, and even the inflection of voice. There are many different types and levels of this experience. Reliving of traumatic childhood experiences involving more than one person is frequently characterized by simultaneous or alternating identification with all the participants; this can give a transpersonal flavor to many otherwise typically personal experiences. In this connection, or independently, the subject can experience identification with his close relatives, friends, acquaintances, teachers, political figures, etc. At other times such identification can involve typical representatives of various professional, ethnic, or racial groups, famous historical figures (such as Genghis Khan, Emperor Nero, Hitler, or Stalin) or religious teachers (such as Jesus or the Buddha).

Group Identification and Group Consciousness

This category of experiences is characterized by further expansion of consciousness; instead of identifying with individuals, the subject experiences identity with typical groups characterized by their race, religion, profession, or destiny. In this way the subject can experience the role of the Jews persecuted through centuries, of the Christians tortured and sacrificed by the Romans, of the victims of the Spanish Inquisition, members of various religious sects such as the Flagellants or the Russian Skopzy,[2] of all the soldiers who have ever died on all the battlefields since the beginning of the world, of all terminal patients or persons dying in accidents, prisoners in concentration camps, members of individual Indian castes or of the total population of India, etc.

Animal Identification

These frequently occurring experiences can be distinguished from the previously described phylogenetic memories by the absence of the feeling that the individual explores his own developmental history. Otherwise, the identification can be in all respects as authentic and convincing as in the case of evolutionary experiences; it contains frequently interesting information about animal psychology, ethology, sexual and breeding habits, etc.

It is necessary to differentiate these experiences also from the much more superficial autosymbolic animal transformations. In the latter experiences, the subject can symbolize his aggression by identification with a predator (such as a tiger, lion, or black panther), his polymorphously perverted instinctual drives by identification with a monkey, his strong sexual drive by identification with a stallion, etc. These experiences lack the experiential authenticity of phylogenetic memories or of animal identification and can be easily recognized by the subject as a symbolic representation of his own emotions and complexes. The subjects who experienced in a series of consecutive sessions all three experiential varieties—animal autosymbolic transformation, animal identification, and phylogenetic memories—can distinguish them easily by their specific experiential flavor.

Plant Identification

The instances of experiencing the consciousness of various plant forms are in general much less frequent than those concerning animal life. The subject may have a unique feeling of witnessing and consciously experiencing the basic life processes of the plants such as germination of the seeds, vegetable growth, pollination, and photosynthesis.

---

[2]Skopzy (Russian expression meaning "rams") is a name given to members of a Russian religious sect whose fanatical members used to automutilate themselves by castration.

As in the case of some previously mentioned experiences, the subjects repeatedly report that the feeling of authenticity and the special experiential flavor of this experience cannot be appreciated by someone who has not had it. It is this experiential character that makes it difficult to discard these identification experiences as mere phantasies. At this point, it seems difficult to offer a plausible explanation of this phenomenon within the framework of the existing commonly accepted paradigms.

Oneness with Life and All Creation

In these experiences, the subject identifies with the totality of life on this planet. He can then experience the complexity of the phylogenetic development of all life forms, problems related to the survival and extinction of species, or to the viability of life as a cosmic phenomenon.

Consciousness of Inorganic Matter

Not infrequently the LSD subjects experience consciousness of inorganic material; the phenomena they can identify with can range from a single atom to various materials such as diamond, granite, or gold. Sometimes the consciousness of particularly stable and durable substances can be experienced as involving an element of sacredness. Some subjects described, for example, that from this point of view the granite statues of the Egyptians and the pre-Columbian golden sculptures do not appear as images of deities, but deities themselves; what was worshipped was the stable, immutable, and undifferentiated consciousness of the material involved. In the light of such experiences, the subjects see consciousness as a basic phenomenon existing throughout the universe; the usual human consciousness appears to be only one of its many outgrowths.

Planetary Consciousness

In this type of experience, the consciousness of the subject seems to encompass all the phenomena of this planet, including both organic and inorganic matter. It is a relatively rare phenomenon occurring usually in advanced sessions of an LSD series.

Extra-Planetary Consciousness

Here the subject experiences phenomena related to celestial bodies other than our planet, existing within our solar system or outside of it. A special type of experience belonging to this category is the consciousness of interstellar space reported independently by several of our subjects. It is characterized by feelings of tranquility, serenity, purity, infinity, and eternity, and unity of all conceivable opposites.

Out-of-Body Experiences, Traveling Clairvoyance, "Space Travel," and Telepathy

The experience of leaving one's own body is a frequent occurrence in psychedelic sessions. The subjects describe that they experience themselves completely detached from their actual physical bodies, hovering above them or watching them from another part of the room. Another typical experience of this kind is that of losing contact with one's body and entering various experiential realms independent of the body and physical processes.

Less frequently does this experience take the form of traveling clairvoyance in which the subject experiences himself at another place in the physical world and can give a detailed description of the situation that he encountered. Attempts to verify such ESP perception can sometimes bring interesting results.

Occasionally, the subject has the feeling that he can actively control such a process, transcend the usual limitations of space, and travel at will to any location he chooses. The following example shows the specific difficulties that can occur if the subject tries to experiment with this unusual condition and put the experience to a rigid test.

> The first three hours of this session were experienced as a fantastic battle between the forces of Light and Darkness; it was a beautiful illustration of the description from the ancient Persian Zend Avesta concerning the fight between the armies of Ahura Mazda and Ahriman. It was fought on all conceivable levels—in the cells and tissues of my body, on the surface of our planet throughout history, in the cosmic space, and on a metaphysical, transcendental level. Occasionally I had a rather convincing feeling that the battle I was witnessing and experiencing had something to do with the relationship between matter and spirit, in particular with the entrapment of spirit in matter.

After this battle was over, I found myself in a rather unusual state of mind; I felt a mixture of serenity and bliss with the naive and primitive faith of the early Christians. It was a world where miracles were possible, acceptable, and understandable. I was preoccupied with the problems of time and space and the insoluble paradoxes of infinity and eternity that baffle our reason in the usual state of consciousness. I could not understand how I could have let myself be "brainwashed" into accepting the simple-minded concept of one-dimensional time and three-dimensional space as being mandatory and existing in objective reality. It appeared to me rather obvious that there are no limits in the realm of spirit and that time and space are arbitrary constructs of the mind. Any number of spaces with different orders of infinities could be deliberately created and experienced. A single second and eternity seemed to be freely interchangeable. I thought about higher mathematics and saw deep parallels between various mathematical concepts and altered states of consciousness.

In this situation, it suddenly occurred to me that I do not have to be bound by the limitations of time and space and can travel in the time-space continuum quite deliberately and without any restrictions. This feeling was so convincing and overwhelming that I wanted to test it by an experiment. I decided to try traveling to the city of my birth, which was several thousand miles away. After visualizing the direction and the distance, I set myself into motion and tried to fly through space to the place of destination. This effort resulted in an experience of flight through space at an enormous velocity, but to my disappointment, I wasn't getting anywhere. I stopped this activity and reconsidered the situation; I could not understand that the experiment would not work in spite of my convincing feeling that such space travel was possible. Immediately, I realized that I was still under the influence of my old concepts of time and space. I continued thinking in terms of directions and distances and approached the task accordingly. It suddenly appeared to me that the proper approach would be to make myself believe that the place of the session was actually identical with the place of destination. When I approached the task in this way, I experienced peculiar and bizarre sensations. I found myself in a strange, rather congested place full of vacuum tubes, wires, resistors, and condensers. After a short period of confusion, I realized that I was trapped in a TV set located in the corner of the room of the apartment in my native city where I spent my childhood. I was trying to use, somehow, the speakers for hearing and the tube for seeing. Suddenly I understood that this experience was a symbolic expression ridiculing the fact that I was still hung up on my previous beliefs concerning space and matter. The only way of transmitting images at long distances that was conceivable and acceptable for me was based on the use of electromagnetic waves such as in the case of television broadcasting. Such a transmission, of course, is restricted by the velocity of the waves involved. At the moment when I realized and firmly believed that I could operate in the realm of free spirit, and did not have to be restricted even by the velocity of light or other types of electromagnetic waves, the experience changed rapidly. I broke through the TV screen and found myself walking in the apartment of my parents. I did not feel any drug effect at that point, and the experience was as sober and real as any other experience of my life. I walked to the window and looked at the clock on the street corner; it showed a five-hour difference from the time in the time zone where the experiment took place. In spite of the fact that this difference reflected the actual time difference between the two zones, I did not find it convincing evidence. I knew the time difference intellectually, and my mind could have easily fabricated this experience.

I felt I needed a much more convincing proof of whether or not what I was experiencing was "objectively real" in the usual sense. I finally decided to perform a test, to take a picture from the wall and later check in correspondence with my parents if something unusual happened at that time in their apartment. I reached for the picture, but before being able to touch the frame, I was overcome by an increasingly unpleasant feeling that it was an extremely risky and dangerous undertaking. I felt suddenly the uncanny influence of evil forces and a touch of something like "black magic"; it seemed as if I were gambling for my soul. I paused and started analyzing what was happening. Images from the world's famous casinos were flashing in front of my eyes—Monte Carlo, Lido, Las Vegas, Reno. . . . I saw roulette balls spiraling at intoxicating speeds, mechanical movements of gambling slot machines, dice jolting on the green surface of the tables during a game of craps, scenes of gamblers involved in baccarat and flickering lights of the keno panels. This was followed by scenes of secret meetings of statesmen, politicians, army officials, and top-notch scientists. I realized that I had not yet overcome my egocentrism and could not resist the temptation of power. The possibility of transcending the limitations of time and space appeared to be intoxicating and dangerously seductive. If I could have control over time and space, an unlimited supply of money appeared to be guaranteed, together with everything that money can buy. All one had to do under those circumstances was to go to the nearest casino, stock market, or lottery office. No secrets would exist for somebody controlling time and space at will; he could eavesdrop on summit meetings of political leaders, read top secret documents, and get hold of the most recent scientific discoveries.

This would open undreamed of possibilities for controlling the course of events in the world.

I started understanding the dangers involved in my experiment. I remembered passages from different books warning against toying with these powers before the individual overcomes his ego limitations and reaches spiritual maturity. There was, however, something that appeared even more relevant. I found out that I was extremely ambivalent in regard to the outcome of my test. On the one hand, it seemed extremely enticing to be able to liberate oneself from the slavery of time and space. On the other hand, however, it was obvious that something like this had far-reaching and serious consequences and could not be seen as an isolated experiment in voluntary control of space. If I could get confirmation that it was possible to manipulate physical environment at a distance of several thousand miles, my whole universe would collapse as a result of this one experiment, and I would find myself in a state of utter metaphysical confusion. The world as I knew it would not exist any more; I would lose all the maps I relied on and felt comfortable with. I would not know who, where, and when I was, and would be lost in a totally new, frightening universe about the laws of which I would have not the slightest notion.

I could not bring myself to carry through the intended experiment and decided to leave the problem of the objectivity and reality of the experience unresolved. This made it possible for me to toy with the idea that I had conquered time and space, while at the same time allowing me, in case the whole thing became too frightening, to see the whole episode as one of many peculiar deceptions due to the intoxication of my brain by a powerful psychedelic drug. The moment I gave up the experiment, I found myself back in the room where the drug session took place.

I never forgave myself for having wasted such a unique and fantastic experiment. The memory of the metaphysical horror involved in this test makes me doubt, however, that I would be more courageous given a similar chance in the future.

Occasionally, telepathic experiences can be observed in psychedelic sessions. The firm feeling the LSD subject has that he can read the minds of the persons present in the session or that he can tune in to people in other parts of the world is more frequently a self-deception than an objectively verifiable fact. Besides gross distortions and misinterpretations there are, however, situations that are strongly indicative of genuine ESP communication. Occasionally the LSD subject can be unusually accurate in his awareness of the sitter's ideation and emotions without even looking at him. Two subjects who have the session at the same time can share many ideas or have parallel experiences without much verbal communication and interchange. Exceptionally, a claim made by an LSD subject about telepathic contact with a distant person can be supported by objective evidence obtained by independent investigation.

Organ, Tissue, and Cellular Consciousness

In this type of experience, the subject reports a feeling of authentically tuning in to the consciousness of a certain part of his body, such as individual organs or tissues (heart, liver, kidney, bone, intestinal mucose membrane, uterine epithelium, etc.) or even individual cells (white and red blood cells, cells of various organs, etc.) The rather frequently reported experience of conscious identification with the germinal cells (sperm, ova) and of the moment of conception belongs to this category. Occasionally this can be associated with interesting insights into biochemical and physiological processes that appear to be beyond the scope of the subject's medical education.

Spiritistic and Mediumistic Experiences

These rare experiences closely resemble phenomena known from spiritistic seances and occult literature. The subject can, for example, exhibit signs of a mediumistic trance; his facial expression is strikingly transformed, his countenance and gestures appear alien, and his voice is dramatically changed. He can speak in a foreign language, write automatic texts, and produce obscure hieroglyphic designs or draw strange pictures and unintelligible squiggles.

Another experience from this category is that of encounter with astral bodies or spiritual entities of deceased persons or extrasensory communication with them. The following episode from an advanced LSD session of a psycholytic series at the Prague Psychiatric Institute can be used as an illustration:

> A patient treated by LSD psychotherapy for a complicated psychoneurosis of an obsessive-phobic nature was reliving in one of her sessions an extremely painful traumatic episode from her childhood. Her father was hospitalized for many years in a mental institution for a psychotic condition. When the patient was ten years old, her father suffered a cerebral hemorrhage and was

discharged from the hospital to die in the home setting. The patient had to witness the deterioration of her father and was even at his bedside at the time of his terminal agony. In this session she literally regressed back to childhood and became a little frightened girl watching the death struggle of her father. At first she watched his terminal agony, but later started experiencing it herself; in full identification with her father, she approached the moment of physical death. When they crossed the threshold of life and death in this peculiar dual unity, she went into a state of almost uncontrollable panic. It was not possible to communicate with her for at least two hours. After the contact was reestablished, she was able to describe her experience in retrospect:

"After we crossed the threshold of life and death, I found myself in an uncanny and frightening world. It was all filled with fluorescent ether of a strangely macabre nature. There was no way of assessing whether the space involved was finite or infinite. An endless number of souls of deceased human beings were suspended in the luminescent ether; in an atmosphere of strange distress and disquieting excitement, they were sending me nonverbal messages through some unidentifiable extrasensory channels. They appeared unusually demanding, and it seemed as if they needed something from me. In general the atmosphere reminded me of the descriptions of the underworld that I had read in Greek literature. But the objectivity and reality of the situation was beyond my imagination—it provoked sheer and utter metaphysical horror that I cannot even start describing. My father was present in this world as an astral body; since I entered this world in union with him, his astral body was as if superimposed over mine. I was not able to communicate with you [the therapist] at all, and it seemed pointless. I was sure that you knew as little about this macabre world as I did, and you could not, therefore, be of any help. It was by far the most frightening experience of my life—in none of the previous LSD sessions did I encounter anything that came close to it."

Experiences of Encounters with Supra-Human Entities

Occasionally LSD subjects report the experience of being in the presence of, or even identifying with, spiritual entities or supra-human beings existing on higher planes of consciousness and higher energy levels. Such beings can appear in the sessions in the role of guides, teachers, and protectors. The subjects can sometimes identify these spiritual entities by name (Jesus, Sri Ramana Maharshi, Ramakrishna, Sri Aurobindo, etc.).

Experiences of Other Universes and of Encounters with Their Inhabitants

These experiences occur extremely rarely in psychedelic sessions. The subjects find themselves in strange and alien universes that do not appear to be part of our cosmos, but exist parallel to it. They report encountering entities inhabiting these alien worlds and experience various dramatic adventures resembling those from science fiction stories and novels.

Archetypal Experiences

Even subjects who have not had any previous exposure to C. G. Jung's books and ideas will experience and describe typical Jungian archetypes, especially in advanced sessions of an LSD series. Most frequently this involves experiences of generalized and universalized social roles, such as that of the Martyr, Fugitive, Outcast, Ruler, Tyrant, Buffoon, etc. Other typical categories of archetypal experiences are sanctified roles and images such as the Great Mother, the Terrible Mother, the Great Hermaphrodite, etc. Occasionally the subjects experience complex archetypal situations—that of the Cosmic Man, Golden Age, or Dark Age, etc.

Experiences of Encounter with Blissful and Wrathful Deities

This category of experiences is closely related to the previous one. In a strictly Jungian sense the encounters and/or identification with various deities would be considered archetypal experiences. Sophisticated professionals acquainted with Jung's theories who volunteered for LSD sessions seemed, however, to distinguish clearly between the archetypes as previously described and experiences involving concrete deities related to specific cultures. The deities occurring in LSD sessions form two rather sharply defined groups: blissful or light deities and wrathful or dark deities. Typical representatives of the former group are Isis, Ahura Mazda, Apollo, and others; the latter group comprises such deities as Kali, Baal, Moloch, Astarte, Huitzilopochtli, etc. The encounter with these deities is usually accompanied by very powerful emotions, ranging from metaphysical horror to ecstatic rapture. The subjects usually do not have the feeling, however, that they are confronted with the Supreme Being or the ultimate force in this universe.

Activation of the Chakras and Arousal of the Serpent Power (Kundalini)

Many experiences in LSD sessions show a striking similarity to those described in various schools of Kundalini yoga as manifestations of activation and opening of the individual chakras.[3] When the subjects are familiar with this Indian concept, they often make specific references to chakras and the Serpent Power (Kundalini). Even in the case of LSD subjects unfamiliar with Indian philosophy and religion, descriptions are often parallel. The system of the chakras seems to provide a useful map of consciousness that is of great help in conceptualizing and understanding many unusual experiences in psychedelic sessions.

An extremely rare and exceptional experience occurring usually in advanced LSD sessions is that which resembles the descriptions of arousal of the Serpent Power (Kundalini) in the sacral parts of the spinal cord and the upward flow of spiritual energy resulting in subsequent opening of all the chakras. This culminates in a profound ecstatic spiritual experience related to the highest chakra, which the Indians refer to as the Thousand-Petal Lotus.

It is interesting to mention in this connection that in a discussion following a paper pointing out the similarities between the LSD experiences and the Indian religions (Grof, 1970a), many of the Indian participants seemed to agree that among all the systems of yoga, the Kundalini yoga bears the closest resemblance to psychedelic psychotherapy. Both techniques can produce profound and dramatic experiences in a relatively short time but involve the greatest potential risk and danger.

Consciousness of the Universal Mind

One of the most profound and total experiences in psychedelic sessions is often described as "consciousness of the Universal Mind." In it, the subject is convinced that he is experiencing the ultimate force in the Universe. This

---

[3]*Chakras* (a Sanskrit term for "wheels") are hypothetical centers of radiation of primal energy (prāna) roughly corresponding to certain levels of the spinal cord and certain body organs. Most systems distinguish seven chakras: (1) anal chakra (mūlādhāra), (2) genital chakra (svadisthana), (3) navel chakra (manipūra), (4) heart chakra (anāhata), (5) throat chakra (vishuddha), (6) brow chakra (ājnā) and (7) crown chakra (sahasrāra). The flow of prāna is mediated by one central conduit (sushumna) and two lateral conduits (ida and pingalā).

experience is typically referred to as ineffable, and subjects complain about the imperfection and inadequacy to the symbolic structure of the language to describe it. The basic attributes of the Universal Mind as experienced by the LSD subjects. can be best expressed by the Sanskrit word *Sat-chit-ānanda;* it suggests infinite existence, infinite wisdom, and infinite bliss. Occasionally the experience of the Universal Mind is associated with interesting insights into the process of the creation of the three-dimensional world and into the Buddhist concept of the Wheel of Death and Rebirth.

The experience of the Universal Mind is closely related to but not identical with the experience of cosmic unity described earlier.

The Supracosmic and Metacosmic Void

It is the experience of primordial Emptiness and Nothingness, which is the ultimate source of all existence. The terms supra- and metacosmic refer to the fact that this Void appears to be both supraordinated to and underlying the world of creation. It is beyond time and space, beyond any change, and beyond polarities such as good and evil, light and darkness, stability and motion, agony and ecstasy. The experience of the Supracosmic Void in its full depth and metaphysical relevance is a rare occurrence in LSD sessions; it is probably close to the Buddhist concept of nirvana. As with the consciousness of the Universal Mind, the Void cannot be described in words, but it can be experienced under special circumstances. It is also possible to attain an experiential and intuitive insight into the emergence of the Universal Mind from the Supracosmic Void and into the initiation of the process of creation.

Being a first attempt at describing transpersonal experiences occurring in psychedelic sessions, this paper is necessarily incomplete and represents only a brief and sketchy outline of vast territories of the human mind as yet unknown to and uncharted by traditional Western science. Transpersonal experiences are so multifaceted and cover such a wide range of phenomena that it is extremely difficult to find a *principium divisionis* and present a simple and comprehensive system for their further classification. Using broad descriptive categories such as mystical, religious, occult, and parapsychological seems to be of questionable practical value and, in addition, results in semantic confusion and an overlapping of categories.

One possibility would be to introduce the concept of "depth" of the unconscious; various categories of these experiences would then refer to the level of the unconscious at which they originate or reflect the degree of difficulty in eliciting them by means of specific tehniques. Such an approach would require a proof that such stratification really exists as well as a reliable system of defining the depth of various experiences.

It might be possible to use one of the existing ancient systems that have developed a detailed map of consciousness, such as the Indian system of the chakras. It is very difficult, however, to clarify these systems and separate them from their underlying ideologies in such a way as to make them acceptable to wide professional audiences in the West.

An interesting possibility would be to choose a system of classification based on the distinction of whether or not the content of the transpersonal experience consists of elements of the phenomenal world (or "objective reality") as we know it from our usual state of consciousness. Some of the transpersonal experiences involve phenomena the existence of which has been generally accepted on the basis of consensual validation, empirical evidence, or scientific research. This is true, for example, for perinatal, intrauterine, ancestral, and phylogenetic experiences or elements of collective unconscious. It is not the content of the experience that is surprising, but the existence of these elements in the human unconscious and the possibility of experiencing them in a rather realistic way. The category of transpersonal experiences of this sort can be further subdivided on the basis of whether the extension of consciousness that they involve can be understood in terms of alteration of the dimension of time or space.

There exists also a group of ESP phenomena that could be classified as transpersonal experiences, the content of which is understandable within the framework of "objective reality." In the case of precognition, clairvoyance, "time travel," out-of-body experiences, traveling clairvoyance, "space travel," and telepathy, it again is not the content of the experiences that is unusual but the way of acquiring certain information or perceiving a certain situation that according to generally accepted scientific paradigms is beyond the reach of the senses.

The second broad category of transpersonal experiences would then involve phenomena that are not part of "objective reality" in the Western sense. This would apply to such experiences as communication with spirits of deceased human beings or suprahuman spiritual entities, encounter or identification with various deities, etc.

The following tentative classification is based on the principle described above:

Transpersonal Experiences

I. Experiential Extension (or Expansion) Within the Framework of "Objective Reality"

A. *Temporal Expansion of Consciousness*

Perinatal Experiences
  Cosmic Unity
  Cosmic Engulfment
  "No Exit" or Hell
  Death-Rebirth Struggle
  Death-Rebirth Experience
Embryonal and Fetal Experiences
Ancestral Experiences
Collective and Racial Experiences
Phylogenetic (Evolutionary) Experiences
"Past Incarnation" Experiences
Precognition, Clairvoyance, and "Time Travels"

B. *Spatial Expansion of Consciouness*

Ego Transcendence in Interpersonal Relations
Identification with Other Persons
Group Identification and Group Consciousness
Animal Identification
Plant Identification
Oneness with Life and All Creation
Consciousness of Inorganic Matter
Planetary Consciousness
Extra-Planetary Consciousness
Out-of-Body Experiences, Traveling Clairvoyance, "Space Travels"
  and Telepathy

C. *Spatial Constriction of Consciousness*

Organ, Tissue, and Cellular Consciousness

II. Experiential Extension (or Expansion) Beyond The Framework of "Objective Reality"

Spiritistic and Mediumistic Experiences
Experiences of Encounters with Supra-Human Spiritual Entities
Experiences of Other Universes and of Encounters with Their Inhabitants
Archetypal Experiences
Experiences of Encounter with Blissful and Wrathful Deities
Activation of the Chakras and Arousal of the Serpent Power (Kundalini)
Consciousness of the Universal Mind
The Supracosmic and Metacosmic Void

It is necessary to bear in mind that transpersonal experiences, in particular in psychedelic sessions, do not always occur in a pure form. It was mentioned before that, for example, perinatal experiences are frequently accompanied by other types of transpersonal experiences, such as identification with other persons, group identification, some archetypal experiences, or encounters with various deities. Similarly, the embryonal experiences can occur simultaneously with phylogenetic memories and with the experience of cosmic unity, etc. This seems to reflect deep intrinsic interrelations between various types of transpersonal phenomena as well as the multilevel nature of the psychedelic experience.

Whatever may prove to be the most fruitful approach to the problem of future classification, it is hoped that the attempt in this paper to define and describe transpersonal experiences on the basis of observations from psychedelic sessions will attract the attention of more professionals to the area of transpersonal experiences. Systematic research of these most unusual phenomena could dramatically change our concepts of man and be of unforeseen relevance to the psychiatry and psychology of the future.

References

Assagioli, R. *Psychosynthesis: A manual of principles and techniques.* New York: Hobbs, Dorman & Co., Inc., 1965.
Freud, S. *Totem and taboo* (ed. James Strachey). New York: W. W. Norton, 1952.

Grof, S. Beyond psychoanalysis: I. Implications of LSD research for understanding dimensions of human personality. Presented at the World Conference on Scientific Yoga, New Delhi, India, December, 1970. Published in *Darshana International* (India), 1970a, *10*, 55.

Grof, S. Beyond psychoanalysis: II. A conceptual model of personality encompassing the psychedelic phenomena. Presented as preprint at the Second Interdisciplinary Conference of Voluntary Control of Internal States, Council Grove, Kansas, April, 1970b.

Grof, S. Beyond psychoanalysis: III. Birth trauma and its relation to mental illness, suicide and ecstasy. Presented as preprint at the Second Interdisciplinary Conference on Voluntary Control of Internal States, Council Grove, Kansas, Arpil, 1970c.

Grof, S. LSD psychotherapy and human culture (Part I). *Journal Study Consciousness,* 1970d, 100. (Part II) *Journal Study Consciousness,* 1971, *4,* 167.

Grof, S., *Theory and practice of LSD psychotherapy.* Philadelphia: University of Pennsylvania Press, in press.

Grof, S., Pahnke, W. N., Kurland, A. A., Goodman, L. E. LSD-assisted psychotherapy in patients with terminal cancer. Presented at the Fifth Symposium of the Foundation of Thanatology, New York City, November 12, 1971.

James, W. *The varieties of religious experience.* New York: Modern Library, 1902.

Jung, C. G. *Collected works,* Bollingen Series. New York: Pantheon, 1959.

Laski, M. *Ecstasy: A study of some secular and religious experiences.* Bloomington, Indiana: Indiana University Press, 1962.

Maslow, A. H. A theory of metamotivation: The biological rooting of the value-life. In A. Sutich and M. A. Vich (Eds.), *Readings in humanistic psychology.* New York: The Free Press, Ltd. 1969.

Maslow, A. H. *Religions, values and peak experiences.* Columbus, Ohio: Ohio State University Press, 1964.

Pahnke, W. N., Richards, W. A. Implications of LSD and experimental mysticism. *J. Religion Health,* 1966, *5,* 176.

Schure, E *The great initiates.* West Nyack, New York: St. George Books, 1961.

Malcolm B. Bowers, Jr., and
Daniel X. Freedman

"Psychedelic" Experiences in Acute Psychoses

The disease which thus evokes these new and wonderful talents and operations of the mind may be compared to an earthquake which, by convulsing the upper strata of our globe, throws upon its surface precious and splendid fossils, the existence of which was unknown to the proprietors of the soil in which they were buried.[1]

THIS PAPER is concerned with subjective experience in the early phases of some psychotic reactions and has been prepared with two problems in mind. First, in the experimental production of altered states of awareness in man, the most common source of information is the self-report; yet when data obtained in this way are compared to clinical conditions it becomes clear that we have very little comparable information from patients. As a result, when studies in experimental psychopathology are related to clinical states, comparisons may be confusing and can give rise to spurious controversy as to whether or not a particular experimental state actually resembles a certain clinical syndrome. Thus precise information about subjective experience in clinical conditions might help to clarify some of these issues. Secondly, altered experiences of self and external world have not been easily accounted for in psychodynamic theories of psychosis. Arlow and Brenner have recently emphasized that some of the observations on which dynamic theories of psychosis have been based require more careful scrutiny,[2] and the observations recorded in this report are a part of such an ongoing attempt.

There are some noteworthy observations in the literature focused on subjective experience in early psychosis. Jaspers, Mayer-Gross, Binswanger, Straus, and Minkowski have written about self-experience interpreted from the viewpoint of existentialist theories or phenomenology.[3,4] McGhie and Chapman have characterized some of the perceptual alterations in early schizophrenia.[5] Their clinical findings have led to several experimental approaches to perceptual and cognitive processes in schizophrenia.[6] Norman Cameron has written in detail about the subjective world of the incipient paranoid psychotic.[7] Arieti has described schizophrenic panic, and his description is similar to many of the cases we will cite.[8]

We have obtained information from two sources. First in clinical work with psychotic patients over a two-year period, an attempt was made to elicit information about their earliest recognition of "changes." This was done either at the time they were acutely disturbed (e.g., "What are you feeling now?") or in retrospect. Whenever possible, a patient was encouraged to write a brief statement describing his earliest subjective experiences when he fell ill. In several instances it turned out that patients had written down their feelings during the early stages of their psychosis, and we asked permission to read these accounts.[9] As our second source, we reviewed most of the available self-reports by psychotic patients in a rather restrictive way.[10,11] That is, we in essence asked of each document the question, "Is there included in this account any clear description of the writer's earliest and/or most consistently experienced alteration in subjectivity?" In a number of instances—some classic, some relatively unfamiliar—we found material pertinent to this question.

Report of Cases

Case 1. —A 38-year-old music teacher, pressed by debts and family problems and concerned with a very real national crisis, began to feel that life was taking on an emotional intensity which was new. He noted a cross on a familiar church for the first time and felt that it had profound, exciting meaning for him. He felt close to nature, emphatically understanding human and subhuman life. A few nights later he described a sensation that "God actually touched my heart. The next day was horror and ecstasy. I began to feel that I might be the agent of some spiritual reawakening." The emotional intensity of the experience became overpowering. Gradually, anxiety and persecutory delusions outstripped the ecstatic elements and the patient made a serious suicide attempt. Even much later in psychotherapy he recalled "the experience" as one of profound meaning for him, one which he would always cherish.

Case 2. —A 21-year-old college student, concerned about his parents and about a love affair, became guilt-ridden after a sexual experience with his girl friend. Soon thereafter, he felt that his life was completely changed. He felt a sense of mission in the world, which he now saw "as a completely wonderful place," and stated, "I began to experience goodness and love for the first time." Life for him took on an intense benevolent quality which he had never felt before. He talked with friends fervently about the "new life" and about the way he could now care for and understand people. The feelings progressed to frank delusions that he was a religious messiah and heralded an acute catatonic psychosis.

Case 3. —Another 21-year-old college student had been ruminating for some time about "personality problems" and difficulties in the choice of a vocation. The following is essentially a verbatim account of the week prior to his admission.

"Before last week, I was quite closed about my emotions; then finally I owned up to them with another person. I began to speak without thinking beforehand and what came out showed an awareness of human beings and God. I could feel deeply about other people. We felt connected. The side which had been suppressing emotions did not seem to be the real one. I was in a higher and higher state of exhilaration and awareness. Things people said had hidden meaning. They said things that applied to life. Everything that was real seemed to make sense. I had a great awareness of life, truth, and God. I went to church and suddenly all parts of the service made sense. My senses were sharpened. I became fascinated by the little insignificant things around me. There was an additional awareness of the world that would do artists, architects, and painters good. I ended up being too emotional, but I felt very much at home with myself, very much at ease. It gave me a great feeling of power. It was not a case of seeing more broadly, but deeper. I was losing touch with the outside world and lost my sense of time. There was a fog around me in some sense, and I felt half asleep. I could see more deeply into problems that other people had and would go directly into a deeper subject with a person. I had the feeling I loved everybody in the world. Sharing emotions was like wiping the shadow away, wiping a false face. I thought I might wake up from a nightmare; ideas were pulsating through me. I became concerned that I might get violent so I called the doctor."

On admission, this patient was severely agitated; delusional and self-referential thoughts were prominent.

Case 4. —A 31-year-old housewife wrote a description of the week prior to her hospitalization for an acute paranoid psychosis.

"Thoughts spun around in my head and everything—objects, sound, events

—took on special meaning for me. I felt like I was putting the pieces of a puzzle together. Childhood feelings began to come back, as symbols and bits from past conversations went through my head. The word *religious* and other words from other past conversations during the fall and summer months came back to me during this week and seemed to take on a new significance. I increasingly began to feel that I was experiencing something like mystical revelations . . . at the gas station, the men smiled at me with twinkles in their eyes, and I felt very good. I saw smiling men's faces in the sky and the stars twinkling in their eyes. I felt better than I ever had in my life."

Case 5. —A 21-year-old student, progressively agitated by homosexual concerns and fears of nuclear disaster, walked all night long with a friend. He described his experience as a "revelation." Sights and sounds possessed a keenness that he had never experienced before. He felt an unusual sense of empathy with this friend and spoke of spontaneous understanding "like that of a little child." Stars in the sky seemed to have special significance, and at one point he felt that his friend resembled Christ. This state proceeded rapidly to an acute catatonic reaction.

Case 6. —A 35-year-old housewife sought psychiatric assistance because of her uneasiness over an impending move to another city. In the course of the evaluation she began to wonder about the "meaning of my whole life." She reported sensations of "being a spectator while the procession of life goes by." Over a two-day period her anxiety mounted as she attempted to deal with her guilt about a long-standing affair of which her husband had no knowledge. Rather abruptly she noted, "My senses were sharpened, sounds were more intense and I could see with greater clarity, everything seemed very clear to me. Even my sense of taste seemed more acute. Things began to fall together and make sense. Words I would repeat had particular significance for my life." She began to feel that God was asking her to give her life to tell other people about religion. These subjective changes were associated with intense fright and acute insomnia.

Case 7. —A 20-year-old artist subsequently followed for seven years in psychotherapy has frequently referred to his states of altered awareness. Such subjective feelings occurred during each of two acute psychotic episodes and throughout psychotherapy. He describes a mystic or "cryptic state" from which the solutions to various problems seem obvious. Colors become impressive to him, they lose their boundaries, and seem to flow. In these states, his sense of communion and community is enhanced; he feels capable of bringing together the arts and sciences, his separated parents, and himself into harmonious "oscillation" with the world. Going without sleep heightens the mystic states and improves his "freedom and vision" in painting. In this state he cannot tell whether he is "thrilled, frightened, pained, or anxious—they are all the same."

Amphetamine and Alcohol Withdrawal States. —We have seen several patients in these categories whose symptomatology suggested similarities to the previous cases. The phenomenon of "amphetamine psychosis" is well known, and our experience suggests that the full-blown syndrome often develops out of a state of hyperawareness.[12] One patient, having taken small doses of amphetamine for only three days in the postpartum period, began to have the subjective feeling that God was trying to help her. Colors and normally trivial observations began to take on ominous significance. Things that would not usually be noticed seemed to be "connected." Another patient, chronically sleepless and taking high doses of amphetamines over several months, phoned and reported he was feeling better, "released," and productive; the world looked beautiful and bright, he could see "how to repair my marriage" and had new ideas for his work. The next day he reported at length that it was fascinating to note "reflections" from polished cars and the following day announced that huge parabolic mirrors were placed on top of a newspaper building and as a hoax were reflecting images of naked women off windows and onto bodies. He thus moved from an absorption in the reflections and in his subjective state of "seeing solutions" to problems, to a full-fledged paranoid psychosis. Another patient who experienced delirium tremens on several occasions noted that prior to the full-blown state he would often become hyperaware of sounds and would find himself suddenly distracted by insignificant items such as a leaf or a bird in a tree. He added that the difference between such a state and delirium tremens was that in the latter he could not "come back."

Case 8. —The final case presented a unique opportunity in that one of us treated for four months a young man who had taken lysergic acid diethylamide (LSD-25) two years prior to his psychotic episode. He frequently compared the two experiences and found a number of similarities. In the following account, the first part was written down after a few weeks of treatment when he was considerably calmer and was reflecting upon the prior LSD-25 experience. The last part is taken from his admission interview.

"In the half hour for the drug to take effect, the drugged person has a psychosomatic terror of madness. He seeks to retain some small part of his former existence unchanged . . . he desires to repeat things for the assurance such repetition gives of a return to normality. The tendency to repeat is compulsive and persistent. There is yet another resistance and that is verbosity. The drugged person, like the insane, feels that weeding out what was previously wrong—an attempt to perfect an earlier feeling—is necessary. There is a paranoid fear of certain places . . . the feeling is that such places are in some way taboo. There are manic feelings under the drug. There are moments when the feeling of omniscience if not omnipotence becomes dominant. The feeling of omnipotence under LSD-25 corresponds directly in intensity to the drugged person's sense of guilt as the drug wears off. The guilt felt afterward can be terribly profound to the point that the depressed person (drugged and/or insane) will do almost anything to bring himself out of the depression. The drugged person, like the insane, is quite vulnerable to suggestion. The experience also involves feelings such as the conviction that one can go through walls. Colors seem to hold great and uncanny significance. All of them are providential and mean something . . . now (on the day hospitalized for psychosis) everything takes on significance and patterns. You feel lost and you try to repeat. I feel surges of warmth and great terror of myself. Walls start to move at the periphery of my vision. I feel my tactile senses are enhanced as well as my visual ones, to a point of great power. Patterns and designs begin to distinguish themselves and take on significance. This is true for the LSD-25 experience also. It's the same now as it was with the drug, only then I knew I was coming back. Now there is nothing to hold onto."

Literary Accounts*

John Custance [13].—First and foremost comes a general sense of intense well-being . . . the pleasurable and sometimes ecstatic feeling tone remains as a sort of permanent background . . . closely allied with this permanent background is . . . the "heightened sense of reality." If I am to judge by my own experience, this "heightened sense of reality" consists of a considerable number of related sensations, the net result of which is that the outer world makes a much more vivid and intense impression on me than usual. . . . The first thing I note is the peculiar appearances of the lights. . . . They are not exactly brighter, but deeper, more intense, perhaps a trifle more ruddy than usual. Certainly my sense of touch is heightened. . . . My hearing appears to be more sensitive, and I am able to take in without disturbance or distraction many different sound impressions at the same time. . . . It is actually a sense of communion, in the first place with God, and in the second place with all

---

*A number of these accounts have been compiled and edited by Kaplan, B. in *The Inner World of Mental Illness,* Harper and Row, Publishers, Inc., 1964.

mankind, indeed with all creation. . . . The sense of communication extends to all fellow creatures with whom I come in contact; it is not merely ideal or imaginative but has a practical effect on my conduct.

Anonymous Account [14].—I experienced a sudden feeling of creative release before my illness, was convinced that I was rapidly attaining the height of my intellectual powers, and that for the first time in my life, I would be able to function up to the level of my ability in this direction. . . . On several occasions my eyes became markedly oversensitive to light. Ordinary colors appeared to be much too bright, and sunlight seemed dazzling in intensity. . . . I also had a sense of discovery, creative excitement, and intense, at times mystical inspiration in intervals where there was relief from fear. . . . My capacities for aesthetic appreciation and heightened sensory receptiveness, for vivid grasp of the qualities of living, and for imaginative empathy were very keen at this time. I had had the same intensity of experience at other times when I was perfectly normal, but such periods were not sustained for as long, and had also been integrated with feelings of well-being and happiness that were absent during the tense disturbed period.

Schreber [15].—Dr. Weber, who was in charge of the asylum where Schreber was hospitalized, wrote the following in his court testimony:

At the beginning of his stay there he (Schreber) mentioned mostly hypochondriacal ideas . . . but ideas of persecution soon appeared in the disease picture, based on hallucinations, which at first appeared sporadically while simultaneously marked hyperesthesia, great sensitivity to light and noise made their appearance. Later the visual and auditory hallucinations multiplied and, in conjunction with disturbances of common sensation, ruled his whole feeling and thinking. . . . Gradually, the delusions took on a mystical and religious character . . . he saw "miracles," heard "holy music" . . . I have in no way assumed a priori the pathological nature of these ideas, but rather tried to show from the history of the patient's illness how the appellant first suffered from severe hyperesthesia, hypersensitivity to light and noise . . . and particular disturbances of common sensation which falsified his conception of things . . . and how from these pathological events, at last the system of ideas was formed which the appellant has recounted . . . in his memoirs.

Clifford Beers [16].—No man can be born again, but I believe I came as near it as ever a man did. . . . It seemed as though the refreshing breath of some kind goddess of wisdom was being gently blown against the surface of my brain. . . . So delicate, so crisp and exhilarating was it that words fail me in my attempt to describe it. Few, if any, experiences can be more delightful. . . . For me, however, this experience was liberation, not enslavement.

Norma McDonald[17].—What I do want to explain, if I can, is the exaggerated state of awareness in which I lived before, during, and after my acute illness. At first it was as if parts of my brain "awoke" which had been dormant, and I became interested in a wide assortment of people, events, places, and ideas which normally would make no impression on me. Not knowing that I was ill, I made no attempt to understand what was happening, but felt that there was some overwhelming significance in all this, produced either by God or Satan, and I felt that I was duty-bound to ponder on each of these new interests, and the more I pondered, the worse it became. The walk of a stranger on the street could be a "sign" to me which I must interpret. Every face in the windows of a passing streetcar would be engraved on my mind, all of them concentrating on me and trying to pass me some sort of message. Now, many years later, I can appreciate what had happened. Each of us is capable of coping with a large number of stimuli invading or being through any one of the senses . . . it is obvious that we would be incapable of carrying on any of our daily activities if even one hundredth of all these available stimuli invaded us at once. So the mind must have a filter which functions without our conscious thought, sorting stimuli and allowing only those which are relevant to the situation in hand to disturb consciousness. And this filter must be working at maximum efficiency at all times, particularly when we require a high degree of concentration. What had happened to me in Toronto was a breakdown in the filter . . . new significance in people and places was not particularly unpleasant, though it got badly in the way of my work, but the significance of the real or imagined feelings of people was very painful. . . . In this state, delusions can very easily take root and begin to grow. . . . By the time I was admitted to hospital I had reached a stage of "wakefulness" when the brilliance of light on a window sill or the color of blue in the sky would be so important it could make me cry. I had very little ability to sort the relevant from the irrelevant. The filter had broken down. Completely unrelated events became intricately connected in my mind.

Comment

Characterization and Comparison.—It will be clear that we have been struck by certain repetitive aspects in these accounts and have abstracted from them to clarify our argument. In brief it seems that these patients are describing a state, early in their illness, in which they recognize an altered way of experiencing themselves, others, and the world. They report having stepped beyond the restrictions of their usual state of awareness. Perceptual modes seem heightened and the emotional response evoked is singularly intense. Such experiences are frequently felt to be a kind of breakthrough, words and phrases such as *release* or *new creativity* being used to characterize them. Individuals experience feelings of getting to the essence of things—of the external world, of others, and of themselves. On the other hand, there is usually a vague disquieting, progressive sense of dread which may eventually dominate the entire experience. In some accounts the experience of perceptual alteration seems to be dominant; others emphasize the intense affectivity, and still others the inner experience of revelation or creative clarification. In most of the accounts—but not in all—the experience comes as a kind of surprise and is apprehended as happening *to the subject* and not *within him.* Others, however, seem to recognize the process as basically an inner change which in turn "makes all things new" (case 3, anonymous account, Beers, McDonald).

Given such an altered *experience,* formal processes of thought and cognition are likely to be altered. Wynn, for example, has suggested that schizophrenia be broadly understood as an "experience disorder," and that formal thought processes are studied as an indicator of altered experience.[18]

When seen from the point of view of subjective experience, early psychotic experiencing becomes less discontinuous with other altered modes of experiencing. For instance, LSD-25 and mescaline may induce a very comparable perceptual and effective condition. It is clearly a multipotential state with many factors influencing the final outcome, which can range from excruciating anxiety and paranoid delusions to an experience of intense self-knowledge. Space does not permit detailed excerpts from the drug literature, but Terrill's summary of "The Nature of the LSD Experience" can serve as a comprehensive statement of the phenomenon.[19] Such characteristics as increased perceptual sensitivity and portentousness, intensification of interpersonal experience, feelings of unique insight into life, and personal clarification—all well-documented in the LSD reaction—are clearly shared by the accounts we have listed. More recent reviews have made it clear that the drugs induce a kind of fluid state in which a number of variables act to fashion the final result along the psychedelic-psychotomimetic continuum. Freedman has characterized this state from the viewpoint of the clinician.[20]

> Psychotomimetic drugs such as d-lysergic acid diethylamide . . . reliably and consistently produce periods of altered perception and experience without clouded consciousness or marked physiological changes; mental processes that are usually dormant and transient

during wakefulness become "locked" into a persistent state. The usual boundaries which structure thought and perception become fluid; awareness becomes vivid while control over input is markedly diminished; customary inputs and modes of thought and perception become novel, illusory, and portentous; and with the loss of customary controlling anchors, dependence on the surroundings, on prior expectations, or on a mystique for structure and support is enhanced. Psychiatrists recognize these primary changes as a background state out of which a number of secondary psychological states can ensue, depending on motive, capacity, and circumstance. This is reflected in the terminology that has grown around these drugs; if symptoms ensue, the term psychotomimetic or psychodysleptic is used; and if mystical experience, religious conversion, or a therapeutic change in behavior is stressed, the term *psychedelic* or mind "manifesting" has been applied.

The drugs and clinical states set up a "search for synthesis," and the motives and capacities of subjects and patients to achieve this are obviously of importance if one is to assess outcomes and compare and contrast these states.

There are other intense self-experiences—unrelated to the use of drugs—which have elements in common with the accounts we have presented. William James' classic study of religious phenomena, for instance, is replete with accounts of conversion experiences that are strikingly similar to the cases we have described and to the experiences of some subjects under LSD-25 and mescaline.[21] James describes the characteristics of the affective experience in religious conversion as follows:

> The central one is the loss of all worry, the sense that all is ultimately well with one, the peace, the harmony, the willingness to be, even though the outer conditions should remain the same. . . . The second feature is the sense of perceiving truths not known before. The mysteries of life become lucid . . . and often the solution is more or less unutterable in words. . . . A third peculiarity of the assurance state is the objective change which the world often appears to undergo. . . . The most characteristic of all the elements of the conversion crisis . . . is the ecstasy of happiness produced.

James himself seems to have been well aware of the similarity between the conversion experience and certain psychotic reactions:

> But more remains to be told, for religious mysticism is only one half of mysticism. The other half has no accumulated traditions

except those which the textbooks on insanity supply. Open any one of these, and you will find abundant cases in which "mystical ideas" are cited as characteristic symptoms of enfeebled or deluded states of mind. In delusional insanity . . . we may have a *diabolical* mysticism, a sort of religious mysticism turned upside down. The same sense of ineffable importance in the smallest events, the same texts and words coming with new meanings, the same voices and visions and leadings and missions, the same controlling by extraneous powers; only this time the emotion is pessimistic: instead of consolations we have desolations; the meanings are dreadful; and the powers are enemies to life. It is evident that from the point of view of their psychological mechanism, the classic mysticism and these lower mysticisms spring from the same mental level, from that great subliminal or transmarginal region of which science is beginning to admit the existence, but of which so little is really known. That region contains every kind of matter: "seraph and snake" abide there side by side. To come from thence is no infallible credential. What comes must be sifted and tested, and run the gauntlet of confrontation with the total context of experience, just like what comes from the outer world of sense.

The significance of religious feeling in psychosis has been earlier explored by Boisen[22] and more recently by Laing.[23] Maslow has described the subjective phenomenology of "peak experiences" and emphasizes new modes of awareness which may be encountered at certain maturational milestones.[24] Similarly, in the course of psychotherapy crisis points and periods of intense insight may also be characterized by exhilaration, expressed new modes of experiencing and perceiving, transient fear mixed with intense happiness, and a sense of acceleration of intrapsychic activity.[25] Mystical experiences occurring as a culmination of intense intrapsychic conflict have recently been presented.[26]

The utility of such insight, the extent to which it is delusional or adaptive, varies not only in psychotherapy but in psychoses, drug states, and religious and mystical states.

Deikman has recently studied mystical practices experimentally and has advanced hyptheses to account for the intrapsychic phenomena in such procedures.[27,28] Further, a number of creative individuals—including Blake, Coleridge, Brahms, and Rilke, to mention only a few—described comparable unique shifts in their subjective experience of perceptual processes which they held to be an integral part of their creative gift.[29-32] Moreover the relationship between genius and insanity has been a provocative question, debated for centuries.[33,34]

Implications

With the advent of psychotomimetic drugs there was renewed interest in the study of altered mental states, but the opportunity to catch "in situ" the formation and genesis of a variety of symptoms and modes of behaving and coping has not been extensively exploited. In part it was doubted that drug-induced experiences were sufficiently related to clinically-encountered dysfunctions to be of interest.[35] Yet it is hardly surprising that temporary and experimentally-induced states do not reproduce all the features characterizing clinical processes; the latter are neither bound as rigorously by time nor circumscribed by the highly socialized safeguards of the conventional laboratory situation. Rather, these differences only highlight those features of clinical disorders which require explanation in terms of developmental factors and restitutive and compensatory sequences. The patient experiencing and functioning in this altered state must cope overtime with a variety of life tasks, family and social interactions; his resilience and overall disposition to represent, identify, and differentiate "inside and outside" and to relate in a reality oriented way, will differentiate him from most experimental subjects.

Similarly, the fact that these drugs produce ecstatic states from which new learning, a shift in values, or subsequent behavior change purportedly ensue, was thought to isolate such states from their "psychotomimetic status" and perhaps to elevate them to a higher level of discourse. Some enthusiasts even appear to argue that this novelty is beyond psychological description and investigation. Yet the variety of contexts in which such mystic states occur includes clinical conditions, as our data have reemphasized. It is also evident that this range of similar states differs not only in outcome but in the extent to which a variety of ego functions are operative—functions such as memory, self-reflective capacity, tolerance for ambiguity, selective attention, the ability to implement wishes and needs in reality, the ability to synthesize, to order, and to serially locate, and to integrate ongoing experiences with past and future. These differentiating features tend to be lost if all such states are described only in terms of loosened ego boundaries, regression in the service of the ego, altered ego autonomy, and deautomatization.[28,36–39] Such descriptions should properly apply only to certain aspects and attributes of certain of the ego operations altered during these conditions. During various phases of the clinical course of a psychosis one frequently can see fluid states in which elements of perceptual instability and psychedelic experience occur preceded or followed by more settled postures in which the patient, through either recognition, insight, withdrawal, or delusion and symptom formation, tends to experience and cope in quite different ways. Similarly, in drug-induced psychedelic states, as the acute and vivid effects subside we and others[40] can observe a variety of paranoid and defensive measures, mild ideas of reference, mood change, and inappropriate or highly imaginative interpretations of the ongoing or previous experience. From a descriptive and theoretical standpoint, then, the clinical and drug-induced psychedelic experience reflects a multipotential mental state which cannot easily be encapsulated or understood without careful scrutiny and study of the sequences of states and differentiation of primary and secondary reactions. It seems apparent that the reaction of the therapist or other significant persons in the environment could crucially affect the course and resolution of such states.

Descriptively, these states of heightened awareness but diminished control over input are frequently characterized by delusional mastery (either shared or idiosyncratic) or (as with dreams) by hallucinatory mastery of the ongoing experience with concomitant euphoria. One is reminded of Freud's "model psychosis." "A dream, then, is a psychosis," he remarked, beginning a chapter in the *Outline of Psychoanalysis.* [41] The absurdities, lapses, hallucinatory mastery, and mental processes of psychoses are evident in dreams, Freud argued. Some of the differences between dream and psychosis cited by him were the short duration of the dream, its useful or adaptive function, and the fact that it is to some degree under the control of the dreamer. In the case of drug-induced states the onset and duration of changes (and to a great extent the intensity of effects) are dependent on dosage. On the other hand, as Freud noted, "The dream is brought about with the subject's consent and is ended by an act of his will." However, this might be translated into the language of ego psychology; the dream as an episode in a sequence of states is implied, as is a normal, overall capacity to integrate this episode into the total fabric of living. Such autonomy or integrative control probably is present in widely varying degrees in the states we have reviewed, and in drug states the role both of altered body chemistry and the milieu is clearly great; all these features require differential assessment.

These states frequently appear almost to compel rationalization or interpretation, as on occasion do dreams or any number of traumatic, infantile, or hypnoid states[42] in which the ongoing intense experiences have yet to "run the gauntlet of confrontation" with total experience. That this is not easy and that delusional outcomes, conversion, or startling change in behavioral patterns can occur is apparent. These outcomes occur with varying degrees of dependence upon persons, groups, or authority. This fact indicates that drug-induced gaps in reality-coping confer a grave responsibility for the bridging of such gaps which should fall heavily upon the therapists using psychotomimetic drugs. One would expect, therefore, to have encountered considerable literature on the need for case supervision and on the characteristic countertransference problems evoked by such treatment, but with a few exceptions[43] this is relatively absent in the psychedelic-treatment literature.

The bearing of the phenomenological accounts such as those presented upon the various psychodynamic theories of psychosis, while complex, deserves at least brief comment. For instance, it is hard to conceive of all of these states as caused and preceded by a simple withdrawal of libidinal investment in the object world. Rather the outside world may be experienced in a highly intensified, albeit personalized manner. This kind of experience is highly narcissistic (in that it is referred to the self), but descriptively certain aspects of relatedness to objects remain and even attain a heightened personal significance; further, such relatedness assumes a heightened importance in regulating ego functions. In the drug experience, subjects characteristically depend on the therapist or "guide" not simply as an object but for elemental ego support—to diminish anxiety and to structure the experience or to sanction participation in it. Patients in acute psychotic states have similar narcissistic needs. From scrutiny of clinical and drug-induced states one might propose that there is a rearrangement of a number of ego functions (of which changes in the control of attention and perception are quite striking); these may lead subsequently *or* concomitantly to a narcissistically enhanced significance of the self and the world. Pious, for example, postulates a sudden ego breach—a "nadir experience," following which characteristic psychotic symptoms ensue.[44] Obviously the question of conceptualizing and observing the sequence of initiating events (libidinal withdrawal or ego disruption or both) requires further differentiation and scrutiny.

The experimental production of experiences of heightened awareness can help both to differentiate and reveal the relatedness of many complex phenomena encountered in clinical psychiatry, with their intricate layering of social, motivational, compensatory, and regressive features. The wide range of contexts in which states of heightened awareness are found to occur and the variety of initiating causes indicate that this mode of functioning and experiencing reflects an innate capacity (like the dream) of which the human mind in a most general sense is capable. These states and the conditions which produce them create a number of unsolved research problems for experimental psychiatry. It is, for example, noteworthy that of the drugs which induce this particular kind of heightened awareness, the indole alkyl amines and certain derivatives of catecholamines are effective, whereas distinctly different pictures are found following other centrally active compounds related to the pharmacology of acetylcholine.[45,46] There are other unresolved research problems. Aside from reconciling the continuity between psychotomimetic and psychedelic experience, a major task is to stipulate the determinants of the various outcomes of both drug-induced and naturally-occurring conditions.

Summary

We have presented accounts of subjective experience in some early psychotic reactions from both our clinical work and the literature and have compared these accounts to certain natural and drug-induced experiences which have a certain experiential characteristic in common—that of heightened consciousness or awareness. *Psychedelic and psychotomimetic phenomena are closely related.* Our hypothesis is that these states demonstrate to varying degrees the subjective phenomena of intrapsychic alteration, that they are fluid states whose outcome is determined by both intrapsychic and environmental factors. There are clearly quantitative, interindividual differences in the way such experiences can be tolerated, interpreted, terminated, and assimilated into the ongoing context of experience. To account for such differences in terms of discrete ego liabilities *and* assets would be to explicate many crucial psychological phenomena, including certain forms of psychosis, therapeutic personality change, and creative insight.

References

1. Rush, B.: *Medical Inquiries and Observations Upon the Diseases of the Mind,* New York: Hafner Publishing Co., 1962.
2. Arlow, J., and Brenner, C.: *Psychoanalytic Concepts and the Structural Theory,* New York: International Universities Press, Inc., 1964.
3. Jaspers, K.: *General Psychopathology,* Chicago: University of Chicago Press, 1964.
4. May, R.; Angel, E.; and Ellenberger, H. F., (Eds.): *Existence,* New York: Basic Books, Inc., 1958.
5. McGhie, A., and Chapman, J. A.: Disorders of Attention and Perception in Early Schizophrenia, *Brit J Med Psychol* 34:103–116, 1961.

6. McGhie, A.; Chapman, J. A.; and Lawson, J. S.: The Effect of Distraction on Schizophrenic Performance, *Brit J Psychiat* 3:383–390, 391–398, 1965.

7. Cameron, N.: "Paranoid Conditions and Paranoia," in Arieti, S. (Ed.): *American Handbook of Psychiatry,* New York: Basic Books, Inc., 1959.

8. Arieti, S.: "Introductory Notes on the Psychoanalytic Therapy of Schizophrenia," in Burton (Ed.): *Psychotherapy of the Psychoses,* New York: Basic Books, Inc., 1961.

9. Bowers, M. B.: The Onset of Psychosis—A Diary Account, *Psychiatry* 28:346–358, 1965.

10. Sommer, R., and Osmond, H.: Autobiographies of Former Mental Patients, *J Ment Sci* 106:648–662, 1960.

11. Sommer, R., and Osmond, H.: Autobiographies of Former Mental Patients—Addendum, *J Ment Sci* 107:1030–1032, 1961.

12. Connell, P. H.: *Amphetamine Psychosis,* London: Oxford University Press, 1958.

13. Custance, J.: *Wisdom, Madness, and Folly,* New York: Farrar, Straus, and Giroux, 1952.

14. Anonymous: An Autobiography of a Schizophrenic Experience, *J Abnorm Soc Psychiat* 51:677–680, 1955.

15. Macalpine, I., and Hunter, R. A.: *Daniel Paul Schreber—Memoirs of My Nervous Illness,* London: William Dawson and Sons Ltd., 1955.

16. Beers, C.: *A Mind That Found Itself,* New York; Longmans, Green, 1908.

17. McDonald, N.: Living With Schizophrenia, *Canad Med Assoc J* 82:218–221, 678–681, 1960.

18. Wynne, L.: Thought Disorder and Family Relations of Schizophrenics, *Arch Gen Psychiat* 9:199–206, 1963.

19. Terrill, J.: The Nature of the LSD Experience, *J Nerv Ment Dis* 135:425–439, 1962.

20. Giarman, N. J., and Freedman, D. X.: Biochemical Aspects of the Actions of Psychotomimetic Drugs, *Pharmacol Rev* 17:1–25, 1965.

21. James, W.: *The Varieties of Religious Experience,* New York: The New American Library of World Literature, Inc., 1958.

22. Boisen, A.: *The Exploration of the Inner World,* New York: Harper and Row, Publishers, Inc., 1952.

23. Laing, R. D.: Transcendental Experience in Relation to Religion and Psychosis. *Psychedelic Rev,* 6:7–15, 1965.

24. Maslow, A. H.: *Toward a Psychology of Being,* New York: D. Van Nostrand Co., Inc., 1962.
25. Carlson, H. B.: The Relationship of the Acute Confusional State to Ego Development, *Int J Psychoanal* 42:517–536, 1962.
26. Freemantle, A. (Ed.): *Protestant Mystics,* New York: New American Library of World Literature, 1965.
27. Deikman, A. J.: Experimental Meditation, *J Nerv Ment Dis* 136:329–343, 1963.
28. Deikman, A. J.: Implications of Experimental Meditation, to be published.
29. Schorer, M.: *William Blake—The Politics of Vision,* New York: Heritage Books, 1959.
30. Abell, A. M.: *Talks With Great Composers,* Garmisch-Partenkirchen: G. E. Schroeder-Verlag, 1964.
31. Leishman, J. B., and Spender, S. T.: *Duino Elegies-Rainer Maria Rilke,* New York: W. W. Norton & Co., Inc., 1963.
32. Kris, E.: On Inspiration, *Int J Psychoanal* 20:377–389, 1939.
33. Mora, G.: One Hundred Years From Lombroso's First Essay-Genius and Insanity, *Amer J Psychiat* 121:562–571, 1964.
34. Lidz, T.: August Strindberg: A Study of the Relationship Between His Creativity and Schizophrenia, *Int J Psychoanal* 45:399–406, 1964.
35. Hollister, L. E.: Drug-Induced Psychoses and Schizophrenic Reactions: A Critical Comparison, *Ann NY Acad Sci* 96:80–92, 1962.
36. Federn, P.: *Ego Psychology and the Psychoses,* New York: Basic Books, Inc., 1952.
37. Kris, E.: *Psychoanalytic Explorations in Art,* New York, International Universities Press, Inc., 1952.
38. Miller, S. C.: Ego-Autonomy in Sensory Deprivation, Isolation, and Stress, *Int J Psychoanal* 43:1–20, 1962.
39. Christensen, C. W.: Religious Conversion, *Arch Gen Psychiat* 9:207–216, 1963.
40. Salvatore, S. and Hyde, R. W.: Progression of Effects of LSD, *Arch Neurol Psychiat* 76:50–59, 1956.
41. Freud, S.: *An Outline of Psychoanalysis,* New York: W. W. Norton & Co., Inc., 1949.
42. Loewald, H.: Hypnoid States—Repression, Abreaction, and Recollection, *J Amer Psychoanal Assoc* 3:201–210, 1955.
43. Savage, C.: Variations in Ego Feeling Induced by LSD-25, *Psychoanal Rev* 42:1–16, 1955.

44. Pious, W.: "A Hypothesis About the Nature of Schizophrenic Behavior," in Burton (Ed.): *Psychotherapy of the Psychosis,* New York: Basic Books, Inc., 1961.
45. Bowers, M. B.; Goodman, E.; and Sim, V.: Some Behavioral Effects in Man Following Anticholinesterase Administration, *J Nerv Ment Dis* **138**:383–389, 1964.
46. Abood, L. G.: A New Group of Psychotomimetic Agents, *Proc Soc* **97**:483–486, 1958.

Julian Silverman

On the Sensory Bases of Transcendental States of Consciousness

When man experiences that certain sequences of mental events
lead to behavior which has, as a matter of fact, survival value, he
calls such mental facts "right." It would be better, however, if
instead of this word some neutral symbol were being used for
those particular events; because the word "right" leads to the
unfortunate notion that some combinations of mental facts are
intrinsically better than others. . . .

Wolfgang Köhler
*The Place of Value
in a World of Facts*

As a scientist, I approach a problem in a particular way. I ask how a
phenomenon occurs; I design experiments to focus on specific aspects of the
phenomenon. I examine data; I draw conclusions from my experiments. They
are how-a-process-works conclusions. They are not what-we should-do-about-
the-process or what-the-process-should be-like conclusions. For example, I can
describe to you, on the basis of laboratory experiments, how a psychoactive
drug like LSD-25 affects sensation, perception, and thought. If you ask me
what we should do with individuals who use this drug, then my scientific
answer is in terms of what I know about how the drug affects sensation,
perception, and thinking. My expertise is in articulating aspects of a process,
not in formulating shoulds. The shoulds about what to do about a process
become obvious when we clearly understand the process.

Part of understanding the process, strange as it may seem, includes understanding how the scientist views it. Every scientific experiment has its origins in a point of view. A point of view influences the way an investigator formulates his experimental problem and chooses his research techniques. It guides him as he sifts through his data in an attempt to summarize his results. How he relates his conclusions to the works of others also depends upon his point of view. Conducting an experiment is not simply a matter of observing a number of facts and then drawing conclusions from them. What is to be observed depends upon the investigator's specific interests and preconceived ideas, on his unique style of organizing and selecting information. This is his way of attending to things; in sum, it is his point of view. There is no such entity as the objective, detached, scientific observer. This is true for every science. I would like, therefore, to begin my presentation on the sensory bases of consciousness with some premises that are basic to my point of view.

Each of us experiences in various modes. We are aware of external ordinary reality, we dream, we imagine, we have semiconscious reveries. Some have visions and hallucinations; they experience faces being transfigured, their bodies being uplifted, disengaged or detached; they see auras, and so on.

Most of us experience the world and ourselves in terms of a consistent identity, a me-here and a you-over-there. We do this in a world stabilized and ordered by constancies: perceptual constancies such as size, shape, brightness, and conceptual constancies including that of the self. Although these constancies exist in physical space-time, the perception of them occurs in sensory-cerebral space-time, inside the organism. We do not perceive what is out there by simply "taking it in"; rather, we *re-present* what is out there. Reality is not intrinsic in man; it is constructed by him. All perceptions are symbolic representations of central nervous system activity. Perception, then, is the interpretation of one's own central nervous system activity (Fischer, 1971*a,b*). If central nervous system activity radically changes, the experience of reality changes.

My aim, therefore, is to formulate an empirical approach to the study of states of consciousness which is rooted in an understanding of sensory and perceptual processes. To do this, I need, first, to lay aside some widely held beliefs regarding stable characteristics of reality.

Nonordinary Experiences in Ordinary People

Until very recently, when studies began to be reported describing spontaneous hallucinations and depersonalization experiences in normal, awake men and women, such occurrences were typically regarded as erupting in psychiatrically disturbed individuals. For example, in a report in the *Journal of Mental Science* in 1960, W. W. Roberts, a psychiatric investigator, was quite unprepared to accept the fact that 39% of a group of college students actually had depersonalization experiences. A depersonalization state is a waking-state occurrence in which there is a significant alteration in the sense of realness of one's experience. The individual feels himself to have lost the familiarity of the real world or he experiences his body as unreal. Everything may seem dreamlike and he may watch his actions and those of others with indifference or detachment.

Conventionally, he would be regarded as abnormal, if he's had that kind of experience. Roberts wrote of his investigation, "it is fairly clear that brief, repetitive, depersonalization *cannot*[1] occur in the general population as frequently as it did in this sample. If it did so, its existence would have been recognized and its incidence acknowledged in the literature [p. 484]." That was in 1960.

Three years later, Dixon (1963) used a different questionnaire procedure for assessing depersonalization and reported a 46% incidence of depersonalization experiences in a group of 112 college students. In a seminar held in Silver Spring, Maryland, for high-caliber student representatives of high schools of five eastern states of the U.S., I also found a 46% incidence of depersonalization (Silverman, unpublished study) in a group of 71 individuals (using the Dixon questionnaire). To the best of my knowledge, the subjects in all of these studies were normal, nonpsychedelic-drug-using, young people.

Taken together, these studies suggest that extraordinary perceptions and sensations of one's environment and of one's self occur in a significant segment of the population who are not turned on, drugged, or so-called behavior-disoriented. Often people simply don't reveal experiences that are conventionally regarded as deviant.

Transcendental States vs. Altered States

There still exists a negative bias on the part of many mental health professionals toward anything but the ordinary waking state of consciousness. And yet normal, waking consciousness—rational consciousness as William James called it—is but one state of consciousness. There are others.

---

[1] italics added

The term "altered states of consciousness" has been applied to states other than the ordinary waking state. "Altered" is, for me, a misleading term. It would be better if, instead of this word, some more neutral symbol were used to denote other states of consciousness, because the word "altered" leads to the unfortunate notion that all other states are deviations from the ordinary waking state. To regard organismic events in this way is, in effect, to judge them rather than merely to describe them. A kind of psychological chauvinism has been the result. It's like saying that the state of California is the best state.

I do not have a thoroughly satisfactory term to substitute for "altered." The one I am presently most comfortable with is "transcendental." *Webster's New Collegiate Dictionary* defines the word "transcendental" as "being beyond the rational, remote from practical affairs or from human comprehension." Any of the nonordinary states of consciousness usually referred to as "altered" fits at least part of this definition.

Sensory Aspects of Transcendental States

In my studies of the reports of religious mystics, Yogi, psychedelic drug–users, meditators, certain acute psychotics, and individuals in other transcendental states of consciousness, I have been impressed by one important similarity. Basic aspects of sensory experiences are remarkably consistent in all of these types.

During ordinary, waking consciousness, simple everyday behaviors are developed and maintained by an ongoing process that continuously and automatically finds ordered relationships in the external environment. Even our usual spatial orientations, however stable they may seem to us, are in the normal course of life brought about and maintained principally by reafferent stimulation (Held & Hein, 1958).[2]

During *non* ordinary states of consciousness, the individual does not respond to stimulation in the same way. For hours or days at a time, he displays such behavioral characteristics as withdrawal and isolation from others, fervent praying, intense mental absorption in a task or thought, prolonged attention to the sound of his breathing, fixation on stationary or moving objects and so on.

Along with the disorganization of psychological structures of ordinary real-

---

[2]Consider also: the isolation experiments of Bexton, Heron and Scott (1954); Freedman et al. (1961); and others. Also the hypnosis studies of Brenman and Gill (1947); the sensory disarrangement experiments of Werner and Wapner (1955); and others.

ity, an increase in sensory intensity and richness occurs. Sensory impressions of low-to-moderate intensity are responded to more strongly; sensory thresholds are lowered. This heightening of sensory awareness in transcendental states has been described with such terms as "the clarity of vision," "seeing the white light," or "cleansing the doors of perception" (Deikman, 1963). The individual may be overwhelmed (literally) by this kind of experience, as St. Paul was, for example. Nearly all mystics known to us describe, at some point in their narrations, their mystical experiences as configurations of lights and sounds (Scholem, 1964). Their sensory experiences are awesome. "At the beginning of their journey, mystics tend to describe their experience in forms drawn from the world of perception. At later stages, corresponding to different levels of consciousness, the world of nature recedes, and these 'natural' forms are replaced by specifically mystical structures [Scholem, 1964, p. 32]." In effect non-sense (meaning) is made out of the initially intense sense experiences.

A change in sensitivity to stimulation is also a primary characteristic of transcendental states labeled as incipient or acute schizophrenia and during psychedelic drug reactions. More than fifty years before Bleuler's classic monograph on the "Group of Schizophrenias" appeared, Connally (1849) wrote of "a sensible excitement of the mind, more or less partial," in psychotic patients; their senses became "disturbed." More recently, investigators such as McGhie and Chapman (1961), Chapman (1966), and Bowers and Freedman (1966), employing specially designed interview techniques, reported that alterations in color and sensory quality precede other perceptual disorder. Many schizophrenic individuals experiencing these changes report that for a time everything around them looks "fascinating, noises all seem to be louder. . . . It's as if someone had turned up the volume." These initial changes in sensory experiences often are regarded as pleasant, and a number of patients at this stage go through a period of mild to marked elation.

> One night I woke up and started feeling good again. . . . I felt alive and vital, full of energy. My senses seemed alive, colors were very bright, they hit me harder. Things appeared clear-cut. I noticed things I had never noticed before [Bowers, 1968, p. 350].

Identical kinds of observations are documented in the literature on subjective reactions to psychedelic drugs (e. g. Bowers & Freedman, 1966; Cohen, 1964; Savage, 1955). In all cases, the individual is acutely aware that he has stepped beyond the bounds of his usual state of awareness. Sensory impressions are awesome and attention is directed, in large measure, *by them*. This "openness" to stimulation is often associated with a fear of being swamped by sensations and images. Laing (1960) terms this the "implosion" of reality— the danger of losing all control, of being hurt, of being obliterated. The natural tendency is to engage in psychological and physical maneuvers which the overwhelmed individual thinks will restore sensory control.[3]

From a strictly clinical viewpoint, these maneuvers are considered to be familiar symptoms of early schizophrenia and of LSD reactions—distractibility, blocking, withdrawal, loss of spontaneity in movment and speech. From the viewpoint presented here, their initial purpose is to reduce the overwhelming intensity of (ordinarily regarded) minimal to moderate intensity stimulation (Silverman, 1968). Indeed, withdrawal from and renunciation of the outside world which occur in various transcendental states can be considered a consequence of neurophysiological adjustments which reduce the experienced intensity of excitation.

Terms like withdrawal, heightened awareness, blocking, and hypersensitivity to stimulation can serve to bridge the gap between transcendental experience and the sensory laboratory study of these phenomena. The scientist need not belabor himself with doubts about the credibility of an individual's report of a transcendental experience. Rather, he can begin his inquiry into such matters by asking a straightforward question: what are the sensory behaviors associated with a report of an extraordinary psychic event?

Sensory Behavior, Attention, and Consciousness

The focus of the empirical studies presented in this paper is on sensory processes and sensory behavior—seeing, hearing, touching and so on—not on what is real or not real.

The theoretical construct used to describe how sensory behavior and consciousness are related is called attention. Attention is a generic term. It refers to the kinds of responses which an organism makes in order to direct his sense receptors to particular inputs and to modify these inputs via central neural processes. Since the term has been applied to a number of quite distinct

---

[3]An experienced LSD guide usually has no difficulty in guiding a subject through such disturbances by encouraging him to "engage in the experience and surrender to it" (Kast, 1967). Comparable techniques are now being used with incipient schizophrenic reactions (Silverman, 1970a.)

sensory and perceptual adjustments, I will need to elaborate presently upon the meaning which "attention" has here.

"Consciousness is awareness, especially of something within oneself; also the state or fact of being conscious of an external object or fact." *(Webster's Seventh New Collegiate Dictionary.)* On the basis of this definition and the existing literature, a number of premises can be formulated.

1. Different states of consciousness are synonymous with different states of awareness.

2. The dynamic structure of awareness is not as an epi-phenomenon of some more basic psychological or biological event. It is a fundamentally important thing in and by itself.

3. Any particular state of awareness and/or consciousness is an emergent phenomenon created out of certain holistic or higher-order patterns of ongoing neural acitivity and organized around the sensory modalities.

4. Any psychologizing regarding qualities or types of awareness can occur without prejudgment as to normal or abnormal.

5. An individual's awareness occurs in utmost privacy. One individual cannot be aware of another's awareness. He can only experience the other's awareness indirectly.

The privacy of awareness is a scientific problem which has been partly overcome in the laboratory. Such tools as the computer and the electroencephalograph (EEG) have allowed us to form a picture of certain patterns characteristic of one or another state of awareness.

Emerging from recent neurophysiological, sensory, and perceptual studies is a model that describes the ways in which various sensory and perceptual responses are organized within an organism. Overall, the individual is viewed as an *active selector of stimuli* rather than as a passive recipient. Given a limited capacity to deal with available stimuli, the individual selects those stimuli that he will become aware of. William James said it a long time ago (1890): "The practical and theoretical life of whole species as well as of individual human beings results from the selection which the habitual direction of their attention involves . . . each of us literally chooses, by his way of attending to things, what sort of universe he shall appear to himself to inhabit [p. 402]." The complex process of stimulus search (preselection) and selection is the process of attention (e.g. Bakan, 1966; Silverman, 1972.)

How an individual attends to his environment—the ways in which he organizes external and internal stimuli—determines what he is aware of. His everyday behavior is maintained by a pattern of attention responses. *If he radically changes this response pattern, he radically changes his consciousness.* [4]

Attention Response Patterns

Attention response patterns are inferred from sensory behavior character-istics. In the model of sensory behavior that I have been working with, the process of attention is considered in terms of three principal factors: intensive-ness, extensiveness, selectiveness (Silverman, 1972)[5]. Originally, the three–factor formulation was elaborated to describe what happens sensorially and perceptually to an individual during the ordinary, waking state, during a psychedelic drug experience or a schizophrenic experience or during sensory deprivation or dreaming sleep. In using this model, we find we have been able to make inferences regarding these and other states of consciousness which are congruent with the literature on religio-mystical experiences reported by Eastern and Western mystics. The model also sheds light on the unusual experiences which I summarized earlier about depersonalization in normal individuals.

Briefly, the intensive aspect of attention concerns how individuals modulate the intensity of a given sensory stimulus (stimulus intensity control). Intensive-

---

[4]Several lines of inquiry have been important to the development and extension of this model of attention response.
   a) Research on the relationships between attention, awareness, and indices of physiological activation (e.g. Fischer, 1971*b*; Lacey, 1966).
   b) Electrophysiological studies of attention which have opened up a whole new technology for the study of psychological functioning (e.g. Buchsbaum and Silverman, 1968; Silverman, 1972).
   c) Research on "styles" of sensory and perceptual information processing employing multivari-ate statistical techniques such as the pioneering factor-analytic and cluster-analytic work of the Menninger group (e.g. Gardner et al., 1959; Gardner, 1961).
   d) Clinical research on attention characteristics in different states of consciousness which have made clear the importance of examining subjective experience (e.g. McGhie and Chapman, 1961; Bowers and Freedman, 1966; Silverman, 1969).

[5]The attention factors have been derived empirically from factor analytic studies of sensory, perceptual, cognitive, and physiological test reponses and from electrophysiological studies of sensory functioning in humans (e.g. Basow, 1970; Buchsbaum & Silverman, 1968; Gardner, 1961; Schooler & Silverman, 1969; Silverman, 1967*a*, 1968, 1972). For each of the factors (intensive-ness, extensiveness, and selectiveness or field articulation), a theoretical construct has been developed. Originally these constructs were elaborated on the basis of analyses of patterns of test correlations with particular factors. Each construct describes both a *response dimension* and a *hypothetical response mechanism* which are postulated to underlie performances on tests which correlate with a factor. A particular constellation of responses on the factors (factor scores) constitutes a person's "attentional style." Habitual styles of paying attention are operationally defined in terms of the three factors.

ness consists of two distinctly different but related kinds of psychological and physiological responses: a) detection and recognition responses to low-intensity stimulation and b) responses to high-intensity stimulation.

Extensiveness of attention refers to the degree to which the environment is scanned for information. It is inferred from certain psychological and physiological laboratory procedures which assess information-search behavior. (For more detailed discussion, see Silverman, 1970*b*).

The third factor, selectiveness of attention (or field articulation), refers to responses that determine which elements in a stimulus field exert a dominant influence on the perceiver. One aspect of this construct describes responses to stimulus configurations on a dimension ranging from differentiated (segmentalizing-analytic) to undifferentiated (global-relational). At one extreme are individuals who perceive elements of a given configuration in a global, diffuse manner; for these individuals there is no distinction among these various elements. At the other extreme are individuals who automatically differentiate between elements in a configuration, who impose their own structure on a stimulus field. The weaker the disposition to segmentalize a stimulus configuration, the more likely an individual is to experience disparate elements in a configuration as related.

A second aspect of the selectiveness or field articulation factor describes the degree of an individual's distractibility; his susceptibility to conflicting or peripheral elements of stimulus configurations.

Figure 1

Dimensions of Attention

1. Stimulus Intensity Control

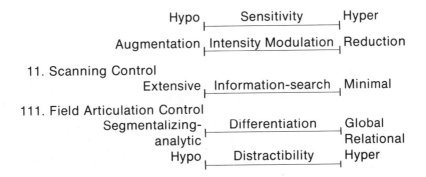

These three factors, then, are the constructs with which individual attention response patterns are formulated.

I consider the factor of intensiveness (stimulus intensity control) to be the primary factor of attention. First, for almost all phyletic levels, behavior is governed in the earliest stages of life by stimulus intensity rather than by stimulus quality (Molz, 1968; Schneirla, 1959). Secondly, individual differences in response to weak and intense stimulation are found at birth and appear to be related to innate differences in sensitivity to stimulation (e.g. Birns et al., 1969; Bridger, 1962). Furthermore, the psychological development of human infants with low-sensory thresholds is different from that of high-sensory threshold infants (e.g. Bergman & Escalona, 1949; Escalona & Heider, 1959; Escalona, 1963; Silverman, 1970*b*). Thirdly, in normal adults, important aspects of personality and intellectual functioning such as introversion and extroversion are found to be correlated with sensory response characteristics (Fischer et al., 1969; Palmer, 1966; Smith, 1968). Last, and most germane to our subject here, is that hypersensitivity to low or moderate intensities of stimulation is an important characteristic of nonordinary states of consciousness.

In regard to the second factor, extensiveness, we find that in nonordinary states of consciousness, scanning of environmental stimulation is minimal relative to the ordinary waking state. Attention is withdrawn from the environment and is focused inside on internal happenings—perhaps on cosmic disorganization or on cosmic unification or on the total chaos that prevails at the beginning of certain of these profound states, or on the illumination that sometimes occurs, and so forth.

In regard to the third factor, selectiveness, we find that an analytic, differentiated experience of an "out-there" is minimal in nonordinary states of consciousness and often ceases to be. Rather, there is a passive, global and diffuse orientation to external stimulation. Since the differentiation of sensory cues is the basis upon which we distinguish hallucinatory states from the normal waking state, minimized field articulation during transcendental states can be seen as a basis for the commonly reported experience of the dissolution of one's self-boundaries.

Hypersensitivity, Overstimulation and Paradoxical Reduction Response

As we have seen, individuals who are hypersensitive to low-intensity stimulation react strongly to ordinary sensory events in the here and now. Experimental studies indicate that these subjects have difficulty in inhibiting responsiveness to irrelevent, non-contextual stimuli when the stimuli are of low to moderate intensity (Palmer, 1966; Silverman, 1968). However, inhibition of response *is* observed in hypersensitive individuals when the intensity of stimulation presented is very strong (Silverman, 1968). Ordinarily painful stimulation is tolerated more easily. Noteworthy here are reports of Yogi, indicating that they are sensitive to low–intensity stimulation and at the same time are capable of such feats as walking on burning hot coals.

An example of this paradoxical inhibition of response can be found in two studies involving LSD. Figure 2 summarizes the results of a study of hearing thresholds of a group of chronic psychedelic drug-users examined at the NIMH Clinical Center. Auditory thresholds were recorded at the time the subjects came into the clinical center. These psychedelic drug-users had lower than normal thresholds on admission. After ingestion of a 50 mcg dosage of LSD, their auditory thresholds became even lower (Henkin et al., 1967).

Figure 2

Effects of LSD-25 on sensory thresholds.
(From Henkin *et al.*, 1967.)

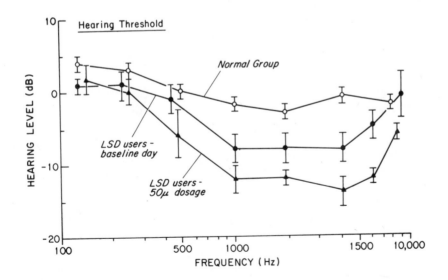

In contrast, response to high–intensity stimulation under the effects of LSD is quite different. Figure 3 summarizes a study by Kast (1967) of a large number of terminally ill patients. Three hours after ingestion of 100 mcg. of LSD, the greater increases in pain tolerance are shown under the effects of LSD as compared with Mepardine or Dilaudid, two conventionally used pain-killers. Also, pain tolerance is sustained for an unusually long period of time under LSD (Silverman, 1971).

In summary, a normal individual, when presented with a stimulus just below his threshold, doesn't hear it. The same individual given 50-100 mcgs of LSD detects such a signal. Yet, while LSD-drugged, an individual doesn't experience pain at levels of stimulation which are painful when not drugged. (Figure 4.)

A similar kind of responsiveness occurs among acute schizophrenics. Figure 5 summarizes a study by Donoghue (1964). Certain schizophrenics appear to tolerate a much higher intensity of stimulation than normal individuals. Other studies indicate that certain types of acute schizophrenics are unusually sensitive to low-intensity stimulation (e.g. Chapman 1966; Rappaport, Silverman et al., 1971; Silverman, 1969, 1972).

The formulation of this kind of mechanism accords beautifully with the teachings of the ancient Yogi. It also accords with the kinds of unusual, often unbelievable experiential reports of people who have been labelled madmen, or shaman, or drug addicts (e.g. Silverman, 1967b, 1969).

Neurophysiological Research

Recently, an electrophysiological procedure has been developed which is especially designed to study responsiveness to strong stimulation. Out of this work a formulation has emerged which emphasizes the importance of an inhibitory sensory modulation system which is the basis for several primal characteristics of transcendental states.

This electrophysiological procedure involves the use of computer averaging of evoked responses for several different intensities of stimulation, ranging from moderate to moderately strong. Average evoked responses (AER) are patterns of electrical response to sensory input which are recorded using a modification of standard electroencephalographic procedure. Evoked responses are usually of such small amplitude (5 to 20 times smaller) as to be completely lost in the random EEG fluctuations. However, we take advantage of the fact that an evoked response is always time-locked to a sensory stimulus, which is not true for random EEG fluctuations. A subject's evoked response

Figure 3

Effects of LSD-25 on pain tolerances of terminally ill patients.

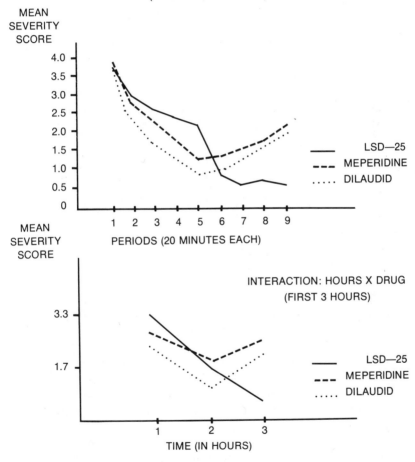

COMPARISON OF MEAN PAIN SCORES THROUGH TIME
(FIRST 3 HOURS ONLY)

Figure 4

Effects of LSD-25 on Auditory Sensory Experience.

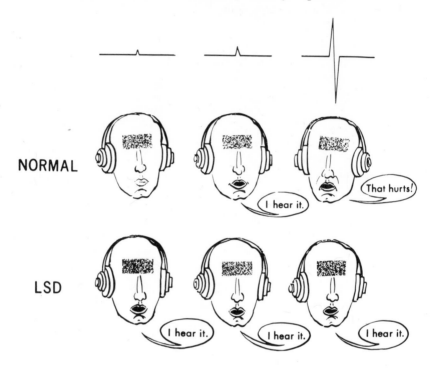

pattern is recorded by presenting him with a long series of stimuli such as light flashes, and for a brief time period after each stimulus, scoring the EEG, using a computer of average transients. An averaged evoked response waveform is produced which is similar from person to person to the extent that specific peaks and latencies of the AER waveform can be named and compared. (In our studies, we have been specifically concerned with the peak-to-trough amplitude from positive peak 3 at 90 msec to negative peak 4 at 120 to 140 msec.)

This procedure can be used with individuals in trance states or hypnotic states, during sleep or with otherwise mute subjects since the subject's active collaboration is not required. Indeed our early studies were conducted on subjects who were instructed to keep their eyes closed throughout the 8–to 9–minute procedure.

Figure 5

Differences in judgments of degree of unpleasantness of stimulation
by Normals, Process Schizophrenics, and Reactive Schizophrenics.

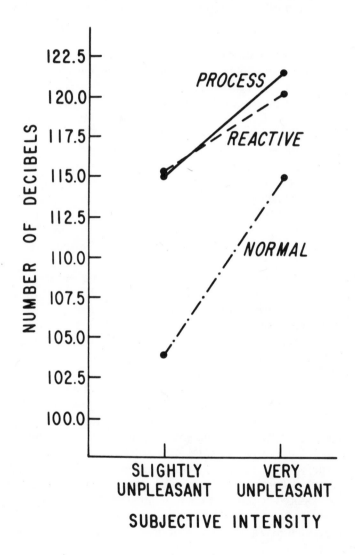

For a given individual, the amplitudes of certain peaks of the AER waveform change systematically with changes in stimulus intensity. In the moderate to high range of stimulus intensities, amplitudes of one particular peak of the waveform (peak 4) are found to change in different ways for individuals with different perceptual characteristics. In brief, subjects who *reduce* the sizes of tactile judgments of width, following a period of tactile stimulation, evidence quite different AER patterns from subjects who *augment* the sizes of tactile judgments following stimulation. Size judgment "reducers" evidence relatively decreased AER amplitudes at the higher stimulus intensities (Buchsbaum & Silverman, 1968). Size judgment "augmenters" show increases in AER amplitudes with increases in stimulus intensity (see Figures 6 and 7).

The reduction effect is found in normal subjects and in certain psychiatric patient and medical patient groups (Silverman, 1972).

The AER reduction curve was found to be pronounced in a group of college-age, essentially schizophrenic "reducer" males (Buchsbaum & Silverman, 1968; see Figure 8).

Comparable findings were reported in a group of schizophrenic subjects by Shagass et al. (1969), employing a different AER procedure to infer reduction responsiveness. An AER reduction curve also was reported by Blacker and his colleagues (1968) for habitual LSD users who had not ingested LSD within 48 hours of the EEG recording (see Figure 9).

Other studies of LSD-drugged subjects, employing rather different AER procedures, have yielded results which are consistent with the hypothesis of reduced responsiveness to strong stimulation (Chapman & Walter, 1964; Rodin & Luby, 1966).

Still other studies have suggested that reduction responsiveness on the AER-procedure is associated with hypersensitivity to low-intensity stimulation. Thus, habitual LSD-users and unmedicated, nonparanoid schizophrenics who evidence AER reduction responsiveness, also evidence hypersensitivity to low-intensity stimulation (e.g. Fischer et al., 1967; Silverman, 1968). In unpublished studies of patients with untreated adrenal-cortical insufficiency, such as Addison's disease, there is a co-occurrence of AER reduction and hypersensitivity to low-intensity stimulation (Henkin, Buchsbaum, & Silverman, unpublished data; see Silverman, et al., 1969). Treatment with carbohydrate active steroids, which corrects this hormone insufficiency, results in a lessening of both pronounced sensitivity to low-intensity stimulation and extreme AER reduction (see also Henkin & Daly, 1968).

The relationship of AER reduction and hypersensitivity to low-intensity stimulation in nonclinical subjects was studied by Silverman, Buchsbaum, and

Figure 6

A series of evoked response wave-forms to four intensities of light
stimulation (ranging from 32 to 980 lumen seconds) for typical
augmenter and reducer subjects.

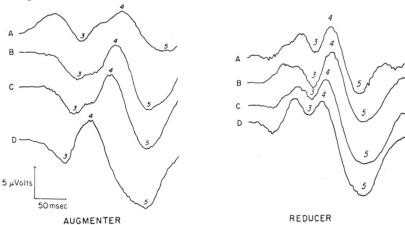

AUGMENTER   REDUCER

Figure 7

Averaged evoked response amplitude-intensity functions of nonpsychiatric (normal) augmenter groups and reducer groups.

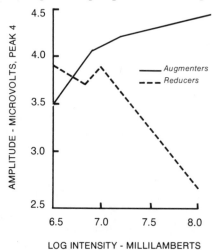

Figure 8

Amplitudes of averaged evoked responses at four intensities for
nonpsychiatric male reducers and schizophrenic male reducers.

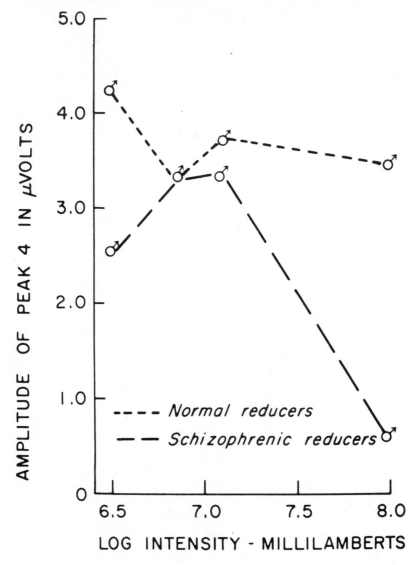

Figure 9

Amplitudes of average evoked responses to five intensities of stimulation for three groups of subjects (from Blacker *et al.*, 1968).

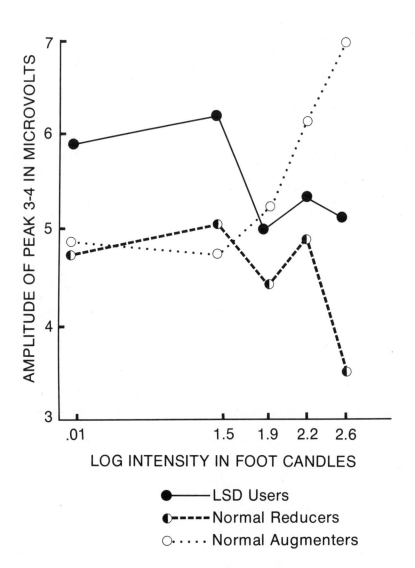

Henkin (1969). A sample of college students was divided into "high-sensitive" and "low-sensitive" groups on the basis of performance on tests of auditory sensitivity, brightness sensitivity, and thermal sensitivity. The testing extended over a six-week period. Among male subjects, AER reduction was found in the "high-sensitive" group; AER augmentation was found in the "low-sensitive" group.

In a study by Hall et al. (1970) using animals, degree of withdrawal behavior evidenced by adult cats was found to correlate significantly with degree of reduction on the AER slope measure (rho $= -.72$, P $< .01$).[6] In contrast, degree of exploration of the environment correlated with AER augmentation and not with reduction. (Ratings of withdrawal and exploratory behavior were made independently by a group of five raters.)

Taken together, these studies suggest that marked reduction responsiveness is a compensatory adjustment to overstimulation or overexcitation in primary sensory pathways of the central nervous system (Silverman, 1972). In this context, the withdrawal which occurs in nonordinary states of consciousness is considered to be a purposeful attempt to reduce the experienced intensity of overstimulation.

Pavlov's work is especially relevant in this regard. He observed that organisms which are hypersensitive to stimulation are most likely to become overstimulated. If overstimulation occurs, he hypothesized that a generalized state of "protective inhibition" is induced in order to protect the nervous system from further stimulation. If further strong stimulation is registered in this state, more protective inhibition is generated; the organism now is observed to evidence reduced responsiveness to strong stimuli. Thus, *hypersensitivity and overstimulation are among the basic precursors of reduced responsiveness to strong stimulation, and reduced responsiveness to strong stimulation is characteristic of subjects in transcendental states* (Silverman 1968).

Transcendental States and Indices of Central Nervous System Excitation

In various transcendental states, central nervous system (CNS) excitation is high. This excitation effect is inferrable from such procedures as the computerized electroencephalogram and fine-eye-movement recording procedures. For example, Table 1 summarizes a series of findings using a particular EEG measure employed by Goldstein and Pfeiffer, 1969. The results indicate a dimen-

---

[6]The correlations reported in the original Hall article are incorrectly presented in some cases. The author will furnish, on request, a corrected summary of the analyses.

sion ranging from extreme relaxation and low excitation to hypertension and high excitation. (Level of EEG variability, expressed as the coefficient of variation of the EEG, is marked at the low-arousal end of the dimension and minimal at the high arousal end.)

In the relaxed state, arousal level is low and there is free muscular activity. In anxiety states, hallucinatory states (either occurring in patients or induced in normals), or in catatonia, there is high excitation and constriction of gross movement in the large muscles.

EEG activity indicative of the high physiologically-aroused transcendental states also is found in stage 1 sleep or dream sleep. This state also shares characteristics with other transcendental states such as minimal motor activity, hallucination, and nonorientation to ordinary waking reality. Besides EEG activity indicative of high excitation, stage 1 dream sleep is distinguished by the occurrence of rapid eye movements (REM). Research on saccadic (fine) movement of the eye which, in the waking state, is essential for clear detailed vision, shows that during certain acute schizophrenic episodes and during psychedelic drug intoxication, an unusually large number of fine eye movements are concentrated in a relatively restricted portion of the visual field. Under these conditions, redundancy of information sampling is pronounced. The combination of minimal scanning and high saccadic rate probably is responsible for reports of an increased intensity of visual experience (Silverman, 1968). Saccadic eye movement is found to be unusually fast (compared to the ordinary waking state) in dream sleep, also. A further relationship between dream sleep and transcendental states is suggested by the fact that ingesting a psychedelic drug results in a subsequent increase in the amount of time spent in stage 1 REM sleep (Green, 1965; Muzio et al., 1966).

Other researchers involving the central nervous system have indicated the importance of understanding the nature of differential excitation in different parts of the brain (Evarts, 1958; Marrazzi & Hart, 1955; Purpura, 1956; Silverman, 1971). The brain is not uniformly excited; excitation in one part of the brain doesn't necessarily cause excitation in other brain areas. For example, animal studies indicate that excitation increases significantly in the primary sensory pathways as a result of the direct application of a minute amount of LSD-25. Increased excitation does not occur if LSD-25 is applied to structures of the nonspecific sensory system of the association cortex; rather, neural inhibition occurs. To repeat, stimulating the primary sensory pathways produces CNS excitation; stimulating association areas of the cortex produces CNS inhibition.

The behavioral analogue of increased excitation in the primary sensory

Table 1

Relationship between Levels of Behavioral Arousal and a Measure of EEG Variability

States of consciousness	Levels of arousal	Levels of EEG variability in coefficient of variation
Catatonia	very high	*7-8
Other types of schizophrenia	high	9-12
Hallucinations (either in patients or induced in normals)	high	10-12
Anxiety states	high	10-12
Creativity (actively engaged)	high	12-15
Normalcy (daily routine)	average	15-25
Euphoria (extreme relaxation)	low	20-35
Drowsiness	very low	25-45
Stage-4 sleep	—	20-25
Stage-1 REM sleep	—	10-15

*lowest variability

pathways of the brain is hypersensitivity to low to moderate sensory stimulation. The behavioral analogue of increased inhibition in the association area of the cortex is increased tolerance of strong stimulation. *This provides an explanation of the paradoxical reports of individuals in transcendental states who experience both hypersensitivity and high-pain tolerance* (Silverman, 1971, 1972.)

Experiential and Sensory Correlates of Transcendental States

There is much to learn from reading about what people experience during unusual states of consciousness. The literature on mysticism (e.g. shamanism, ecstatic states in saints, Yogi experience, etc.) contains much that is compatible with the kind of sensory formulation being outlined here. "A mystic," states Gershom Scholem (1964), "is a man who is favored with an immediate and to him real experience of the divine, of ultimate reality, or who at least strives to attain such experience. It may come to him through sudden illumination, or it may be the result of long and often elaborate preparations [p.31]." The primary aim of this type of individual is to transcend the limitations of corporal reality.

Mircea Eliade (1957), an outstanding authority in the field of shamanism and yoga, has noted that the development of the shaman state of mystical sensitivity requires a major change in the way sensory functioning occurs. All traditional shaman practices pursue the same end: to destroy the profane, to eliminate ordinary sensibility. This is done by monotonous chants, endlessly repeated refrains, fatigue, fasting, dancing, narcotics, and so forth. These techniques serve to create a sensory condition that is wide open to the "supernatural." The senses are bombarded with highly intense forms of stimulation: painful friction on the skin, massage with liquids, dancing on tightropes of various heights, swinging suspended in air. The focus of attention is narrowed to a fine point.

In the course of their ascetic and contemplative labors, the Yogi come to a plane of experience on which extraordinary (i.e. extrasensory) experience occurs. If one reads the yoga text attentively, one can follow the successive stages leading to a radical alteration of the apprentices' sensibility. It is the apparent breakdown in the structures of profane sensibility which makes extrasensory response possible. The exercises of *hatha* yoga refine the sensory awareness and make possible realms of experience which are ordinarily inaccessible. "The insensibility to heat and the incombustibility are obtained by prayer and fasting: 'faith' plays the essential part and sometimes the walk over the embers is achieved in ecstasy [Eliade, 1957, p.95]."

"Thus there exists a perfect continuity of these mystical techniques, from cultures at the paleolithic stage right up to the modern religions. . . . The 'mastery of fire' and the insensibility both to extreme cold and to the temperature of live embers are material expressions of the idea that the shaman and the Yogi have surpassed the human condition and already participate in the condition of the spirits [p.95]." In this way, Eliade describes the sensory basis of these mystical quests.

Radically modify the patterns of stimulation which an individual is accustomed to (e.g. by narrowing attention onto certain sensory inputs, by sensory

Figure 10

Model of Psychobiological Effects of Psychedelic drugs.

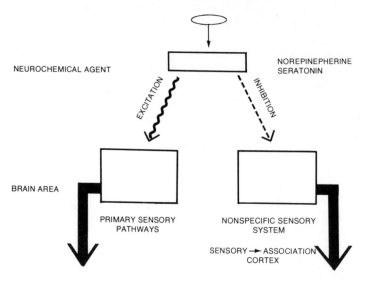

PSYCHEDELIC AGENT
(LSD, MESCALINE, PSILOCYBIN)

NEUROCHEMICAL AGENT

NOREPINEPHERINE
SERATONIN

EXCITATION

INHIBITION

BRAIN AREA

PRIMARY SENSORY
PATHWAYS

NONSPECIFIC SENSORY
SYSTEM

SENSORY → ASSOCIATION
CORTEX

BASIC
BEHAVIORAL
EFFECTS

HYPERSENSITIVITY TO

LOW-TO-MODERATE

INTENSITY STIMULATION

INCREASED TOLERANCE

OF HIGH INTENSITY

STIMULATION

DISTURBANCES IN INTEGRATION

OF SENSORY INFORMATION

CLINICAL
SYNDROME

DISTRACTIBILITY, THOUGHT-DISORDER, BLOCKING,
HALLUCINATIONS OR PSEUDO-HALLUCINATIONS, WITHDRAWAL,
CHANGES IN FIGURE-GROUND RELATIONSHIPS,
LOSS OF SPONTANEITY IN MOVEMENT AND SPEECH

isolation), precipitate a chemical imbalance (e.g. through fasting), and you change dramatically the perceptual experience. With this "old knowledge," extraordinary individuals throughout history cultivated noetic qualities by means of exercises which altered the organization of sensory information in the central nervous system.

A classical example of this process is found in the New Testament, St. Luke, Chapter 4. "And Jesus was led by the Spirit into the wilderness being forty days tempted of the Devil and in those days he did eat nothing. . . . And when the Devil had ended all the temptations he departed from him for a season, and Jesus returned in the power of the Spirit to Galilee. And there went out a fame of him through all the region roundabout, and he taught in their synagogues being glorified by all [1-2 . . . 13–15]."

Now in terms of the formulation presented here, Jesus left his ordinary sensory environment and went out into an isolated, sensorially restricted environment. On top of that he fasted for a long period of time, which induced hyperglycemia. In this radically different internal and external environment, his consciousness changed. Many things were revealed to him which he never knew before that wilderness "trip." In effect, he undertook a journey away from the ordinary and mundane, in order to make manifest his transcendental nature.

Psychopathology and Religious Consciousness

Religious consciousness is something quite different from a religious creed. Jung in his book, *Psychology and Religion* (1938), wrote: "Religion . . . is a careful and scrupulous observation of what Rudolf Otto aptly termed the numinosum, that is, a dynamic existence or effect, not caused by an arbitrary act of the will. On the contrary, it seizes and controls the human subject which is always rather its victim than its creator. The numinosum is an involuntary condition of the subject whatever its cause may be [p.4]." The subject is, as it were, gripped by something wholly other which he experiences with overwhelming intensity. The experience contains a tremendous sense of awesomeness. "Religion, it might be said, is the term that designates the attitude peculiar to a consciousness which has been altered by the experience of the numinosum [Jung, 1938, p.6]."

When one examines the available literature on eminent religious figures throughout history, it turns out that they were in considerable emotional turmoil prior to and during their profound "realization" experiences. St. Paul, George Fox (founder of the Quakers), St. Teresa, the old Hebrew prophets, Ezekiel and Jeremiah, and many others were markedly dis-eased. Gautama Siddhartha, founder of Buddhism, left his family at the time of his child's birth and wandered off in turmoil to do battle with the forces of darkness, and so on.

Mental dis-ease in these individuals was marked; depersonalization and derealization were common. Yet, in retrospect, such episodes can be looked upon as problem-solving experiences rather than medically treatable disease. Observations bearing out this point of view can be found in the book *Exploration of the Inner World* by Anton Boisen, founder of pastoral psychology in the United States. He was a minister, a psychologist, and several times in his life he was blatantly schizophrenic in a classically acute manner (Boisen, 1936).

In his research conducted at Worcester, Boisen studied individuals who did and did not reconstitute after going through schizophrenic episodes. He found three characteristics that distinguished individuals who went through psychotic episodes and actually became well. (Karl Menninger described such individuals as "weller than before.") For individuals in whom the dis-ease actually appeared to serve a healing function, ideas of cosmic catastrophe, cosmic identification, death, and rebirth were predominant. These same characteristics are commonly reported during LSD experiences which have positive repercussions (e.g. Caldwell, 1968); they predominate as well in the reports of religious mystics throughout history (e.g. Gopi Krishna, 1967; Silverman, 1967*b*; Wallace, 1956).

On the basis of his studies of religious figures and of numerous mental hospital cases, Anton Boisen formulated an association between religio-mystical experiences and so-called psychopathology. He wrote, "the explanation is to be found in the principle that religious concern and religious consciousness tend to appear wherever men are facing the issues of life and are seeking to become better. Wherever this involves severe conflict, pathological features are likely also to appear. In some cases, the charge of pathology applied to religious experience is due simply to the failure to recognize that such phenomena as hallucinations spring from the tapping of the deeper levels of the mental life and that as such they are not necessarily symptomatic of mental disorder but may be creative and constructive. But in a large number of cases, the association of the mystical and the pathological is due to the fact that a fundamental reorientation is a necessary stage in the development of the individual [p.82]."

Boisen's observations accord with the neurological and sensory formulations of psychological structure and the breakdown of psychological structure being developed here. The formulation can be reiterated as follows: perceptual and conceptual structures require the "nutriment" of their accustomed stimuli in order to exist; prolonged minimal scanning and minimal differentiation of the environmental field weaken and disrupt these ordinarily stable psychological structures. The individual's functioning no longer is stabilized by constancies, such as size and shape, which have served to form his interpretations of his central nervous system activity. Under these conditions, reality—ordinary perceptual and conceptual reality—breaks down. Previous experiences and accepted standards do not apply now. New and awesome meanings abound. The individual becomes aware of psychic processes beyond the scope of everyday awareness.

Out of this disorganization or de-automatization of psychological structure arises unusual experience. The sensory basis of the entire process is neatly summarized by Freedman et al. (1961) in their report on the psychological effects of so-called "sensory deprivation": "our data imply that these effects (perceptual and cognitive abnormalities) are produced by the release of tendencies inherent in the primitive process but held in check by a process of stabilizing of the visual (sensory) field [pp.70–71]."

Positive Aspects of Psychological Disorganization

There is mounting evidence (Silverman, 1974), that some of the most profound psychotic disorganizations can be regarded as preludes to impressive reorganization and personality growth—not so much breakdown as breakthrough. Kazimierz Dabrowski (1964) has termed such a process "positive disintegration." It is a natural reaction to severe stress, a spontaneous process into which persons may enter when their usual problem-solving techniques fail to solve such basic life crises as occupational or sexual inadequacy. If it is interrupted (in certain individuals) by well-intended psychiatric therapies, the effect may be to detour the individual away from a process as natural and benign as fever. The effect can be most unfortunate—it can rob him of his natural problem-solving potential. The basic hypothesis here is that the organism's *natural* wisdom is greater than our current limited intellectual appreciation of it. The demonic symptoms can be essentially benign responses to the deeper trials of life that the individual never solves if a therapist encourages escape or drugs him into a permanent state of psychic helplessness (Silverman, 1970a).

Concluding Remarks

In the course of this presentation, I have shifted back and forth between two perspectives for the study of transcendental states of consciousness: the experiential (or subjective) and the experimental. I have attempted to present, in "broad strokes," a way of asking questions about the various transcendental states, which is rooted in an empirically testable orientation—consciousness organized around the sensory modalities.

Until recently, transcendental states have been most difficult to investigate in the laboratory. This is because the kinds of performance procedures that experimental psychologists and psychiatrists employ in their examinations often implicitly require that an individual be in one particular state—the ordinary waking state of consciousness. Thus, for example, in order to demonstrate hypersensitivity, the scientist used to need to have the subject performing with some modicum of efficiency on a sensory threshold procedure. However, if an individual did not scan and articulate the experimental stimuli in a "normal" manner, he obviously could not register and analyze them. Hence the scientist's techniques for studying sensory behavior could tell us nothing about the *actual* sensitivity of the subject. With the advent of more sophisticated electrophysiological techniques and computer analytic techniques, it has become possible to allow individuals to be in whatever state of consciousness they happen to be in and to interfere minimally with their "space."

Under these new experimental conditions, more accurate information can be obtained about organismic functioning in transcendental states. In all likelihood, these new kinds of information will turn out to be far more compatible with the "data" presented by the ancient mystics than has been the case until now. One day soon, scientists will be able to consider the mystical nature of man in much the same way as they now consider such effects as gravity. A major reformulation of the nature of mental disease will be one of the important consequences of this approach to the study of mind.

References

Bakan, P. (Ed.). *Attention.* New York: Van Nostrand, 1966.

Basow, S. A factor analysis of attention. Unpublished Master's thesis, Brandeis University, New York.

Bergman, P. and Escalona, S. K. Unusual sensitivities in very young children. In W. Hoffer et al. (Eds.) *Psychoanalytic study of the child.* Vols. 3,4. New York: International University Press, 1949.

Bexton, W. H., Heron, W. and Scott, T. H. Effects of decreased variation in the sensory environment. *Canadian Journal of Psychology,* 1954, 8, 70–76.

Birns, B., Garten, S. and Bredger, W. H. Individual differences in temperamental characteristics of infants. *Transactions of New York Academy of Science,* 1969, 31, 1071–1082.

Blacker, K. H., Jones, R. T., Stone, G. C., and Pfefferbaum, D. Chronic users of LSD: 'The acidheads'. *American Journal of Psychiatry,* 1968, 125, 341–351.

Boisen, A. T. *The exploration of the inner world.* New York: Harper & Row, 1936.

Bowers, M. B. Pathogenesis of acute schizophrenia psychoses: an experimental approach. *Archives of General Psychiatry,* 1968, 19, 348–355.

Bowers, M. B. and Freedman, D. X. Psychedelic experiences in acute psychoses. *Archives of General Psychiatry,* 1966, 15, 24, 248.

Brenman, M. and Gill, M. M. *Hypnotherapy.* New York: International Universities Press, 1947.

Bridger, W. H. Sensory discrimination and autonomic function in newborn. *Journal of the American Academy of Child Psychiatry,* 1962, 1, 1962.

Buchsbaum, M. and Silverman, J. Stimulus intensity control and the cortical evoked response. *Psychosomatic Medicine,* 1968, 30, 12–22.

Caldwell, W. V. *LSD psychotherapy: an exploration of psychedelic and psycholytic therapy.* New York: Grove Press, 1968.

Chapman, J. The early symptoms of schizophrenia. *British Journal of Psychiatry,* 1966, 122, 225–251.

Chapman, L. F. and Walter, R. D. Actions of lysergic acid diethylamide on averaged human cortical evoked responses to light flash. In J. Wortis,

(Ed.) *Recent advances in biological psychiatry.* Vol VII. New York: Plenum Press, 1964.

Cohen, S. *The beyond within: the LSD story.* New York: Atheneum, 1964.

Connally, J. *The Croonian lectures* (1849). Southall, England: St. Bernard's Hospital, 1960.

Dabrowski, K. In J. Aronson (Ed.), *Positive disintegration.* Boston: Little, Brown, 1964.

Deikman, A. J. Experimental meditation. *Journal of Nervous and Mental Diseases,* 1963, **136,** 329–343.

Dixon, J. C. Depersonalization phenomena in a sample population of college students. *British Journal of Psychiatry,* 1963, **109,** 371–375.

Donoghue, J. R. Motivation and conceptualization in process and reactive schizophrenia. Unpublished doctoral dissertation, University of Nebraska, 1964.

Eliade, M. *Myths, dreams and mysteries.* New York: Harper & Row, 1967.

Escalona, S. K. Patterns of infantile experience and the developmental process. In W. Hoffer et al. (Eds.), *Psychoanalytic studies of the child.* New York: International Universities Press, 1963.

————, and Heider, G. M. *Prediction and outcome.* New York: Basic Books, 1959.

Evarts, E. V. Neurophysiological correlates of pharmacologically-induced behavioral disturbances. In H. C. Solomon, S. Cobb, and W. Penfield (Eds.), *The brain and human behavior.* Baltimore: William & Wilkins, 1958.

Fischer, R. The "flashback": arousal-state bound recall of experience. *Journal of Psychedelic Drugs,* 1971a, **3,** 31–39.

————. A cartography of ecstatic and meditative states. *Science,* 1971b, **174,** 31–39.

————. On creative, psychotic, and ecstatic states. In I. Jakob (Ed.), *Proceedings of the American Society of Psychopathology of Expression.* Basel, Switzerland: Karger, 1969.

————, and Kaebling, R. Increase in taste acuity with sympathetic stimulation: the relation of a just-noticeable taste difference to systemic psychotropic drug dose. *Recent Advances in Biological Psychiatry,* 1967, **9,** 183–195.

Fischer, R., Risetine, L. P., and Wisecupt, P. Increases in gustatory acuity and hyperarousal in schizophrenia. *Biological Psychiatry,* 1969, **1,** 209–218.

Freedman, S. J., Grunebaum, H. U., and Greenblatt, M. In P. Solomon et al. (Eds.), *Harvard medical school symposium on sensory deprivation.* Cambridge, Mass.: Harvard University Press, 1961.

Freud, S. Beyond the pleasure principle. In *The complete works of Sigmund Freud.* London: Hogarth Press, 1955.

Galambos, R. Suppression of auditory nerve activity by stimulation of efferent fibers to the cochlea. *Federal Proceedings of the Federation of American Societies for Experimental Biology,* 1955, 14, 53.

Gardner, R. W. Cognitive controls of attention deployment as determinants of visual illusions. *Journal of Abnormal Social Psychology,* 1959, I, No. 4.

————, Holzman, P. S., Klein, G. S., Linton, H. B., and Spence, D. P. Cognitive control: a study of individual consistencies in cognitive behavior. *Psychological Issues,* 1959, I, No. 4.

Goldstein, L. and Pfeiffer, C. C. Quantitative electroencephalographic correlates of the psychological status in schizophrenics. In D. V. Siva Sankar (Ed.), *Schizophrenia: current concepts and research.* New York: P.J.D. Publications, 1969.

Green, W. J. The effect of LSD on the sleep-dream cycle. *Journal of Nervous and Mental Diseases,* 1965, 140(6), 417–426.

Hall, R. A. Rappaport, M., Hopkins, H. K., Griffin, R., and Silverman, J. Evoked response and behavior in cats. *Science,* 1970, 170, 998–1000.

Hebb, D. The American revolution. *American Psychologist,* 1960, 15, 735–745.

Held, R., and Hein, A. Adaptation of disarranged hand-eye coordination contingent upon reafferent stimulation. *Perceptual and Motor Skills,* 1958, 8, 87–90.

Henkin, R., Welpton, D., Zahn, T., Wynne, L., and Silverman, J. Physiological and psychological effects of LSD in chronic users. *Clinical Research,* 1967, 15, 484.

Henkin, R. I., and Daly, R. L. Auditory detection and perception in normal man and in patients with adrenal cortical insufficiency. *Journal of Clinical Investigation,* 1968, 47, 1269–1280.

James, W. *Principles of psychology.* Vol I. New York: Henry Holt, 1890.

Jung, C. G. *Psychology and religion.* New Haven, Conn.: Yale University Press, 1938.

Kast, E. C. Attenuation of anticipation:; a therapeutic use of lysergic acid diethylamide. *Psychiatric Quarterly,* 1967, 41.

Krishna, Gopi, *Kundalini,* New Delhi, India: Ramadhar & Hopman, 1967.

Lacey, J. I. Somatic response patterning and stress: some revisions of activation theory. In M. H. Appley & R. Turnbull (Eds.), *Psychological Stress: Issues in Research.* New York: Appleton-Century, 1966.

Laing, R. D. *The divided self.* London: Tavistock, 1960.

Marrazzi, A. S., and Hart, E. R. Evoked cortical responses under the influences of hallucinogens and related drugs. *Electroencephalography and Clinical Neurophysiology,* 1955, 7, 146.

McGhie, A. and Chapman, J. Disorders of attention and perception in early schizophrenia. *British Journal of Medical Psychology,* 1961, **34**, 103–116.

Molz, H. An epinetic interpretation of the imprinting phenomenon. In Newton and Levins (Eds.), *Early experience and behavior.* Springfield, Ill.: Thomas, 1968.

Muzio, J. N., Howard, J. A., Ruffwarg, P. and Kaufman, E. Alterations in the nocturnal sleep cycle resulting from LSD. *Electroencephalography and Clinical Neurophysiology,* 1966, **21**, 313–324.

Palmer, R. D. Visual acuity and excitement. *Psychosomatic Medicine,* 1966, **28**, 364–374.

Pavlov, I. P. *Experimental psychology and other essays.* New York: Philosophical Library, 1957.

Purpura, D. P. Electrophysiological analysis of psychotogenic drug action II. General nature of lysergic acid diethylamide (LSD) action on central synapses. *Archives of Neurology and Psychiatry,* 1956, **75**, 132–143.

Rappaport, M., Silverman, J., Hopkins, H. K., and Hall, K. Phenothiazine effects on auditory signal detection in paranoid and nonparanoid schizophrenics. *Science,* 1971, **174**, 723–725.

Roberts, W. W. Normal and abnormal depersonalization. *Journal of Mental Science,* 1960, **106**, 478–493.

Rodin, E., and Luby, E. Effects of LSD-25 in the EEG and photic evoked responses. *Archives of General Psychiatry,* 1966, **14**, 435–441.

Savage, C. Variations in ego feeling induced by D-Lysergic acid diethylamide (LSD-25). *Psychoanalytical Review,* 1955, **42**, 1–16.

Schneirla, T. A. An evolutionary and developmental theory of biphasic processes underlying approach and withdrawal. In R. M. Jones (Ed.), *Nebraska symposium on motivation.* Lincoln: University of Nebraska Press, 1959.

Scholem, G. Religious authority and mysticism. *Commentary,* 1964, 5(11), 31–39.

Schooler, C., and Silverman, J. Perceptual styles and their correlates among schizophrenic patients. *Journal of Abnormal Psychology,* 1969, **74,** 459–470.

Shagass, C., Overton, D. A., and Bartolucci, G. In D. V. S. Sankor (Ed.), *Schizophrenia: current concepts and research.* New York: PJD Publications, 1969.

Sherrington, C. S. *The integrative action of the nervous system.* New Haven, Conn.: Yale University Press, 1906.

Silverman, J. Variations in cognitive control and psychophysiological defense in the schizophrenias. *Psychosomatic Medicine,* 1967a, **29**(3), 225–251.

———. Shamans and acute schizophrenia. *American Anthropologist,* 1967b, **69**(2), 21–31.

———. A paradigm for the study of altered states of consciousness. *British Journal of Psychiatry,* 1968, **14,** 1201–1218.

———. Perceptual and neurophysiological analogues of "experience" in schizophrenic and LSD reaction. In D. V. S. Sankar (Ed.), *Schizophrenia: current concepts and research.* New York: PJD Publications, 1969.

———. Acute schizophrenia: disease or dis-ease? *Psychology Today,* 1970a, **4,** 62–65.

———. Attentional styles and the study of sex differences. In D. Mostofsky (Ed.), *Attention: contemporary theory and analyses.* New York: Appleton-Century, 1970b.

———. Research with psychedelics. *Archives of General Psychiatry,* 1971, **25,** 498–510.

———. Stimulus intensity modulation and psychological dis-ease. *Psychopharmacologia,* 1972, **24,** 42–80.

———. "Altered" states of consciousness: positive and negative outcomes. Paper presented at the 19th Annual Meeting of the American Academy of Psychoanalysis, 1974.

———, Buchsbaum, M., and Henkin, R. Stimulus sensitivity and stimulus intensity control. *Journal of Perceptual and Motor Skills,* 1969, **28,** 71–78.

Smith, S. L. Extraversion and sensory threshold. *Psychophysiology,* 1968, **5,** 293–299.

Titchener, E. B. *Lectures on the elementary psychology of feeling and attention.* New York: Macmillan, 1908.

Wallace, A. F. C. Stress and rapid personality changes. *International Record of Medicine and General Practitioner Clinics,* 1955, **62,** 130–138.

Werner, H., and Wapner, S. The Innsbruck studies on distorted visual fields in relation to an organismic theory of perception. *Psychological Review,* 1955, **62,** 130–135.

Index